Handbook of Neurologic
Rating Scales

Handbook of Neurologic Rating Scales

Edited by

Robert M. Herndon, M.D.

demos vermande ❖

Library of Congress Cataloging-in-Publication Data

Handbook of neurologic rating scales / edited by Robert M. Herndon.
    p.   cm.
    ISBN 1-888799-07-2
    1. Neurologic examination—Handbooks, manuals, etc.
  2. Psychiatric rating scales—Handbooks, manuals, etc.   I. Herndon,
Robert M.
    [DNLM: 1. Nervous System Diseases—diagnosis.   2. Neurologic
Examination—methods.   3. Psychological Tests.   WL 141 H23648 1997]
RC348.H296   1997
616.8′0475—dc21
DNLM/DLC
for Library of Congress   97–23208
                                                                 CIP

Demos Vermande, 386 Park Avenue South, New York, New York 10016

Made in the United States of America

Contents

**10.   Rehabilitation Outcome
       Measures   225**

*Linda Coulthard-Morris, Jack S. Burks, and
  Robert M. Herndon*

Preface

This volume is a reference work that provides, in a straightforward standardized format, information on most of the scales that are widely used in neurology and in neurologic clinical trials. It provides a starting point for those interested in locating and evaluating scales for clinical trial planning or for simply following disease progression in a standard fashion.

The prevalence and economic consequences of chronic neurologic diseases have increased dramatically in the past half century and can be expected to continue to increase for decades to come. The incidence of senile dementia of Alzheimer's type, Parkinson's disease, stroke, progressive supranuclear palsy, and multi-infarct dementia increase dramatically with age. Even those with a fairly early average age of onset such as multiple sclerosis increase in prevalence with age because of the now nearly normal life span.

These diseases have become a major public health problem and the cost of care, both medical and custodial, is in the billions of dollars each year, to say nothing of the human cost. The majority of patients in nursing homes are there because of neurologic illnesses. For most, treatment is palliative and of limited effectiveness. Since even modest improvements in the condition of these patients can have a large impact both in quality of life and economically, symptomatic and rehabilitative therapies have become increasingly important and clinical trials to test drugs designed to slow disease progression and for symptomatic and rehabilitative therapy have expanded enormously.

As a result, accurate measurement of disease progression and improvement has become increasingly important. Additionally, outcomes research has begun to play an important role in clinical therapy, and this also depends largely on measurement of disease status and change. Neurologists, like most other specialists, will have to produce outcomes data demonstrating the effectiveness of neurologic care if the specialty is to survive and certainly if it is to thrive.

The marked increase in clinical trials has resulted in a proliferation of scales to measure complex neurologic functions and quantitate disease status. Most of these scales are specific to a limited range of neurologic problems but a few, such as the quality of life scales, are intended for broad application over a range of diseases. To date, there has been no good general reference on neurologic scales. Derick Wade's excellent volume *Measurements in Neurologic Rehabilitation* (1992) has excellent discussions of a substantial number of neurologic scales but is applicable primarily to rehabilitation. However, scales designed and validated for rehabilitation purposes are frequently ill-suited for clinical trials.

As more clinicians have become involved in clinical research and have begun to look at noncurative and symptomatic treatment for neurologic disorders, the development of better methods of measuring changes in patient status has become increasingly important. Clinical trials now routinely use scales to measure disease severity, rate of progression, and rate of improvement. These scales are routinely referred to in the clinical trials literature but such reference usually mentions the meaning of the scale only by reference to other publications and often by reference to secondary sources.

This book arose out of the my frustration in trying to find out the meaning of changes on an obscure self-administered functional scale in a multiple sclerosis trial. After a half day in two different libraries tracking down references in journals that were difficult to locate, it finally turned out that the scale had never been published. There was no way to go beyond the author's comments on the meaning of the scale, no evidence that it had ever been validated in any way, and one was left with the author's word on the conclusions. Other scales have been published in clinical reports where nothing in the title or abstract indicates that it includes the scale description so that it is extremely difficult to find. In my attempts to keep up with the neurologic literature, I frequently have occasion to read clinical trials articles only to be frustrated by a lack of familiarity with the scales being used.

Scales vary enormously in complexity from simple, straightforward ones like the ambulation index or timed gait to complex scales such as the Kurtzke EDSS or the Functional Independence Measure (FIM). They also vary in how closely they relate to pathology ranging from scales that directly relate to the pathology or pathophysiology to quality of life scales. Indeed, some treatments may slow the disease process but at a significant and sometimes unacceptable cost in quality of life.

In this volume, each chapter is structured with an introductory overview describing the area covered and any problems specific to the area in question. This is followed by the most commonly used scales given in a standard format: (1) the purpose for which the scale was developed along with current uses if they differ from the original purpose; (2) a description of the scale; (3) information on scale validation; (4) how and by whom the scale is administered or scored and time required to administer it; (5) the scale itself or, if it is very long or copyrighted, a reference that includes the scale; (6) any special considerations regarding the scale or its administration; (7) advantages; (8) disadvantages; and (9) a summary. The clinical trials and outcomes research arena has expanded dramatically in recent years and can be expected to continue to expand to fill the demand for information on which to base medical decisions.

It is hoped that this volume will provide a valuable reference work for those interested in locating and evaluating scales for clinical trial planning or who simply wish to follow patients' disease progression in a standard fashion.

Robert M. Herndon, M.D.

CHAPTER **1** Introduction to Clinical
Neurologic Scales

Robert M. Herndon, M.D.

"One's knowledge of science begins when he can measure what he is speaking about and express it in numbers." *Lord Nelson*

Formal measurement of the effects of neurologic disease and treatment effects, beyond the description of changes on the standard neurologic examination, is a relatively recent development. Neurologic rating scales began to appear around 1950 and their number has increased dramatically in the last few decades. Medicine is progressively changing from the empirical art it was at the beginning of the twentieth century to an information-based, more scientific enterprise. A surprising amount of medical therapy does remain empirical but this is changing rapidly. Although much of the change is due to the uncontrolled increase in medical costs and the pressures brought about by managed care in attempting to control them, medicine was changing and becoming more scientific before these pressures arose. Controlled clinical trials and outcomes research are at the heart of information-based medicine, and neurologic scales are essential tools in clinical trials designed to provide the information. As much as we dislike the idea, in this era of managed care if we cannot demonstrate objectively

that treatment is effective, it will not be reimbursed. Even effective therapies are likely to fall by the wayside if studies to prove their effectiveness are not done.

The earliest reported controlled trial appears to be that of Dr. James Lind. In 1747 he assessed the value of various popular remedies for scurvy aboard a Royal Navy ship. He took twelve scorbutic sailors and put them all on the same diet with the exception of the experimental treatment. He put two each on the following remedies:

1. a quart of cider a day;
2. 25 drops of vitriol three times a day;
3. two spoonfuls of vinegar three times a day on an empty stomach;
4. two spoonfuls of vinegar three times a day with vinegar used to spice their food;
5. a half pint of sea water a day;
6. two oranges and one lemon a day.

After six days, one of those who had received the oranges and lemon was back at work and the other was much improved. Those who received the cider were a little better, and the others were not improved. Given the dramatic response, one won-

1

ders if a controlled trial was really necessary. Despite the obvious effectiveness of the therapy, it was decades before it was widely used even in the Royal Navy. Of interest is the fact that prevention of scurvy in the Royal Navy had a major impact on the Battle of Trafalgar, since the British fleet had been at sea long enough that the opposing forces expected the British sailors to have diminished effectiveness because of the well-known extremely high frequency of scurvy after long periods at sea and its profound effect on the crews.

Controlled trials remained rare and did not become common until after World War II. Controlled trials became more common with the development of the National Institutes of Health and their training and research grant programs. This approach became still more common in the late 1960s, following the Kefauver committee report and related changes in the FDA, which resulted in the requirement that efficacy as well as safety be established before a new drug could be approved for marketing.

The number of controlled trials of new therapies for agents affecting neurologic function has expanded exponentially over the last two decades following the explosion of new information in immunology and transmitter/receptor physiology and chemistry. With this enormous expansion, a plethora of new scales to measure neurologic function have been developed. These range from very simple and straightforward scales that directly measure the function of interest, such as the ambulation index, to scales quite remote from the pathology, such as those that measure quality of life. Some are well-designed and carefully validated, whereas others are used without much thought as to what is actually being measured, the efficiency or reliability of the measurement, or the validity of the scale being used.

This book provides a resource for clinicians and clinical investigators in the broad field of neurology and neurologic rehabilitation to help them (1) evaluate the clinical trials literature by providing information on the scales being used; (2) evaluate and select appropriate and efficient scales for clinical trials and outcomes research; and (3) provide information that will help them to develop new scales or measures or to improve existing ones.

This book is not intended as a clinical trials book, and the reader is referred to some of the excellent books on trial design and methodology, such as Curtis L. Meinert's *Clinical Trials, Design, Conduct and Analysis*, for further information

regarding trial design and planning. Nevertheless, to understand the purposes and uses of neurologic scales, it is necessary to understand some of the basics of clinical trials.

Outcomes research involves the systematic comparison of preexisting risk factors, treatment, and outcome. This has been done effectively with some surgical procedures such as coronary artery bypass grafts and balloon angioplasty, where systems have been developed that make it possible to put in such factors as age, weight, ejection fraction, diabetes, smoking, and so on, and thus derive an overall risk of various surgical complications. Although it is generally more difficult to do in neurologic disease, it is being done in a variety of illnesses and injuries, particularly head and spine trauma and stroke. Outcomes research is also important in establishing the effectiveness and cost-effectiveness of treatment. Outcomes research requires efficient scales.

There are many types of clinical trials. The most common are (1) open trials, in which both the patient and the investigator know what each patient is receiving; (2) single blind trials, in which the investigator knows what treatment the patient is receiving but the patient does not know; (3) double blind trials, in which neither the patient nor the investigator knows who is receiving which treatment; and (4) modified double blind trials, in which the patient and an examining physician do not know what the patient is receiving but there is a monitor or treating physician who either knows from the outset what the patient is receiving or who is in a position to make an educated guess as to who is receiving which therapy because of the drug's side effects or laboratory abnormalities. While many trials are placebo-controlled, comparison trials are more usual when an effective treatment already exists, and these trials also can be open or blinded.

Open trials are often used early in the investigation of a new drug, in what are commonly known as phase I trials. Here the investigator is trying to determine safety, whether or not there is enough indication of efficacy to warrant further trial, and what dosage might be both safe and effective. Open trials may also be used after definitive trials to assess safety and toxicity in a larger population than that in the initial trial to detect rare side effects and complications prior to marketing. Outcomes research is also a form of open trial. Sometimes single blind trials are used in phase I, often with a crossover design. This can help to adjust for placebo effects and suggestibility and may give a clearer picture of the nature of the drug effects and nature and severity of side effects. When one is dealing with a drug that is clearly rapidly curative, such as penicillin for lobar pneumonia, one does not need a controlled trial to establish effectiveness. Controlled trials become essential when dealing with therapies that have a palliative or limited effect in a chronic disease or when comparing two treatments of somewhat similar effectiveness.

Phase II trials are designed to demonstrate safety and something of efficacy and are typically double blind or "double masked." They are typically larger than phase I trials and may provide clear evidence of efficacy; they generally lack the power to provide definitive evidence of safety and efficacy.

Phase III trials, often referred to as pivotal trials, are larger trials designed to establish both safety and efficacy and are generally required for FDA approval. Phase III trials are almost invariably double blind or modified double blind controlled trials.

The World Health Organization (WHO) model is widely used as a theoretical base for developing and evaluating scales. While it has its uses, it also has serious limitations. In the opinion of the author, *the most important question in designing or choosing a scale is how well it is suited to the task at hand in terms of validity, efficiency, sensitivity, and specificity*, not how well it agrees with some theoretical construct. Nevertheless, an understanding of the theory behind the International Classification of Impairments, Disabilities, and Handicaps (ICIDH) is of value in understanding the organization and design of many scales.

The World Health Organization (WHO) Model

The World Health Organization model was developed as an attempt to standardize classification and terminology relating to the consequences of disease. According to this model, any disease can be evaluated at four defined levels—pathology, impairment, disability, and handicap. The WHO classification is known as the International Classification of Impairments, Disabilities, and Handicaps (ICIDH). For purposes of evaluating and understanding scales and their meaning, it is important to understand the technical definition of each of these words in this context, which differs somewhat from their meaning in casual usage.

Pathology is defined in its traditional medical sense; that is, the structural damage done to the body, organ, or organ system caused by the disease process.

Impairment is the functional consequence of the underlying pathology and is usually interpreted to include pathophysiology.

Disability is ". . . any restriction or lack of ability to perform an activity within the range considered normal for a human being."

Handicap refers to the effects of the disorder on the individual's function in society. It reflects the social and societal consequences of the disease process for the individual.

While these definitions present a sometimes useful framework, they also present significant problems. Many of the boundaries are fuzzy. Impairment is presumed to include pathophysiology since its definition is "the functional (i.e., physiologic) consequence of the underlying pathology." If this is so, can we have impairments without pathology? Epilepsy, for example, may or may not in an individual case have a recognizable structural abnormality, but it certainly has a pathophysiology, or is the electrical abnormality seen on EEG pathology? What about bipolar disease and schizophrenia? Is a central scotoma an impairment or a disability?

Similarly, the other definitions have fuzzy overlapping borders. A stroke is a pathology, a resulting paralysis of a leg is an impairment, whereas the consequence, inability to walk, is a disability. If we measure gait, presumably that is a measure of disability, but it is also an indirect measure of impairment. The restriction that this places on the individual's ability to function in society, such as inability to work or inability to do routine activities, represents handicap.

While it may be desirable for purposes of classification and rehabilitation to use measures that fall at a single level, it is not always possible or even desirable to limit scales in this way for clinical trials or outcomes research. There are many situations in which a surrogate measure is a much more efficient and sometimes more accurate and sensitive way to get the information desired. Although this has been decried as measurement at different levels, in most neurologic disorders it is not possible to directly measure pathology, so one is already using a surrogate measure. It makes sense to use the simplest and most efficient measure that will accomplish the task. In some situations it may be desirable to use a measure of impairment, but it is often far more efficient to use a few simple functional tests, such as timed tandem gait or Hauser's ambulation index (Hauser et al., 1983) and the nine hole peg test and box and blocks test, as opposed to separate measures of sensation, motor strength, and coordination in each extremity to assess motor function and coordination for a clinical trial. The gait and upper extremity measures are more sensitive to change, have no significant interrater variability, and are much more sensitive to real change than is the standardized neurologic examination of the upper and lower extremity, in which judgment as to whether something is mild, moderate, or severe must be made. In multiple sclerosis magnetic resonance imaging (MRI) has been used as a more or less direct measure of pathology, but it correlates rather poorly with impairment and disability and thus is not a satisfactory surrogate for pathology.

The most difficult neurologic disease as far as scale development is concerned is probably multiple sclerosis. The Kurtzke (1983) extended disability status scale (EDSS) has been the most widely used scale, but it is clearly not satisfactory. The EDSS has been heavily criticized because it includes functional systems that are primarily impairments, yet it depends on disability measures in more advanced patients. Although it is misnamed according to the present definition of disability, it has proven useful, but it does need replacement. Criticism of the scale because it does not fit a theoretical construct developed at a later date seems inappropriate. It deserves criticism for its ambiguity, for the relatively high interobserver and even intraobserver variability, and its inefficiency, particularly if, as you should do at the intermediate scale levels, you walk the patient to see how far she can go before her legs cease to function. Additionally, patients have a bimodal distribution in the hands of most investigators. Clearly, it needs to be superseded. Clinical trials that use it need pages of clarifying rules detailing its application. One recent trial had 15 pages of clarification. Gauging items on the examination as mild, moderate, or severe is extremely crude and without clear boundaries. If we are to have a scale that is efficient, sensitive to change, reproducible, and applicable to the whole range of the disease, we have to look at everything from minor impairments, such as mild facial weakness that causes no disability or handi-

cap, to severe upper and lower extremity impairment resulting in severe disability. In measuring advanced limb impairments, it is much simpler and more efficient to look at ambulation and mobility than to use crude subjective measures of leg strength, sensation, and coordination. In this case, ambulation is a surrogate for impairment in leg motor, sensory, and coordination functions. Ambulation is sensitive to all of these impairments and in most MS patients dominates the impairment and disability picture as the disease advances, with minor items such as facial weakness or a partial internuclear ophthalmoplegia fading into relative insignificance as far as disability is concerned. Nevertheless, if one is interested in disease activity, then any new neurologic finding not explained by fever or other causes unrelated to the disease process can be considered evidence of new disease activity.

Mobility is a better measure of leg impairment in the disease than is weakness or incoordination or sensory impairment or a combination of these. In the early stages there are often a number of minor symptoms and impairments that have very little impact on function and would not even register on a disability scale but are detectable and represent a real underlying pathology. In the later stages, with ataxia, paraplegia, or quadriplegia, one has impairments, disability, and handicap. One could use a combination of ambulation measures and upper extremity measures, but this ignores other important functions such as vision, which can be used to detect changes. *The determining factor in evaluating the usefulness of a scale is how well it accomplishes the task at hand.* By this measure, the Kurtzke EDSS scale has served fairly well for three decades; it has been the *de facto* standard for clinical trials in the absence of better scales. That is not to say that it cannot or should not be improved or superseded, but the fact that no other scale has supplanted it suggests that despite its flaws it has fulfilled a need reasonably well.

Characteristics of Useful Scales

A useful measure or scale should have the following characteristics:

1. It should be appropriate to the task.
2. It should be valid; that is, it should measure what it purports to measure.

3. It should be reliable.

4. It should be reproducible.

5. It should be efficient and easy to use with little special training.

6. It should be sensitive to change in the underlying condition yet relatively insensitive to symptom fluctuation.

1. The scale should be appropriate to the task. Many scales are used for tasks other than the one for which they were designed. It would generally not be appropriate to use a handicap scale to assess pathology or to use an impairment scale to assess rehabilitation. Some scales, such as the quality of life scales, are intended to cover a broad range of diseases. Others are appropriate only for a very limited range of problems. A scale that is being used for a purpose other than the one for which it was designed will usually require validation for the new use.

2. The scale should have demonstrated validity. A valid scale or measure is one that reliably measures what it purports to measure. Several terms are used to describe various types and aspects of validity.

Face validity is the apparent congruence between what is to be measured and the measurement. Wade (1992) describes this as the "apparent sensibility of the measure and its components." Face validity is only rarely adequate. The Hauser ambulation index has obvious face validity for the assessment of mobility. It is, in fact, a simple direct assessment of the person's mobility and requirement for mobility aids. On the other hand, the ambulation index would not have face validity as a measure of urinary function, although it might be shown to have some predictive value.

Construct validity is the extent to which results from the measure concur with results predicted from the theoretical model. If it is assumed that weakness and spasticity in the legs will impair gait, then independent measures of strength and spasticity should correlate with gait impairment. If there is no correlation, the measure is probably not valid for the purpose. If the correlation is perfect, the measure is redundant.

Criterion related validity is the extent to which a measure agrees with some external criterion. This may be another widely accepted measure or the opinion of experts. Unfortunately, there is not always a "gold standard" available. For example, while the Kurtzke extended disability status scale is widely regarded as inadequate and outdated, it remains the standard for clinical research in MS, and until a better measure is devised and accepted, any new proposed scale will be measured against this standard.

Content validity is the extent to which a measure with multiple items covers all aspects of the model and avoids irrelevancies. For example, the Hauser ambulation index is a valid measure of mobility in multiple sclerosis but would not be valid as an overall measure of disability in MS since it ignores upper extremity function, vision, and other systems frequently affected by the disease.

Ecological validity is the validity of the measure in the context in which it is to be used. For example, the ability of a wheelchair-bound patient with MS to prepare a meal in a kitchen designed for the handicapped may have little validity if she only has access to a kitchen designed for the physically able that has not been modified.

3. Scale results should be reliable. An individual whose condition has not changed should always receive the same score. There should be minimal intra- or interobserver variability. Since borders between levels on a given scale are rarely sharp, this is a difficult but important standard. Some measures such as timed gait, walking distance, requirement for walking aids, and timed upper extremity functions, such as the nine hole peg test and box and blocks test, can have clear, fairly well defined, and consistent boundaries. On the other hand, with items like weakness or coordination scored as mild, moderate, or severe, different observers will have different boundaries and the same observer may define the boundaries differently on different days.

4. Scale results should be reproducible. In the absence of change in the disease, the same patient should receive the same score from either the same or a different examiner.

5. It should be efficient. Many measures fall by the wayside because they require too much time to administer or score. A busy clinician often will try to take a shortcut. For example, in the middle range of the Kurtzke scale, a great deal depends on how far the patient can walk without a rest. Accurate determination requires walking the patient but it is quite common for the examiner to simply ask the patient how far he or she can walk, which is simply not adequate for reliable determination. Efficiency is important even if the measure is self-administered or administered by a technician. Patients do not want to spend long periods of time filling out questionnaires, technicians must be paid, and since clinical studies usually require a substantial number of patients, time savings from using efficient measures mean that more individuals can be studied in the same time or with the same amount of money. Additionally, for outcomes research in which the assessment is commonly made during a routine office visit, efficiency is imperative.

6. It should be sensitive to change in the underlying condition yet relatively insensitive to day-to-day symptom fluctuation. Sensitivity is very important for clinical trials in chronic diseases, in which change in clinical condition may occur very slowly. A number of studies in MS have failed to show an effect on disease progression despite effects on number of attacks. This is almost certainly not because there was no effect but rather because the effect was too small to show on the Kurtzke scale, which is insensitive to small changes in some parts of its range. This problem is also seen in other degenerative diseases such as parkinsonism, in which marked fluctuation in patient performance occurs even minute to minute. In this case, the frequency and severity of the fluctuations themselves may be represented on the scale. Care must be taken to avoid identifying spurious improvement or worsening that results from fluctuation in symptoms rather than change in the underlying disease.

Scale Selection

Selection of a scale or scales is one of the most important steps in planning a clinical research project. The scales and the related statistical methods will determine, to a very large extent, how many patients you need to achieve a specified statistical power, what kind of statistics you can use, how much time and effort will be required to gather the essential data, and how many personnel you will need to help with the study.

In some instances, measures other than the main scale on which a trial depends will be needed. For example, in the interferon beta–1a (Avonex®) trial for MS, attack frequency was used even though the investigators considered it a poor measure. It was included because it had been used in other critical trials and there was a need to be able to compare this trial with the interferon beta–1b

(Betaseron®) and copolymer–1 (Copaxone®) trials. Similarly, despite the fact that there are better measures, it is still almost imperative that the Kurtzke extended disability scale be included in any multiple sclerosis trial so results can be compared with previous trials.

Whatever scales are chosen, it is important that they have demonstrated validity for the purpose for which they are being used. It would not be appropriate, for example, to use a Parkinson's scale in a stroke trial, or even in another movement disorder, without first demonstrating that it has some validity for that purpose.

The efficiency of the scale(s) selected for a trial is important. When possible, the most efficient scale(s) that will do the job should be selected. Efficiency is important whether the examiner is a physician, a psychologist, a medical assistant, or the patient filling out extensive questionnaires. Patients become impatient with extended testing and may drop out rather than put up with testing that fatigues them or takes too much of their time. Unfortunately, the need for comparison with earlier trials and to use well-validated scales often limits one's ability to use only the more efficient measures.

There are thousands of scales that are used in neurologic diseases, and it is not possible to include them all in a single volume. In this handbook, we emphasize public domain scales that have been validated and are reliable and efficient.

References

Bollet AJ. The purpura nautica, or low C on the high seas. In: *Plagues and poxes*. New York: Demos,1987:1–8.

Hauser SL, Dawson DM, Lehrich JR, et al. Intensive immunosuppression in progressive multiple sclerosis: a randomized three-arm study of high dose intravenous cyclophosphamide, plasma exchange and ACTH. *N Engl J Med* 1983;308:173–80.

Kurtzke JF. Rating neurologic impairment in multiple sclerosis: an expanded disability status scale (EDSS). *Neurology* 1983;33:1444–52.

Meinert CL. *Clinical trials, design, conduct and analysis.* New York: Oxford University Press, 1986.

Wade DT. *Measurement in neurological rehabilitation.* New York: Oxford Medical Publications, 1992:38.

CHAPTER 2 Pediatric Developmental Scales

Roger A. Brumback, M.D.

Many of the scales that have been developed in clinical neuroscience for the evaluation of adults can be adapted for use in children, such as the Mini-Mental State Examination (Ouvrier et al., 1993; Folstein et al., 1975). However, the unique aspect of pediatric neurology is the developmental changes that occur in children. Many scales have been developed to assess development for a variety of functions. Many of these are used routinely by pediatricians as well as by pediatric neurologists. One of the most important scales is the simple measurement of the fronto-occipital head circumference. Growth charts for plotting head circumference (as well as height and weight) are widely available in all hospitals with pediatric services and in the offices of pediatricians. Many of the scales for evaluating children are proprietary and copies must be purchased or permission obtained from various companies or individuals for their use (see also Spreen & Strauss, 1991; Raskin, 1985; Hammill et al., 1992).

Adaptive Behavior Inventory

Assessment of adaptive behavior is an important part of the evaluation of mental retardation.

Description

This scale can be used to measure the skills of daily living. The inventory consists of five scales: self-care skills, communication skills, social skills, academic skills, and occupational skills, which together yield a summary adaptive behavior quotient. Administration requires about 20 to 25 minutes. Norms are available for ages 6 to 18 years (Brown & Leigh, 1986).

American Association on Mental Deficiency Adaptive Behavior Scale

Adaptive behavior is now considered an important part of the diagnosis of mental retardation (Grossman, 1983), which requires subnormal functioning in both intelligence and adaptive behavior. Thus, the American Association on Mental Deficiency published a scale for use in the assessment of adaptive behavior (Fogelman, 1974; Nihira et al., 1969)

Description

The American Association on Mental Deficiency Adaptive Behavior Scale consists of two parts. The Part I behavioral domains are developmentally

7

organized and measure basic survival skills and behaviors that are important for independent living, whereas the Part II domains assess maladaptive behaviors. Administration requires about 15 to 30 minutes. Norms are available down to age 3 years.

Part I   *Behavioral Domains*
   Independent Functioning
   Physical Development
   Economic Activity
   Language Development
   Number and Time Concepts
   Domestic Activity
   Vocational Activity
   Self-Direction
   Responsibility
   Socialization
Part II   *Behavioral Domains*
   Violent and Destructive Behavior
   Antisocial Behavior
   Rebellious Behavior
   Untrustworthy Behavior
   Withdrawal
   Stereotyped Behavior and Odd
      Mannerisms
   Inappropriate Interpersonal Manners
   Unacceptable or Eccentric Habits
   Unacceptable Vocal Habits
   Self-Abusive Behavior
   Hyperactive Tendencies
   Sexually Aberrant Behavior
   Psychological Disturbance

Bayley Scales of Infant Development

The Bayley Scales of Infant Development (BSID) is now one of the most widely used measures for infant development (Bayley, 1970, 1993; Damarin, 1978; Lehr et al., 1987)

Description

This test measures mental and motor development. It consists of three parts: Mental Scale (sensory-perceptual acuity, discrimination, object constancy, memory, learning, problem solving, vocalization, early verbalization, and early abstract thinking);

Motor Scale (body control, coordination, and finger manipulation); and Behavior Rating Scale (affective behavior, motivation, and interest). Items are numbered according to difficulty (age level), and all items are tested between a basal level at which all items are passed and a ceiling level at which no items are passed. Items at many levels utilize similar test situations; for example, item 3 is response to the sound of a rattle, item 36 is the child playing with the rattle, item 48 is turning the head to the sound of the rattle, and item 59 is the child finding the rattle after it has been taken away. Scoring results in a Mental Development Index (MDI) and Psychomotor Development Index (PDI). These scores can also be converted to age equivalents. Age range of the test is from 2 months to 2 years. Administration time is approximately 30 to 40 minutes.

The BSID has been standardized on a large sample (> 1,000) of normal children. However, the predictive value of this test for later intelligence scores is not completely settled (Ramey et al., 1973).

Bellevue Index of Depression (BID)

In 1973 Weinberg and colleagues published criteria for establishing the diagnosis of depression in children. Subsequently, Petti (1978) used these criteria to develop a semistructured interview questionnaire termed the Bellevue Index of Depression, which is administered separately to the child and the parent or caretaker.

Description

The Bellevue Index of Depression consists of 40 items in 10 categories. Each item is to be rated on a four-part scale of "not at all," "a little," "quite a bit," or "very much," and for duration of "less than 1 month," "1 month to 6 months," "6 months to 2 years" or "always." The items are administered on a written form for parents and in a semistructured interview format with the child. A summary score is obtained from both the child's answers and the parent's form, with the higher of the summary scores considered the total score for the test purposes. The total score above a cut-off value is considered evidence of depression, with greater severity of depression relating to higher scores. Age range is from 6 to 12 years. Completion requires about 15 to 30 minutes.

Interrater reliability is good, it is relatively easy to administer, and it can be used to identify changes with therapy (Petti & Law, 1982; Petti & Conners, 1983)

I. Dysphoric mood
 1. Statements or appearance of sadness, loneliness, unhappiness, hopelessness, and/or pessimism
 2. Mood swings, moodiness
 3. Irritable, easily annoyed
 4. Hypersensitive, cries easily
 5. Negative, difficult to please
II. Self-deprecatory ideation
 6. Feelings of being worthless, useless, dumb, stupid, ugly, guilty
 7. Beliefs of persecution
 8. Death wishes
 9. Suicidal thoughts
 10. Suicidal attempts
III. Aggressive behavior (agitation)
 11. Difficult to get along with
 12. Quarrelsome
 13. Disrespectful of authority
 14. Belligerent, hostile, agitated
 15. Excessive fighting or sudden anger
IV. Sleep disturbance
 16. Initial insomnia
 17. Restless sleep
 18. Terminal insomnia
 19. Difficulty awakening in the morning
V. Change in school performance
 20. Frequent complaints from teachers ("daydreaming," "poor concentration," "poor memory")
 21. Loss of usual work effort in school subjects
 22. Loss of usual interest in nonacademic school activities
 23. Much incomplete school work
 24. Much incomplete homework
 25. A drop in usual grades
 26. Finds homework difficult
VI. Diminished socialization
 27. Less group participation
 28. Less friendly, less outgoing
 29. Socially withdrawing

 30. Loss of usual social interests
VII. Change in attitude toward school
 31. Does not enjoy school activities
 32. Does not want or refuses to attend school
VIII. Somatic complaints
 33. Non-migraine headaches
 34. Abdominal pain
 35. Muscle aches or pains
 36. Other somatic complaints or concerns (specify)
IX. Loss of usual energy
 37. Loss of usual personal interests or pursuits (other than school, e.g., hobbies, playing)
 38. Decreased activity level; mental and/or physical fatigue
X. Unusual change in appetite and/or of weight
 39. Anorexia or polyphagia
 40. Unusual weight change in past four months

Brazelton Neonatal Behavioral Assessment Scale (NBAS)

The Brazelton Scale was originally introduced in 1973 as a means of evaluating the behavior of infants, particularly the ability of infants to interact with the environment (Brazelton, 1973, 1984; Brazelton & Nugent, 1995).

Description

The Brazelton Scale includes 28 behavioral items (scored on a 9-point scale), 18 reflex items (scored on a 4-point scale), and 7 supplementary items (scored on a 9-point scale) of particular value in assessing frail premature infants. Items assessed are:

Behavioral Items

Response decrement to light

Response decrement to rattle

Response decrement to bell

Response decrement to tactile stimulation of foot

Orientation—inanimate visual

Orientation—inanimate auditory

Orientation—inanimate visual and auditory
Orientation—animate visual
Orientation—animate auditory
Orientation—animate visual and auditory
Alertness
General tonus
Motor maturity
Pull-to-sit
Defensive movements
Activity level
Peak of excitement
Rapidity of build-up
Irritability
Lability of states
Cuddliness
Consolability
Self-quieting
Hand-to-mouth
Tremulousness
Startles
Lability of skin color
Smiles

Reflex Items

Plantar grasp
Babinski
Ankle clonus
Rooting
Sucking
Glabella
Passive movements—arms
Passive movements—legs
Palmar grasp
Placing
Standing
Walking
Crawling
Incurvation (Gallant response)
Tonic deviation of head and eyes
Nystagmus
Tonic neck reflex
Moro

Supplementary Items

Quality of alertness
Cost of attention

Examiner facilitation
General irritability
Robustness and endurance
State regulation
Examiner's emotional response

This scale has been used in a variety of obstetric and neonatal research studies to ascertain effects on newborns (Stjernqvist & Svenningsen, 1990; Dixon et al., 1984; Field et al., 1986).

Children's Depression Inventory (CDI)

The popular 21-item Beck Depression Inventory (Beck, 1967) was modified for use in children as the Children's Depression Inventory (Kovacs, 1980-1981).

Description

The CDI is a 27-item self-report scale that evaluates a range of depressive symptoms. Each item is rated with three choices of severity (scored from 0 to 2). The total score correlates with severity of depressive symptomatology and can be used to follow changes in severity. Age range is from 6 to 16 years. The test requires a first grade reading level (Kazden & Petti, 1982). Completion requires about 15 minutes.

Children's Depression Rating Scale— Revised (CDRS-R)

The Children's Depression Rating Scale can be used as a clinical screening device for depression and as a measure of change with treatment (Poznanski et al., 1979, 1984, 1985).

Description

The CDRS-R consists of 17 items administered in a semistructured interview. Fourteen of the items are rated on the basis of the answers by the child during the interview and three are rated by the examiner on the basis of observation of the child's nonverbal behavior. Severity ratings for each item reflect both intensity and frequency of the symptom. The total score above a cut-off value is considered evidence of depression, with greater severity relating to higher scores. Age range is from 6 to 12 years. Testing requires about 20 to 30 minutes.

Conners Parent Rating Scale

The Conners Parent Rating Scale is one of the most widely used scales for assessment of childhood behavioral disturbances in psychopharmacologic studies. Two versions exist, the original version introduced by Conners (1970) and a shorter revised version by Goyette and colleagues (1978).

Description

The original version has 93 questions (the revised version has only 48 questions). The test is completed by the parent or caretaker of the child for the symptoms that are currently evident (previous symptoms—i.e., not present during the past month—are not to be rated). Areas assessed by the questionnaire include conduct problems, hyperactivity, inattention, aggression, anxiety, somatic complaints, fears, obsessive-compulsive behavior, and school adjustment problems. Each item is to be rated by the parent on a four-part scale of "not at all," "just a little," "pretty much," or "very much," with scores of 0, 1, 2, 3 for these respective responses:

Problems of Eating

1. Picky and finicky
2. Will not eat enough
3. Overweight

Problems of Sleep

4. Restless
5. Nightmares
6. Awakens at night
7. Cannot fall asleep

Fear and Worries

8. Afraid of new situations
9. Afraid of people
10. Afraid of being alone
11. Worries about illness and death

Muscular Tension

12. Gets stiff and rigid

13. Twitches, jerks, etc.
14. Shakes

Speech Problems

15. Stuttering
16. Hard to understand

Wetting

17. Bed wetting
18. Runs to bathroom constantly

Bowel Problems

19. Soiling self
20. Holds back bowel movements

Complains of Following Symptoms Even Though Doctor Can Find Nothing Wrong

21. Headaches
22. Stomachaches
23. Vomiting
24. Aches and pains
25. Loose bowels

Problems of Sucking, Chewing, or Picking

26. Sucks thumb
27. Bites or picks nails
28. Chews on clothes, blankets, or other items
29. Picks at things such as hair, clothing, etc.

Childish or Immature

30. Does not act his age
31. Cries easily
32. Wants help doing things he should do alone
33. Clings to parents or other adults
34. Baby talk

Trouble with Feelings

35. Keeps anger to himself
36. Lets himself get pushed around by other children
37. Unhappy
38. Carries a chip on his shoulder

Over-Asserts Himself

39. Bullying

40. Bragging and boasting
41. Sassy to grown-ups

Problems Making Friends

42. Shy
43. Afraid they do not like him
44. Feelings easily hurt
45. Has no friends

Problems with Brothers and Sisters

46. Feels cheated
47. Mean
48. Fights constantly

Problems Keeping Friends

49. Disturbs other children
50. Wants to run things
51. Picks on other children

Restless

52. Restless or overactive
53. Excitable, impulsive
54. Fails to finish things he starts—short attention span

Temper

55. Temper outbursts, explosive and unpredictable behavior
56. Throws himself around
57. Throws and breaks things
58. Pouts and sulks

Sex

59. Plays with own sex organs
60. Involved in sex play with others
61. Modest about his body

Problems in School

62. Is not learning
63. Does not like to go to school
64. Is afraid to go to school
65. Daydreams
66. Truancy
67. Will not obey school rules

Lying

68. Denies having done wrong
69. Blames others for his mistakes
70. Tells stories which did not happen

Stealing

71. From parents
72. At school
73. From stores and other places

Fire-Setting

74. Sets fires

Trouble with Police

75. Gets into trouble with police

Perfectionism

76. Everything must be just so
77. Things must be done same way every time
78. Sets goals too high

Additional Problems

79. Inattentive, easily distracted
80. Constantly fidgeting
81. Cannot be left alone
82. Always climbing
83. A very early riser
84. Will run around between mouthfuls at meals
85. Demands must be met immediately—easily frustrated
86. Cannot stand too much excitement
87. Laces and zippers are always open
88. Cries often and easily
89. Unable to stop a repetitive activity
90. Acts as if driven by a motor
91. Mood changes quickly and drastically
92. Poorly aware of surroundings or time of day
93. Still cannot tie shoelaces

Summary scores and factor scores can be obtained. Age range is from 6 to 14 years. Completion requires about 10 to 15 minutes.

This test has been shown to have a relatively consistent practice effect on successive administrations, resulting in lower scores (Werry &

Sprague, 1974); thus, several baseline administrations are necessary before beginning any therapeutic trials.

Conners Teacher Rating Scale

The Conners Teacher Rating Scale is the most widely used scale in assessing stimulant drug effects in hyperactive children. There is the original version, which was introduced in 1969, and a shortened revised version; the original version has been more extensively utilized and standardized (Trites et al., 1982).

Description

The original version has 39 items (the revised version has 28). The test is completed by the homeroom teacher. Items are divided into three groups—classroom behavior, group participation, and attitude toward authority. Each item is to be rated on a 4-part scale of "not at all," "just a little," "pretty much," or "very much," with scores of 0, 1, 2, 3 for these respective responses:

Classroom Behavior

1. Constantly fidgeting
2. Hums and makes other odd noises
3. Demands must be met immediately—easily frustrated
4. Coordination poor
5. Restless or overactive
6. Excitable, impulsive
7. Inattentive, easily distracted
8. Fails to finish things he starts—short attention span
9. Overly sensitive
10. Overly serious or sad
11. Daydreams
12. Sullen or sulky
13. Cries often and easily
14. Disturbs other children
15. Quarrelsome
16. Mood changes quickly and drastically
17. Acts "smart"
18. Destructive
19. Steals

20. Lies
21. Temper outbursts, explosive and unpredictable behavior

Group Participation

22. Isolates himself from other children
23. Appears to be unaccepted by group
24. Appears to be easily led
25. No sense of fair play
26. Appears to lack leadership
27. Does not get along with opposite sex
28. Does not get along with same sex
29. Teases other children or interferes with their activities

Attitude Toward Authority

30. Submissive
31. Defiant
32. Impudent
33. Shy
34. Fearful
35. Excessive demands for teacher's attention
36. Stubborn
37. Overly anxious to please
38. Uncooperative
39. Attendance problem

Summary scores and factor scores can be obtained. Age range is from 6 to 17 years. Completion requires about 5 to 10 minutes.

Denver Developmental Screening Test

The Denver Developmental Screening Test was introduced in 1969 by Frankenburg and Dodds and almost immediately became a favorite technique for pediatricians to quickly assess the developmental level of infants and young children (Frankenburg et al., 1988a, 1988b; Frankenburg & Camp, 1975). The current revision of the test underwent extensive restandardization and is now know as the Denver-II (Frankenburg et al., 1992) (Figure 2-1).

Description

The Denver Developmental Screening Test measures four domains of behavior: Personal-

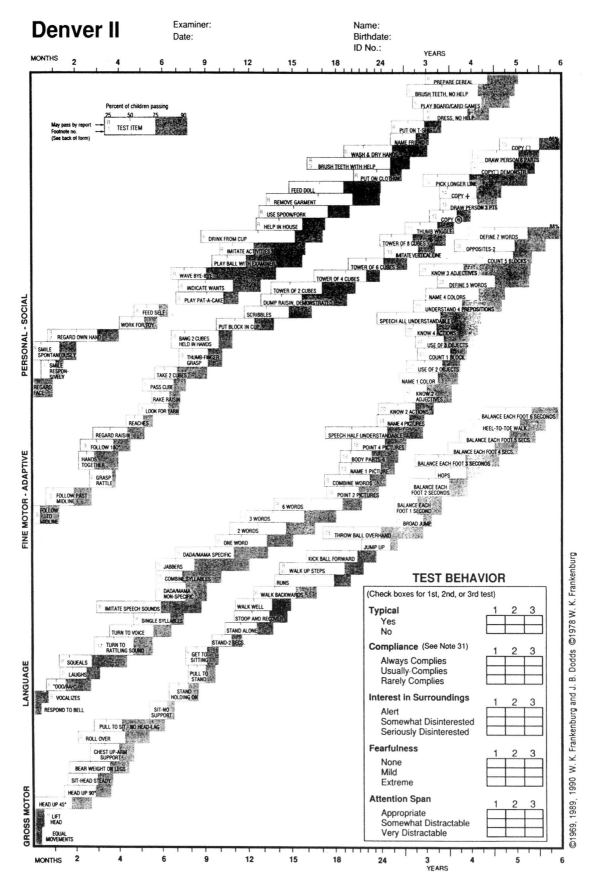

Figure 2-1

14

DIRECTIONS FOR ADMINISTRATION

1. Try to get child to smile by smiling, talking or waving. Do not touch him/her.
2. Child must stare at hand several seconds.
3. Parent may help guide toothbrush and put toothpaste on brush.
4. Child does not have to be able to tie shoes or button/zip in the back.
5. Move yarn slowly in an arc from one side to the other, about 8" above child's face.
6. Pass if child grasps rattle when it is touched to the backs or tips of fingers.
7. Pass if child tries to see where yarn went. Yarn should be dropped quickly from sight from tester's hand without arm movement.
8. Child must transfer cube from hand to hand without help of body, mouth, or table.
9. Pass if child picks up raisin with any part of thumb and finger.
10. Line can vary only 30 degrees or less from tester's line.|/
11. Make a fist with thumb pointing upward and wiggle only the thumb. Pass if child imitates and does not move any fingers other than the thumb.

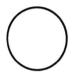

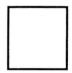

12. Pass any enclosed form. Fail continuous round motions.

13. Which line is longer? (Not bigger.) Turn paper upside down and repeat. (pass 3 of 3 or 5 of 6)

14. Pass any lines crossing near midpoint.

15. Have child copy first. If failed, demonstrate.

When giving items 12, 14, and 15, do not name the forms. Do not demonstrate 12 and 14.

16. When scoring, each pair (2 arms, 2 legs, etc.) counts as one part.
17. Place one cube in cup and shake gently near child's ear, but out of sight. Repeat for other ear.
18. Point to picture and have child name it. (No credit is given for sounds only.)
   If less than 4 pictures are named correctly, have child point to picture as each is named by tester.

 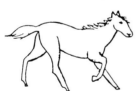 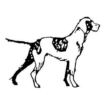 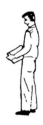

19. Using doll, tell child: Show me the nose, eyes, ears, mouth, hands, feet, tummy, hair. Pass 6 of 8.
20. Using pictures, ask child: Which one flies?... says meow?... talks?... barks?... gallops? Pass 2 of 5, 4 of 5.
21. Ask child: What do you do when you are cold?... tired?... hungry? Pass 2 of 3, 3 of 3.
22. Ask child: What do you do with a cup? What is a chair used for? What is a pencil used for?
   Action words must be included in answers.
23. Pass if child correctly places and says how many blocks are on paper. (1, 5).
24. Tell child: Put block on table; under table; in front of me, behind me. Pass 4 of 4.
   (Do not help child by pointing, moving head or eyes.)
25. Ask child: What is a ball?... lake?... desk?... house?... banana?... curtain?... fence?... ceiling? Pass if defined in terms of use, shape, what it is made of, or general category (such as banana is fruit, not just yellow). Pass 5 of 8, 7 of 8.
26. Ask child: If a horse is big, a mouse is __? If fire is hot, ice is __? If the sun shines during the day, the moon shines during the __? Pass 2 of 3.
27. Child may use wall or rail only, not person. May not crawl.
28. Child must throw ball overhand 3 feet to within arm's reach of tester.
29. Child must perform standing broad jump over width of test sheet (8 1/2 inches).
30. Tell child to walk forward, ᴐᴑᴐᴑᴐᴑ➤ heel within 1 inch of toe. Tester may demonstrate.
   Child must walk 4 consecutive steps.
31. In the second year, half of normal children are non-compliant.

OBSERVATIONS:

Figure 2-1 *(continued)*

social, Fine motor-adaptive, Language, and Gross motor. The test consists of 125 items arranged in order of difficulty. Test forms give the ages at which 25%, 50%, 75%, and 90% of children will correctly pass each item. The age equivalent developmental level for each of the domains is determined by the last item the child successfully completes. Some test items can be passed by report of a caretaker. Age range is from birth to 6 years (the age scale conforms to the American Academy of Pediatrics Health Supervision Visit Schedule). Administration requires about 20 minutes.

Developmental Test of Visual-Motor Integration

The Developmental Test of Visual-Motor Integration (VMI) is a copying test that is modeled after the visual perception test of Frostig (Frostig et al., 1966) and is similar to the Bender-Gestalt test (Armstrong & Knopf, 1982). The VMI was originally introduced in 1967 (Beery & Buktenica, 1967) but has since been revised (Beery 1982, 1989).

Description

This test consists of 24 designs of progressive difficulty, from a vertical line to a three-dimensional cube that the child is told to copy into a blank space directly below the stimulus figure. The test is in two forms—the short form with only the first 15 designs for use in ages 2 to 8 years, and the long form with all designs for use up to age 14 11/12 years. Scoring results in a standard score and an age equivalent. Completion requires about 20 minutes.

Although the original normative data were criticized on ethnic and socioeconomic grounds (Martin et al., 1977), the restandarization in over 3,000 children for the revision has overcome this problem (Beery 1982, 1989).

Dubowitz Scale

The Dubowitz Scale uses a series of 10 neuromuscular criteria to assess gestational age of a newborn infant (Dubowitz et al., 1970). These neuromuscular criteria in combination with 12 physical criteria can be used to determine gestational age from 26 to 44 weeks (Dubowitz & Dubowitz, 1981). Ballard (1991) reduced the neuromuscular items to 6 and the physical maturity items to 6 to define a scale that accurately assesses infants from 20 to 44 weeks gestational age (Ballard et al., 1991).

Description

The original Dubowitz scale has 10 neuromuscular items, but the New Ballard Score adaptation includes only the 6 most reproducible neuromuscular items (Figure 2-2). The evaluation must be performed within the first 12 hours of life.

Posture: Observed with infant quiet and in supine position. Score 0: arms and legs extended; 1: beginning of flexion of hips and knees, arms extended; 2: stronger flexion of legs, arms extended; 3: arms slightly flexed, legs flexed and abducted; 4: full flexion of arms and legs.

Square Window: The hand is flexed on the forearm between the thumb and index finger of the examiner. Enough pressure is applied to get as full a flexion as possible, and the angle between the hypothenar eminence and the ventral aspect of the forearm is measured and graded according to diagram. (Care is taken not to rotate the infant's wrist while doing this maneuver.)

Arm Recoil: With the infant in the supine position, the forearms are first flexed for 5 seconds, then fully extended by pulling on the hands, and then released. The sign is fully positive if the arms return briskly to full flexion (Score 2). If the arms return to incomplete flexion or the response is sluggish it is graded as Score 1. If they remain extended or are only followed by random movements the score is 0.

Popliteal Angle: With the infant supine and his pelvis flat on the examining couch, the thigh is held in the knee-chest position by the examiner's left index finger and thumb supporting the knee. The leg is then extended by gentle pressure from the examiner's right index finger behind the ankle and the popliteal angle is measured.

Scarf Sign: With the baby supine, take the infant's hand and try to put it around the neck and as far posteriorly as possible around the opposite shoulder. Assist this maneuver by lifting the elbow across the body. See how far the elbow will go across. Score 0: elbow reaches opposite axillary line; 1: elbow between midline and opposite axillary line; 2: elbow reaches midline; 3: elbow will not reach midline.

Heel to Ear Maneuver: With the baby supine, draw the baby's foot as near to the head as it will go without forcing it. Observe the distance between the foot and the head as well as the degree of extension at the knee. Note that the knee is left free and may draw down alongside the abdomen.

Neuromuscular Maturity

	-1	0	1	2	3	4	5
Posture							
Square Window (wrist)	>90°	90°	60°	45°	30°	0°	
Arm Recoil		180°	140°-180°	110°-140°	90-110°	<90°	
Popliteal Angle	180°	160°	140°	120°	100°	90°	<90°
Scarf Sign							
Heel to Ear							

Physical Maturity

Skin	sticky friable transparent	gelatinous red, translucent	smooth pink, visible veins	superficial peeling &/or rash, few veins	cracking pale areas rare veins	parchment deep cracking no vessels	leathery cracked wrinkled
Lanugo	none	sparse	abundant	thinning	bald areas	mostly bald	
Plantar Surface	heel-toe 40-50mm: -1 <40mm: -2	>50mm no crease	faint red marks	anterior transverse crease only	creases ant. 2/3	creases over entire sole	
Breast	imperceptible	barely perceptible	flat areola no bud	stippled areola 1-2mm bud	raised areola 3-4mm bud	full areola 5-10mm bud	
Eye/Ear	lids fused loosely:-1 tightly:-2	lids open pinna flat stays folded	sl. curved pinna; soft; slow recoil	well-curved pinna; soft but ready recoil	formed & firm instant recoil	thick cartilage ear stiff	
Genitals male	scrotum flat, smooth	scrotum empty faint rugae	testes in upper canal rare rugae	testes descending few rugae	testes down good rugae	testes pendulous deep rugae	
Genitals female	clitoris prominent labia flat	prominent clitoris small labia minora	prominent clitoris enlarging minora	majora & minora equally prominent	majora large minora small	majora cover clitoris & minora	

Maturity Rating

score	weeks
-10	20
-5	22
0	24
5	26
10	28
15	30
20	32
25	34
30	36
35	38
40	40
45	42
50	44

Figure 2-2

Kaufman Assessment Battery for Children (K-ABC)

The K-ABC is the newest of the intelligence tests and uses a different theoretical model than the two standard tests, the Stanford-Binet and the Wechsler Scales. The theoretical model is of sequential and simultaneous processing of information, which is presumably based on the theories of Luria (Das et al., 1979; Luria, 1980). It incorporates 6 achievement tests and 10 mental process subtests, 7 of which are "simultaneous" and 3 "sequential." Six subtests are considered nonverbal and suitable for children with language problems (Kaufman et al., 1987).

Description

The K-ABC consists of 16 subtests. Although the test is designed for ages 2 6/12 to 12 6/12, not all subtests are administered to all ages. Subtests are as follows:

1. Magic Window (15 items; simultaneous; age 2 6/12 to 4 11/12)—child must name an object (such as a car) rotated behind a narrow slit

that only allows part of the object to be seen at any one time.

2. Face Recognition (15 items; simultaneous; age range 2 6/12 to 4 11/12)—child briefly views picture of face and must pick same face with different pose out of a group photograph.

3. Hand Movements (21 items; sequential; all ages)—child must copy exact sequence of taps on table with fist, palm, or side of hand.

4. Gestalt Closure (25 items, simultaneous; all ages)—child must name or describe an incomplete ink drawing.

5. Number Recall (19 items; sequential; all ages)—a digit repetition task.

6. Triangles (18 items; simultaneous; age range 4 0/12 to 12 6/12)—child assembles identical rubber triangles (blue on one side, yellow on other side) to match an abstract design.

7. Word Order (20 items; sequential; age range 4 0/12 to 12 6/12)—child points to outlines of common objects in same order as named by examiner.

8. Matrix Analogies (20 items; simultaneous; age range 5 0/12 to 12 6/12)—child selects from an array the design that matches the test design.

9. Spatial Memory (21 items; simultaneous; age range 5 0/12 to 12 6/12)—child has to recall location of pictures arranged randomly on page.

10. Photo Series (17 items; simultaneous; age range 6 0/12 to 12 6/12)—child arranges photographs in proper time sequence.

11. Expressive Vocabulary (24 items; achievement; age range 2 6/12 to 4 11/12)—child names photographed objects.

12. Faces and Places (35 items; achievement; all ages)—child identifies fictional characters and famous persons and places (such as Santa Claus).

13. Arithmetic (38 items; achievement; age range 3 0/12 to 12 6/12)—various tasks such as counting, recognizing shapes, identifying numbers, and solving verbal arithmetic problems.

14. Riddles (32 items; achievement; age range 3 0/12 to 12 6/12)—child must infer name from characteristics (such as "What has fur, wags its tail, and barks?").

15. Reading/Decoding (38 items; achievement; age range 5 0/12 to 12 6/12)—child identifies letters and reads words.

16. Reading/Understanding (24 items; achievement; age range 7 0/12 to 12 6/12)—child must act out printed commands.

Testing involves sequential administration of each item from a basal level to a ceiling level (last item correctly answered), with raw score consisting of the ceiling item minus errors. This score can be translated into a scaled score and age-appropriate standard scores. In addition to a mental processing composite score, scores for four scales are available (Sequential Processing Scale, Simultaneous Processing Scale, Achievement Scale, and Nonverbal Scale). Average administration time ranges from 30 minutes for 3-year-olds to 75 minutes for 12-year-olds.

The K-ABC has been well standardized (Kaufman & Kaufman, 1983). A disadvantage of the test is that it is not equivalent to the Wechsler Scales or the Stanford-Binet test (the K-ABC overestimates IQ by up to 8 points), but it does offer additional information supplementary to these tests (Naglieri, 1985).

KeyMath Diagnostic Arithmetic Test

The KeyMath Diagnostic Arithmetic Test assesses mathematical skills (Connolly et al., 1976)

Description

The test consists of 14 subtests divided into three areas. The Content area has three subtests—Numeration, Fractions, and Geometry and Symbols—which evaluate the understanding of basic arithmetic operations. The Operations area has 6 subtests—Addition, Subtraction, Multiplication, Division, Mental Computation, and Numerical Reasoning—which evaluate computational abilities. The Applications area contains 5 subtests—Word Problems, Missing Elements, Money, Measurements, and Time—which evaluate the ability to use arithmetic in everyday life. The test items of increasing difficulty are presented orally as an open-ended question by the examiner. For most items the child must respond orally, although for a few of the more difficult items, written computation may be necessary. Results are expressed as subtest scores, areas scores, and a composite grade equivalent score. Age range is preschool through grade 6. Administration requires 30 to 40 minutes.

The KeyMath Test is a grade equivalency test and does not allow for age comparisons (Price, 1984). It is a particularly useful test for evaluating individuals with poor reading and writing skills since these skills are not required.

Neurologic Examination for Subtle Signs

Subtle neurologic signs ("soft signs") are frequently evident in children with a variety of neurologic, learning, and behavior problems. The Physical and Neurological Examination for Soft Signs (PANESS) was developed to quantitate these findings (Camp et al., 1978; Holden et al., 1982). It was subsequently revised and renamed the Neurological Examination for Subtle Signs (NESS) (Denckla, 1985)

Description

The Neurological Examination for Subtle Signs consists of 21 items that test lateral preferences, gait and station, and coordination (10 of the items are timed). Items include various walking (on the heels, on the toes, and on the sides of the feet), rapid alternating movement, and balancing tasks. Age range is about 4 to 15 years. Administration requires approximately 15 to 20 minutes.

While norms have been published from the National Institutes of Health sample for some of the timed tasks, this examination is observer-dependent, so norms need to be established for each investigator on his or her own population. The test does provide a systematic method for reproducibly examining and detecting subtle neurologic signs in children.

Peabody Picture Vocabulary Test—Revised (PPVT-R)

This is a multiple-choice test designed to evaluate receptive vocabulary. It was originally introduced in 1965 and revised in 1981 (Dunn & Dunn, 1981). The test requires no reading ability. Two equivalent alternate forms are available.

Description

The child is asked to pick 1 of 4 pictured items that depict the word spoken by the examiner. There are 5 training questions and 175 test questions of increasing difficulty. The test is stopped after failures on 6 out of 8 consecutive questions. The score is the total number of items passed that can be translated into a standard score or age equivalent. (Note that in the original test these translations of the score were termed *IQ* and *mental age,* implying that the PPVT was a test of verbal intelligence). Average administration time is 10 minutes. Age range is from 2 years to adulthood.

The PPVT was standardized on a sample ranging in age from 2 1/2 years to 40 years. Retest reliability is very high with readministration within 2 weeks using the alternate form or with the same form after several months. (Tillinghast et al., 1983)

Stanford-Binet Intelligence Scale—Revised

In 1905 in France, Binet introduced an intelligence test that was subsequently introduced in North America by Terman in 1916. Subsequent revisions were introduced in 1937, 1960, and 1986. The current form is the fourth edition (Thorndike et al., 1986a, 1986b).

Description

The Stanford-Binet Intelligence Scale consists of 15 subtests. The vocabulary subtest is administered first to obtain a basal level for beginning items in all the other subtests. The basal level for each test is established where two consecutive items are passed, while the ceiling level is established by four consecutive failures. The only timed subtest is pattern analysis (subtest 5). The subtests are as follows:

1. Vocabulary (46 items)—child names pictures (to item 14) and gives word definitions.
2. Comprehension (42 items)—child answers questions (such as "Give two reasons why there are commercials on television").
3. Absurdities (32 items)—child must point out incongruities in pictures (such as girl writing on a piece of paper with a fork).
4. Verbal Relations (18 items)—child is shown cards each containing four words and is instructed to describe how the fourth word differs from the other three words (such as boy, girl, man, dog).
5. Pattern Analysis (42 items)—child must properly place blocks in holes (to item 10) and arrange up to nine blocks in a design.
6. Copying (28 items)—child must copy the arrangement of four blocks shown by the examiner (to item 12) and copy geometric shapes shown on cards.

7. Matrices (26 items)—child must chose correct geometric design or letter pattern to fill empty box in 2 X 2 and 3 X 3 matrices.

8. Paper Folding and Cutting—child is asked to pick which pattern of folded paper would produce the paper form shown as the test item.

9. Quantitative (40 items)—child must correctly arrange blocks with varying numbers of dots, count, and perform simple arithmetic.

10. Number Series (26 items)—child determines the next two numbers in various number series.

11. Equation Building (18 items)—child must arrange numbers and arithmetic symbols to produce equations.

12. Bead Memory (42 items)—child must pick the correct bead or arrange beads on a stick after being shown a card for 5 seconds.

13. Memory for Sentences (42 items)—child repeats sentences ranging in length from 2 words to 22 words.

14. Memory for Digits (26 items)—child must repeat in correct order and in reverse order 3 to 9 digits.

15. Memory for Objects—child must find 2 to 8 objects in correct sequence as shown previously on cards.

The subtests are grouped into four broad areas—Verbal Reasoning, Abstract/Visual Reasoning, Quantitative Reasoning, and Short-Term Memory—and a composite score is derived from the area scores. These Standard Age Scores (equivalent to IQ scores) have a mean of 100 and standard deviation of 16. The test is designed for ages 2 to 23 years. Administration requires an average of 60 to 90 minutes.

Vineland Adaptive Behavior Scales

The purpose of the Vineland Adaptive Behavior Scales is to evaluate the various social adaptive behaviors normally important in daily living (Evan & Bradley-Johnson, 1988). This test is an extensive revision of the original Vineland Social Maturity Scales (Doll, 1935)

Description

The test is not administered to the subject, but to the caretaker or person most familiar with the subject. The test items are administered in a semi-structured interview. For example, for the item "speaks in full sentences," the examiner must ask the caretaker about this with probing questions in such a way as to be certain of the correct understanding and response by the caretaker. Considerable training and skill on the part of the examiner are necessary to accurately administer this test.

The survey form consists of 297 items and the expanded form has an additional 280 items. There are 4 domains (and multiple subdomains) of behavior assessed with this test: Communication (receptive, expressive, and written); Daily Living Skills (personal, domestic, and community); Socialization (interpersonal relationships, play and leisure time, and coping skills); and Motor Skills (gross motor and fine motor). Scoring of each item is: 2 points for activity satisfactorily performed often, 1 point for new or sometimes correctly performed activities, and 0 for no performance of the activity. Scoring yields an Adaptive Behavior Composite Score, individual domain and subdomain scores, and age equivalents. An optional set of questions covers maladaptive behaviors such as bed wetting, impulsiveness, etc. Age range is birth to 19 years (which is presumably an adult ceiling for adaptive behavior). Administration time is about 20 to 40 minutes for the survey form and 60 to 90 minutes for the expanded form.

Standardization of the test involved administration to 3,000 normals (Sparrow et al., 1984). This is an advantage since correlations have been made with other tests. The disadvantage of the test is that it requires extensive training of examiners. Administration time can be greatly increased with poorly informed or uneducated caretakers.

Wechsler Intelligence Tests

The Wechsler intelligence tests have three forms for different age ranges—the Wechsler Preschool and Primary Scale of Intelligence—Revised (WPPSI-R) for ages 3 to 7 3/12 years, the Wechsler Intelligence Scale for Children—Third Edition (WISC-III) for ages 6 to 16 11/12 years, and the Wechsler Adult Intelligence Scale—Revised (WAIS-R) for ages 16 to 74 years. They are individually administered tests that provide a measure of general intelligence and are the most popular tests used for such evaluation (Kaufman et al., 1986; Kaufman 1979; Wechsler 1989, 1991).

Description

The test consists of a series of subtests dihotomized as to Verbal or Performance subtests. The WISC-III consists of five Verbal subtests and five Performance subtests (plus one optional subtest in the Verbal and two optional subtests in the Performance categories):

1. Information (Verbal)—child is asked questions such as "How many days are there in a week?" or "Who discovered America?" to assess the basic fund of knowledge.

2. Similarities (Verbal)—child is told to describe how two objects go together or are alike (for example, "cat" and "mouse"), which assesses higher order conceptual abilities and language facility.

3. Arithmetic (Verbal)—child is asked to count objects or compute simple word problems without assistance of paper and pencil (for example, "If I cut an apple in half, how many pieces will I have left?").

4. Vocabulary (Verbal)—child is asked to define words (for example, "bicycle," "nail," "affliction"), which assesses receptive vocabulary.

5. Comprehension (Verbal)—child is asked questions that require practical reasoning (for example, "What is the thing to do when you cut your finger?," "Why should a promise be kept?").

6. Digit Span (Verbal; optional test)—child repeats series of three to nine numbers forward and series of two to eight numbers backward, which assesses attention and short-term memory (although anxiety and difficulties with sequential organization can impair performance).

7. Picture Completion (Performance)—child is asked to identify what parts are missing in a series of pictures (for example, "leg of an elephant," "slot in a screw"), which assesses part–whole relationships.

8. Picture Arrangement (Performance; timed)—child is asked to arrange a set of jumbled pictures in order to tell a story, which assesses visual sequencing, social awareness, planning, and appreciation of the relationships of events.

9. Block Design (Performance; timed)—child must recreate designs using blocks with sides that are all red, all white, or half red/half white, which assesses visual-motor coordination.

10. Object Assembly (Performance; timed)—child must assemble puzzle pieces to produce five objects (for example, child, horse, car, human face, ball), which assesses visual-motor coordination.

11. Coding (Performance; timed)—this is a substitution task in which the child must fill a blank row of squares above a row of shapes (Coding A) or numbers (Coding B) with the appropriate symbol keyed to the same number or shape, which assesses visual motor coordination and motor efficiency.

12. Symbol Search (Performance; optional; timed)—child must determine whether the example shapes are included in a group of test shapes, which assesses visual-motor coordination.

13. Mazes (Performance; optional; timed)—child must draw a line from the middle of the maze to the exit without entering any blind alleys, which assesses visual-motor skills and planning.

The WPPSI-R is similar to the WISC-III, with five Performance subtests, five Verbal subtests (plus one optional subtest in both Verbal and Performance categories). Nine subtests (Information, Similarities, Arithmetic, Vocabulary, Comprehension, Picture Completion, Block Design, Object Assembly, and Mazes) are the same in both the WPPSI-R and the WISC-III, but the versions are simpler in the WPPSI-R. The Sentences subtest is an optional subtest that substitutes for Digit Span in the Verbal category. The Animal Pegs subtest is an optional subtest in the Performance category that substitutes for the coding subtest. The Geometric Design subtest in the Performance category has no counterpart in the WISC-III.

1. Sentences (Verbal; optional)—child must repeat verbatim a sentence read aloud by the examiner (for example, "Fish swim."), which assesses short-term memory and attention.

2. Animal Pegs (Performance; optional)—child must place a colored peg next to a picture of an animal according to a key.

3. Geometric Design (Performance)—consists of two parts: in the Visual Recognition/Discrimination items, child must identify an example shape among a group of test shapes; in the Drawing items, child must copy a series of figures, which assesses visual-motor coordination.

Scoring produces subtest scaled scores, composite scores for the Verbal and Performance sec-

Table 2-1. Weinberg Screening Affective Scale (WSAS)

Instructions—"We would like to ask you some very serious and very important questions. We want to know how you feel about yourself. If you agree with the statement, circle yes. If you do not agree with the statement, circle no. We consider these questions and your answers very important."

1. I will try to give my honest feelings on these questions.	yes	no
2. I feel dumb and stupid too much of the time.	yes	no
3. I can't do my homework anymore.	yes	no
4. I wish that I could stay in bed all day.	yes	no
5. I can't do anything right.	yes	no
6. Sometimes I wish I were dead.	yes	no
7. I don't like other people.	yes	no
8. I don't like school anymore.	yes	no
9. I feel sad too much of the time.	yes	no
10. I can't do my school work anymore, it's too hard.	yes	no
11. It's hard to have any fun anymore.	yes	no
12. School makes me feel sick.	yes	no
13. I have too many bad moods.	yes	no
14. This is not a good world.	yes	no
15. I don't like to eat anymore.	yes	no
16. I feel lonely too much of the time.	yes	no
17. I have too much trouble remembering things.	yes	no
18. Nothing is ever done the way I like it.	yes	no
19. I eat too much.	yes	no
20. I am not as good as other people.	yes	no
21. It seems like I'm always in trouble for fighting and that is not fair.	yes	no
22. I have gained too much weight.	yes	no
23. I have too many headaches.	yes	no
24. I don't want to go to school anymore.	yes	no
25. I don't have fun playing with my friends anymore.	yes	no
26. I feel too tired to play.	yes	no
27. It seems like some part of my body always hurts me.	yes	no
28. It makes me feel good to tease other people.	yes	no
29. People are always talking about me when I'm not there.	yes	no
30. I can't sit still and that is a problem for me.	yes	no
31. My friends don't want to be with me anymore.	yes	no
32. I'm too hard to get along with.	yes	no
33. I can't concentrate on my work.	yes	no
34. I daydream too much in school.	yes	no
35. I never seem to be able to finish my work in school.	yes	no
36. I have too many stomach aches.	yes	no
37. I have too many aches and pains in my muscles.	yes	no
38. I don't want to get out of bed in the morning.	yes	no
39. I talk too much and that causes a problem for me.	yes	no
40. I'm always grouchy and that's bad.	yes	no
41. It's hard to fall asleep and that bothers me.	yes	no
42. My friends don't like me anymore.	yes	no
43. When I wake up at night, it is hard to go back to sleep.	yes	no

Table 2-1.   *(continued)*

44. I am losing too much weight.	yes	no
45. I cause trouble for everybody.	yes	no
46. I don't want to be with my friends anymore.	yes	no
47. Everybody picks on me.	yes	no
48. I get angry easily.	yes	no
49. School makes me feel nervous.	yes	no
50. I cry a lot.	yes	no
51. I talk back to grown-ups.	yes	no
52. I wake up too early in the morning and it is hard to go back to sleep.	yes	no
53. I can't have any fun anymore.	yes	no
54. I think a lot about killing myself.	yes	no
55. My answers are how I have been feeling most of the time.	yes	no
56. These answers represent my honest feelings.	yes	no

Score Sheet

Criteria for depression by self-report

   A. I and II plus four (4) or more of III–X.

   B. Two or more positive items per major symptom category: I–X.

   C. "Yes" response on Question 55.

	Number of Positive Items	***Criteria***	
I: 9,13,14,16,18,40,48,50	_____	yes	no
II: 2,5,6,20,21,29,31,42,47,54	_____	yes	no
III: 28,32,45,51	_____	yes	no
IV: 38,41,43,52	_____	yes	no
V: 3,10,17,33,34,35	_____	yes	no
VI: 7,25,46	_____	yes	no
VII: 8,12,24,49	_____	yes	no
VIII: 23,27,36,37	_____	yes	no
IX: 4,11,26,53	_____	yes	no
X: 15,19,22,44	_____	yes	no
TOTAL:	_____		

Total number of positive categories

I II III IV V VI VII VIII IX X:	_____		
Response to Question 55:		yes	no
DEPRESSION BY SELF-REPORT:		yes	no
Death wish—positive on item 6:		yes	no
Suicidal ideation—positive on item 54:		yes	no

The WSAS has been used in one study to survey a school population for evidence of depression (Emslie et al., 1990).

tions (Verbal IQ and Performance IQ), and an over-all score (Full Scale IQ). Administration requires an average of 90 minutes.

The Wechsler Scales are probably the most widely used intelligence tests in the United States and have been extensively studied; the previous version, the WISC-R, was the most extensively cited test in the psychology literature (Kaufman, 1979, 1990). In addition to correlations with the Verbal, Performance, and Full Scale IQ scores, many factor analyses have been performed on the various subtests (Wechsler, 1991).

Weinberg Screening Affective Scale (WSAS)

In 1973 Weinberg and colleagues published criteria for establishing the diagnosis of depression in children. Weinberg subsequently developed a questionnaire that can be used to screen for depression in individual settings or with group administration (Weinberg & Emslie, 1988)

Description

The WSAS (Table 2-1) is used as a screening measure for evidence of depression in children and adolescents. The test consists of 56 "yes-no" items.

References

Armstrong BB, Knopf KF. Comparison of the Bender-Gestalt and Revised Developmental Test of Visual-Motor Integration. *Percept Motor Skills* 1982;55:164–66.

Ballard J, Khoury JC, Wedig K, Wang L, Eiler-Walsman BL, Lipp R. New Ballard Score, expanded to include extremely premature infants. *J Pediatr* 1991;119:417-23.

Bayley N. Development of mental abilities. In: Mussen PH (ed.). *Carmichael's manual of child psychology*, 3rd ed. New York: John Wiley, 1970.

Bayley N. *Bayley Scales of Infant Development*, 2nd ed. San Antonio: The Psychological Corporation, 1993.

Beck AT. *Depression: clinical, experimental, and theoretical aspects.* New York: Harper & Row, 1967.

Beery KE, Buktenica NA. *Developmental Test of Visual-Motor Integration.* Chicago: Follett Publishing, 1967.

Beery KE. *Revised Administration, Scoring, and Teaching Manual for the Developmental Test of Visual-Motor Integration.* Cleveland: Modern Curriculum Press, 1982

Beery KE. *Developmental Test of Visual-Motor Integration.* Austin, TX: Pro-Ed, 1989.

Brazelton TB, Nugent JK. *Neonatal Behavioral Assessment Scale,* 3rd ed. Clinics in Developmental Medicine No. 137. London: MacKeith Press, 1995.

Brazelton TB. *Neonatal Behavioral Assessment Scale.* Clinics in Developmental Medicine No. 50. London: Spastics International Medical Publications, 1973.

Brazelton TB. *Neonatal Behavioral Assessment Scale,* 2nd ed. Clinics in Developmental Medicine No. 88. London: Spastics International Medical Publications, 1984.

Brown L, Leigh JE. *Adaptive Behavior Inventory.* Austin, TX: Pro-Ed, 1986.

Camp JA, Bialer I, Sverd J, Winsberg BB. Clinical usefulness of the NIMH Physical and Neurological Examination for Soft Signs. *Am J Psychiatry* 1978;135:362–64.

Conners CK. *The Conners' Rating Scales.* Austin, TX: Pro-Ed, 1985.

Conners CK. Symptom patterns in hyperkinetic, neurotic, and normal children. *Child Development* 1970;41:667–82.

Conners CK. A teacher rating scale for use in drug studies with children. *Am J Psychiatry* 1969;126:884–88.

Connolly AJ, Nachtman W, Pritchett EM. *The KeyMath Diagnostic Arithmetic Test.* Circle Pines, MN: American Guidance Service, 1976

Damarin F. Bayley Scales of Infant Development. In: Buros OK (ed.). *The eighth mental measurement yearbook, Vol 1.* Highland Park, NJ: Gryphon, 1978:290–93.

Das JP, Kirby JR, Jarman RF. *Simultaneous and successive cognitive processes.* New York: Academic Press, 1979.

Denckla MB. Revised neurological examination for subtle signs. *Psychopharmacol Bull* 1985;21:773–800.

Dixon SD, Synder J, Holve R, Bromberger P. Behavioral effects of circumcision with and without anesthesia. *Develop Behav Pediatr* 1984;3:246–50.

Doll EA. A genetic scale of social maturity. *Am J Orthopsychiatry* 1935;5:180-88.

Dubowitz LMS, Dubowitz V, Goldberg C. Clinical assessment of gestational age in the newborn infant. *J Pediatr* 1970;77:1–10.

Dubowitz L, Dubowitz V. *The neurological assessment of the preterm and fullterm newborn infant.* London: Spastics International Medical Publications, 1981.

Dunn LM, Dunn LM. *Peabody Picture Vocabulary Test—Revised.* Circle Pines, MN: American Guidance Service, 1981.

Emslie GJ, Weinberg WA, Rush AJ, Adams RM, Rintelmann JW. Depressive symptoms by self-report in adolescence: phase I of the development of a questionnaire for depression by self-report. *J Child Neurol* 1990;3:114–21.

Evans LD, Bradley-Johnson S. A review of recently developed measures of adaptive behavior. *J Clin Psychol* 1988;44:276–87.

Field T, Schanberg SM, Scafidi F, Bauer CR, Vega-Lahr N, Carcia R, Nystrom J, Kuhn CM. Tactile/kinesthetic stimulation effects on preterm neonates. *Pediatrics* 1986;77:654–58.

Fogelman C (ed.). *Manual for the AAMD Adaptive Behavior Scales,* 1974 Revision. Washington, DC: American Association on Mental Deficiency, 1974.

Folstein MF, Folstein SE, McHugh PR. "Mini-Mental State." A practical method for grading the cognitive state of patients for the clinician. *J Psychiatr Res* 1975;12:189–98.

Frankenburg WK, Camp BW (eds.). *Pediatric screening tests.* Springfield, IL: Charles C. Thomas, 1975.

Frankenburg WK, Chen J, Thornton SM. Common pitfalls in the evaluation of developmental screening tests. *J Pediatr* 1988a;113:1110–13.

Frankenburg WK, Dodds J, Archer P, Shapiro H, Bresnick B. The Denver II: a major revision and standardization of the Denver Developmental Screening Test. *Pediatrics* 1992;89:91–97.

Frankenburg WK, Ker CY, Engelke S, Schaefer ES, Thornton SM. Validation of key Denver Developmental Screening Test items: a preliminary study. *J Pediatr* 1988b;112:560–66

Frostig M, Lefever DW, Whittlesey JRB. *Administration and scoring manual for the Frostig Developmental Test of Visual Perception.* Palo Alto: Consulting Psychologists Press, 1966.

Goyette C, Conner CK, Ulrich R. Normative data on revised Conners parent and teacher rating scales. *J Abnorm Child Psychol* 1978;6:221–36.

Grossman HJ. *Manual on terminology and classification in mental retardation,* Rev ed. Washington, DC: American Association on Mental Deficiency, 1983.

Hammill DD, Brown L, Bryant BR. *A consumer's guide to tests in print,* 2nd ed. Austin, TX: Pro-Ed, 1992.

Holden EW, Tranowski KJ, Prinz RJ. Reliability of neurological soft sign in children: reevaluation of the PANESS. *J Abnorm Child Psychol* 1982;10:163–72.

Kaufman AS. *Intelligent testing with the WISC-R.* New York: John Wiley, 1979.

Kaufman AS. *Assessing adolescent and adult intelligence.* Boston: Allyn and Bacon, 1990.

Kaufman AS, Kaufman NL. *K-ABC: Kaufman Assessment Battery for Children.* Circle Pines, MN: American Guidance Service, 1983.

Kaufman AS, Long SW, O'Neal MR. Topical review of the WISC-R for pediatric neuroclinicians. *J Child Neurol* 1986;1:89–98.

Kaufman AS, O'Neal MR, Avant AH, Long SW. Introduction to the Kaufman Assessment Battery for Children (K-ABC) for pediatric neuroclinicians. *J Child Neurol* 1987;2:3–16.

Kazdin AE, Petti TA. Self-report and interview measures of childhood and adolescent depression. *J Child Psychol Psychiatry* 1982;23:437–57.

Kovacs M. Rating scales to assess depression in school-aged children. *Acta Paedopsychiatr* 1980–1981;46:305–15.

Lehr CA, Ysseldyke JE, Thurlow ML. Assessment practices in model early childhood special education programs. *Psychology in the Schools* 1987;24:390-99.

Luria A. *Higher cortical function in man,* 2nd ed. New York: Basic Books, 1980.

Martin R, Sewell T, Manni J. Effects of race and social class on pre-school performance of the Developmental Test of Visual-Motor Integration. *Psychology in the Schools* 1977;14:466–70.

Naglieri JA. Use of the WISC-R and the K-ABC with learning disabled, borderline mentally retarded, and normal children. *Psychology in the Schools* 1985;22:133–41.

Nihira K, Foster R, Shelihaas M, Leland H. *Adaptive behavior scales.* Washington, DC: American Association on Mental Deficiency, 1969

Ouvrier RA, Goldsmith RF, Ouvrier S, Williams IC. The value of the Mini-Mental State Examination in childhood: a preliminary study. *J Child Neurol* 1993;8:145–48.

Petti TA. Depression in hospitalized child psychiatry patients: approaches to measuring depression. *J Am Acad Child Psychiatry* 1978;17:49–59.

Petti TA, Conners CK. Changes in behavioral ratings of depressed children treated with imipramine. *J Am Acad Child Psychiatry* 1983;22:355–60.

Petti TA, Law W. Imipramine treatment of depressed children: a double-blind study. *J Clin Psychopharmacol* 1982;2:107–10.

Poznanski EO, Cook SC, Carroll BJ. A depression rating scale for children. *Pediatrics* 1979;64:442–50.

Poznanski EO, Freeman LN, Mokros HB. Children's Depression Rating Scale—Revised. *Psychopharmacol Bull* 1985;21:979–89.

Poznanski EO, Grossman JA, Buchsbaum Y. Preliminary studies of the reliability and validity of the Children's Depression Rating Scale. *J Am Acad Child Psychiatry* 1984;23:191–97.

Price PA. A comparative study of the California Achievement Test (Forms C and D) and the KeyMath Diagnostic Arithmetic Test with secondary LH students. *J Learn Disabil* 1984;17:392–96.

Ramey CT, Campbell FA, Nicholson JE. The predictive power of the Bayley Scales of Infant Development and the Stanford-Binet Intelligence Test in a relatively constant environment. *Child Development* 1973;44:790–95.

Raskin A (ed.). *Psychopharmacol Bull* 1985;21(4):713–1124.

Sparrow SS, Balla DA, Cicchetti DV. *Vineland Adaptive Behavior Scales.* Circle Pines, MN: American Guidance Service, 1984.

Spreen O, Strauss E. *A compendium of neuropsychological tests: administration, norms, and commentary.* New York: Oxford University Press, 1991.

Sternqvist K, Svenningsen NW. Neurobehavioural development at term of extremely low-birthweight infants (less than 901 g). *Develop Med Child Neurol* 1990;32:679–88.

Thorndike RL, Hagen EP, Sattler JM. *Technical manual: Stanford-Binet Intelligence Scale,* 4th ed. Chicago: Riverside Publishing, 1986b.

Thorndike RL, Hagen EP, Sattler JM. *Stanford-Binet Intelligence Scale,* 4th ed. Chicago: Riverside Publishing, 1986a.

Tillinghas BS, Morrow JE, Uhlig GE. Retest and alternate form reliability of the PPVT-R with fourth, fifth, and sixth grade pupils. *J Education Res* 1983;76:243–44.

Trites RL, Blouin AG, Ferguson HB, Lynch GW. The Conners Teacher Rating Scale: an epidemiological inter-rater reliability and follow-up investigation. In: Gadow K, Loney J (eds.). *Psychosocial aspects of drug treatment for hyperactivity.* Boulder, CO: Westview Press, 1982a.

Trites RL, Blouin AGA, Laprade K. Factor analysis of the Conners Teacher Rating Scale based on a large normative sample. *J Consult Clin Psychol* 1982b;50:615–23.

Wechsler D. *Manual for the Wechsler Intelligence Scale for Children,* 3rd ed. San Antonio: The Psychological Corporation, 1991.

Wechsler D:. *Manual for the Wechsler Preschool and Primary Scale of Intelligence—Revised.* San Antonio: The Psychological Corporation, 1989.

Weinberg WA, Rutman J, Sullivan L, Penick EC, Dietz SG. Depression in children referred to an educational diagnostic center: diagnosis and treatment. *J Pediatr* 1973;83:1065–72.

Weinberg WA, Emslie GJ. Weinberg screening affective scales (WSAS and WSAS-SF). *J Child Neurol* 1988;3:294–96.

Werry JS, Sprague RL. Methylphenidate in children—effect of dosage. *Aust NZ J Psychiatry* 1974;8:9–19.

CHAPTER 3 Amyotrophic Lateral Sclerosis Clinimetric Scales—Guidelines for Administration and Scoring

Benjamin Rix Brooks, M.D.

Amyotrophic lateral sclerosis (ALS) is a progressive degeneration of corticobulbar, corticospinal, brainstem, and spinal cord motor neurons whose clinical manifestations are weakness, muscle atrophy, hyperreflexia, and spasticity. Employing the World Health Organization model for disease consequences, the *pathology* of ALS may be measured by motor neuron pathologic change, motor neuron loss, and corticospinal tract degeneration (Table 3-1). Disease-related *impairment* is defined by strength loss, respiratory insufficiency, spasticity, loss of fine motor coordination, and speech and swallowing difficulties. These impairments are measured by elements of the neurologic examination including manual muscle testing and functional testing (Brooks et al., 1989; Caroscio et al., 1987; Fallat et al., 1979; Fallat, 1994). These impairments result in *disability* that may be measured by a number of clinimetric scales (Table 3-2). The initial clinimetric scale employed to evaluate the course of ALS was developed to assess the ergotropic effects of guanidine (Norris et al., 1974). It actually included both impairments and disabilities in five domains (bulbar, respiratory, arm, trunk, and leg) to weight the different regional involvement of the nervous system in ALS. The evolution of clinimetric scales resulted in more quantitation of impair-

ments and addition of further measures of disability maintaining the same regional weighting (Appel et al., 1987). In an attempt to define clinical impairment before it could be ascertained by manual muscle testing, isometric muscle testing was incorporated into clinimetric scales for the evaluation of the clinical course of ALS (Munsat et al., 1988; Ringel et al., 1993). Recent clinical trials of new therapies for ALS have employed both the Appel scale and composite evaluations measuring impairments of isometric muscle strength or timed bulbar, respiratory, arm and leg function (ALS CNTF Treatment Study (ACTS) Phase I-II Study Group, 1995a, 1995b, 1996, (ALS CNTF Treatment Study (ACTS) Phase II-III Study Group, 1996, Miller et al., 1996). More importantly, the new composite evaluations have separated impairments from disabilities and permit separate evaluation of the effects of the ALS on impairments and the disabilities resulting from impairments due to ALS (Table 3-2). The *handicap* to individual patients is in direct proportion to the accumulation of these ALS-related disabilities and results in a decreased quality of life leading ultimately to accelerated death.

Muscle strength, pulmonary function, and mortality are being used in current clinical trials of treatments for ALS to measure the effects of treat-

Table 3-1. World Health Organization Disease Consequences—Amyotrophic Lateral Sclerosis

Domain	Substrate	Measurement
Pathology	Motor Neuron Pathologic Change	Ubiquitin (+) Motor Neurons
		Neurofilament (+) Motor Neurons
	Motor Neuron Loss	
	Corticospinal Tract Degeneration	Glial Fibrillary Acidic Protein(+) Corticospinal Tract Staining
Impairment	Strength Loss Arm Leg	Manual Muscle Testing Maximal Voluntary Isometric Contraction (MVIC)
	Breathing	Respiratory Rate Vital Capacity (Forced, Slow) Peak Inspiratory Flow Rate
	Spasticity	Ashworth Spasticity Scale Walking Velocity
	Fine Coordination Loss	Ashworth Spasticity Scale
Disability	Function Loss	
	Speech	Intelligibility, PaTa velocity Speech ALS FRS
	Swallow	Deglutition, Swallowing ALS FRS
	Breathing	Breathing ALS FRS
	Arm	Arm ALS FRS
	Leg	Leg ALS FRS
Handicap	Independence Loss	Quality of Life Scales
	Work Social Integration Self-care	Sickness Impact Profile (SIP) Short-Form 36 (SF-36)
	Death	Survival

Table 3-2. Comparison of Impairments and Disabilities in Norris Scale, Appel Scale, and ACTS ALS Evaluation

	Norris ALS Scale	Appel ALS Scale	ACTS ALS Evaluation
BULBAR Impairments			
	Fasciculations/atrophy	—	Speech PaTa
	Fatigue	—	—
	Jaw jerk	—	—
	Labile emotions		
Disabilities			
	Speech	Speech	Speech ALS FRS
	Swallowing	Diet	Swallow ALS FRS
	Chewing	—	Salivation ALS FRS
RESPIRATORY Impairments			
	—	Vital capacity	Vital capacity
Disabilities			
	Breathing	—	Breathing ALS FRS
	Cough	—	—
ARM Impairments			
	Fasciculations/atrophy	Deltoid, biceps, triceps,	Deltoid, biceps, triceps,
	Fatigue	Wrist extensor/flexor	Isometric strength
	Biceps, brachialradialis	Finger extensor/flexor	—
	Triceps tendon reflexes	Manual muscle strength	—
	—	Grip isometric strength	Grip isometric strength
	—	Pinch isometric strength	—
	—	Timed propelling wheelchair	—
	—	Timed large block board	—
	—	Timed cutting theraplast	—
	—	Timed pegboard	Timed pegboard
Disabilities			
	Change arm position	Dressing	Dressing ALS FRS
	Grip, lift self	Feeding	Feeding ALS FRS
	Lift book, lift utensil	—	—
	Writing	—	Writing ALS FRS
	Buttons, zipper	—	—
TRUNK Impairments			
	Fasciculations/atrophy	—	—
	Fatigue	—	—
Disabilities			
	—	—	Turning in bed ALS FRS

Table 3-2.   *(continued)*

		Norris ALS Scale	*Appel ALS Scale*	*ACTS ALS Evaluation*
LEG Impairments				
		Fasciculations/atrophy	Timed walk 20 ft	Timed walk 15 ft
		Fatigue	Timed stand from lying	—
		Quadriceps, adductor, Achilles tendon reflexes	Timed stand from chair	—
			Timed climb stairs	—
		Plantar responses	—	—
		Leg rigidity	—	—
Disabilities		Climb stairs		Climbing stairs ALS FRS
		Walk one block unassisted	AFO/cane/walker	Walking ALS FRS
		Walk one room unassisted	Occasional/constant wheelchair	—
		Stand	Climb stairs unassisted	—
		Change leg position	—	—

ment on ALS-determined impairments; however, the impact of potential new therapies on the activities of self-care must be captured by a disease-specific assessment of activities of daily living in patients with ALS. Previous clinimetric scales in ALS have combined measurements of impairments with measures of disability or handicap (Appel et al., 1987; Brooks et al., 1990, 1991, 1994; Norris et al., 1974). Mixture of impairment and disability elements in the same clinimetric scale leads to difficulty with regard to interpretation of the dynamic range of the total score or subscores of the clinimetric scale as measures of the health status in individuals or groups of individuals with ALS being studied and to difficulty concerning the statistical behavior of the total score or subscores of the clinimetric scale in individuals or groups of individuals over time (Feinstein, 1987; Streiner & Norman, 1989). Disease impairments may occur early in the disease process but the time course of change in the degree of impairment may be quite different from the time course of change in the degree of disability (Brooks et al., 1990, 1991, 1994; Brooks, 1996). Both the Norris scale and the Appel scale have mixed impairments and disabilities in varying proportions (Table 3-2). The Norris scale weights reflexes, fasciculations, and weakness as impairments and other self-reported items as disabilities in bulbar : respiratory : arm : trunk : leg domains in the ratio 3 : 1 : 5 : 2 : 5. The Appel scale weights bulbar : respiratory : arm : leg domains in the ratio 5 : 5 : 8 : 8. The different weighting of respiratory relative to other domains between the Appel and Norris scales is problematic. Moreover, within the Appel scale there is duplication of the scale with respect to rating lower extremity function and use of aids. This duplication indicates that the same clinical information is added to the total scale more than once, causing increased autocorrelation (Feinstein, 1987; Streiner & Norman, 1989). Additionally, the total Appel scale demonstrates nonlinearity over time during the early and late stages of the disease. This effect is amply demonstrated in several studies (Brooks et al., 1991; Italian ALS Study Group, 1993; Lange et al., 1996). Weighting of the five domains is arbitrary, but guidelines have now been developed to establish the elements measuring impairment, disability, and handicap that should be employed in clinical trials of therapies for ALS (Subcommittee on Motor Neuron Diseases, 1995).

Recent and current clinical trials include the ALS Functional Rating Scale (ALS FRS), a new clinimetric scale developed specifically to measure disease-related disability alone in ALS. This scale was developed because currently employed clinimetric scales were contaminated with impairment measurements, did not measure the broad range of disabilities that result from ALS, and did not lend themselves to subscore analysis that was based entirely on disability components (Feinstein, 1987; Louwerse et al., 1990; Streiner & Norman, 1989). The ALS FRS is a synthesis of five elements from the Unified Parkinson's Disease Rating Scale (UPDRS), four elements from the ALS Severity Scale (ALSSS), and a new element concerning the breathing state of the ALS patient (ALS CNTF Treatment Study (ACTS) Phase I-II Study Group, 1996; Hillel et al., 1989, 1990). The ALS FRS was developed as an internally consistent, reliable, valid measure of disability in ALS patients as part of the (ALS CNTF Treatment Study (ACTS) Phase I-II Study Group, 1996). The ability of the ALS FRS to be responsive to change in the clinical status of ALS patients was evaluated cross-sectionally and prospectively over time in phase I and phase II studies of CNTF in ALS (ALS CNTF Treatment Study (ACTS) Phase I-II Study Group, 1995a, 1995b, 1996; ALS CNTF Treatment Study (ACTS) Phase II-III Study Group, 1996).

Administration of Norris ALS Scale

The Norris ALS Scale was developed to follow clinical change in ALS patients after treatment (Norris et al., 1974; Brooks, 1994). This scale (Figure 3-1) measures both impairments and disabilities in a single patient. Both are regionally grouped under the *bulbar, respiratory, arm, trunk, leg,* and *general* domains. The Norris scale has evolved since its introduction in 1974 and can be performed with minimum equipment in a number of clinical situations by neurologists or well-trained research nurses (Table 3-3).

Administration of Appel ALS Scale

The total Appel ALS scale score (Figure 3-2) consists of five domain subscores: *bulbar, respiratory, muscle strength, lower extremity function* and *upper extremity function* (Table 3-4). The patients are graded in ALS clinic. Those involved in the actual grading of the patients may include the neurologist

Norris ALS Scale

	3 Normal	2 Impaired	1 Trace	0 No Use
1. Hold up neck				
2. Chewing				
3. Swallowing				
4. Speech				
5. Roll over in bed				
6. Do a sit-up				
7. Bowel/bladder pressure				
8. Breathing				
9. Coughing				
10. Write name				
11. Work buttons, zippers				
12. Feed self				
13. Grip/lift self				
14. Grip/lift book/tray				
15. Grip/lift fork/pencil				
16. Change arm position				
17. Climb stairs – 1 flight				
18. Walk – 1 block				
19. Walk – 1 room				
20. Walk – assisted				
21. Stand up from chair				
22. Change leg position				

	Normal	Hyper/Hypo	Absent	Clonic
23. Stretch reflexes – arms				
24. Stretch reflexes – legs				

	Absent	Present	Hyperactive	Clonic
25. Jaw jerk				

	Flexor	Mute	Equivocal	Extensor
26. Plantar response – right				
27. Plantar response – left				

	None/Rare	Slight	Moderate	Severe
28. Fasciculation				
29. Atrophy – face, tongue				
30. Atrophy – arms, shoulders				
31. Atrophy – legs, hips				
32. Labile emotions				

		0 to Mild		Moderate to Severe
33. Fatigability				
34. Leg rigidity				

				PATIENT TOTAL SCORE
Patient Subtotals				
Normal Subtotals	96	4		

Figure 3-1.   Norris ALS Scale rating form.

Table 3-3.	Guidelines for Administration/Scoring Norris ALS Scale	
Item	*Description*	*Score*
1	Hold up head (test)—no problem	3
	Droops when tired, or unable to complete chin-test	2
	Always droops without support collar, only clears pillow supine	1
	Cannot clear pillow when supine	0
2	Chewing (history)—No problem	3
	Requires some soft or blenderized foods, some rest periods	2
	Completely soft/blenderized foods, frequent rest periods	1
	Food must be pushed to back of mouth	0
3	Swallowing (test)—No problem	3
	Aspirates some water but not saliva during entire examination	2
	Aspirates saliva occasionally, drools frequently	1
	Water runs out of mouth, aspirates saliva frequently	0
4	Speech (test)—Normal throughout visit	3
	Any problem during visit	2
	Barely understandable simple phrases	1
	Grunts, groans, rare intelligible sounds	0
5	Roll over (test)—Turn readily to at least one side from supine on examination table	3
	Any problems (may be due to severe arm weakness but score here also	2
	Barely turns with great effort to just one side	1
	Needs assistance to turn	0
6	Sit up (test)—Sit to full vertical form supine on examination table	3
	Clears head, shoulders, but not trunk, without pulling	2
	Clears head, but not shoulders, without pull/lift	1
	Requires lift of both head, trunk	0
7	Bowel/bladder pressure (history)—No apparent problem	3
	Problem bearing down; needs laxative or stool softener every week	2
	Needs laxative or softener more often, occasional enema	1
	Enema needed more often than not	0
8	Breathing (test)—No problem during entire visit	3
	Dyspnea arriving at office or during strength test	2
	Dyspnea in ordinary conversation	1
	Respiratory distress	0
9	Cough (test)—Examiner unable to restrain lower chest in coughing (hold from behind)	3
	Cough effective but examiner able to restrain chest	2
	Cough usually ineffective, e.g., multiple shallow coughs after aspiration	1
	Cough ineffective	0
10	Write (test)—Write name, address; spouse confirms normalcy	3
	Any legibility problem with name, address	2
	Unable to complete name, address, or mainly illegible	1
	Only able to make marks	0
11	Buttons, zippers (test)—Button shirt; may use both hands, time not limited but no assist devices, pull zipper closed	3
	Unable to complete above without aid	2

Table 3-3. *(continued)*

Item	Description	Score
	Only able to do two buttons with assist devices, half of zipper	1
	Unable to perform above, near-full assistance needed	0
12	Feeding (history)—No problem or needs simple assist devices only, large handle	3
	Requires help cutting meat or needs more assist devices, finger splints, arm slings/pivots, etc.	2
	Unable to cut or use fork but can raise food to mouth	1
	Must be fed	0
13	Grip/lift self (test)—Pulls self erect from supine position with one hand	3
	Above with great effort or both grips necessary	2
	Above using trunk flexors (examiner palpates abdomen)	1
	Requires lift or pull by examiner	0
14	Grip/lift book, tray (test)—Lifts large book from lap to face level	3
	Clears lap but cannot lift to face	2
	Lifts paperback book from lap to face	1
	Clears lap with paperback book but cannot lift to face	0
15	Grip/lift fork, pencil (test)—Holds pencil to write, legibility not considered	3
	Lifts pencil but unable to grip enough to mark	2
	Lifts pencil clear of table only briefly	1
	May move pencil but cannot lift clear	0
16	Change arm position (test)—Lift both arms over head from lap	3
	Arms clear lap but not shoulders	2
	Moves both arms from lap to arm rests	1
	Wiggles arms but not enough to move from lap	0
17	Climb stairs (test)—Climbs one flight without pausing or pulling	3
	Climbs one flight but resting or pulling on rail required	2
	Climbs two or more steps unaided	1
	Climbs less than two steps, probably needs lift onto examination table	0
18	Walk (test)—Walks one block (office corridor four times without pause), may wear favorable shoes, ankle brace, etc., < 5 min	3
	Completes the distance with problems of any type or needs > 5 min	2
	Completes only with assist or multiple rests	1
	Cannot complete	0
19	Walk one room (test 15 ft)—Completes without difficulty	3
	Any problems	2
	Completes but needs minimal assist or is exhausted	1
	Cannot complete without substantial aid including cane/crutch	0
20	Walk assisted (test only if assist required above, score three if item 19 scores one or better)—Completes one room using cane/crutch or holding examiner's arm	3
	Cannot complete without assistance	2
	Takes steps in transfer from chair to examination table	1
	Legs drag in assisted transfer	0
21	Stand (test)—Stands readily from standard chair, no pushing with arms	3
	Any problem	2
	Actively assists but needs lift to complete rise	1

Table 3-3.   *(continued)*

Item	Description	Score
	Needs lifting throughout	0
22	Change leg position (test)—Raises each leg to 45°in supine position	3
	Clears table but one leg cannot reach 45°	2
	Only clears table briefly, on one leg completely paralyzed	1
	Only ineffective wiggles	0
23	Biceps, brachioradialis, triceps muscle stretch reflexes (test)—	
	All within the broad range of normal and symmetrical	3
	Asymmetry or at least one clearly abnormal	2
	Any three absent, the remaining three only trace responses	1
	Any three clonic	0
24	Quadriceps, Achilles, internal hamstring muscle stretch reflexes (test)—as in item 23	
25	Jaw jerk (test)—Absent	3
	Present	2
	Hyperactive	1
	Clonic	0
26,27	Plantar responses (test)—Flexor	3
	Mute	2
	Equivocal	1
	Extensor	0
28	Fasciculation (observe throughout examination), patient stripped to standard underwear, no T-shirt; no neuromuscular function drugs, i.e., pyridostigmine, during the previous 24 hours	
	None/rare	3
	Slight	2
	Moderate	1
	Severe	0
29–31	Wasting—atrophy (observe)—Normal bulk	3
	Mild loss of bulk	2
	Moderate loss of bulk	1
	Marked loss of bulk	0
32	Labile emotions (history and observation)—No problem, spouse confirms	3
	Occasional inappropriate weeping or giggling	2
	At least daily lability	1
	Weeping (rarely laughter) with most stimuli, entering office	0
33	Fatigability (test)—No abnormality ranging to occasional reduction in strength during examination with rapid recovery in minutes	2
	Frequent reduction in strength during examination or general decline in function with time	0
34	Leg rigidity (test)—Muscle tone normal or slightly increased in both legs, or normal in one but moderate (resists gravity) in the other; no muscle relaxant in last 24 hours	2
	Moderate rigidity in both, or board-like rigidity in one, or worse	0

Adapted with permission from Brooks, 1994

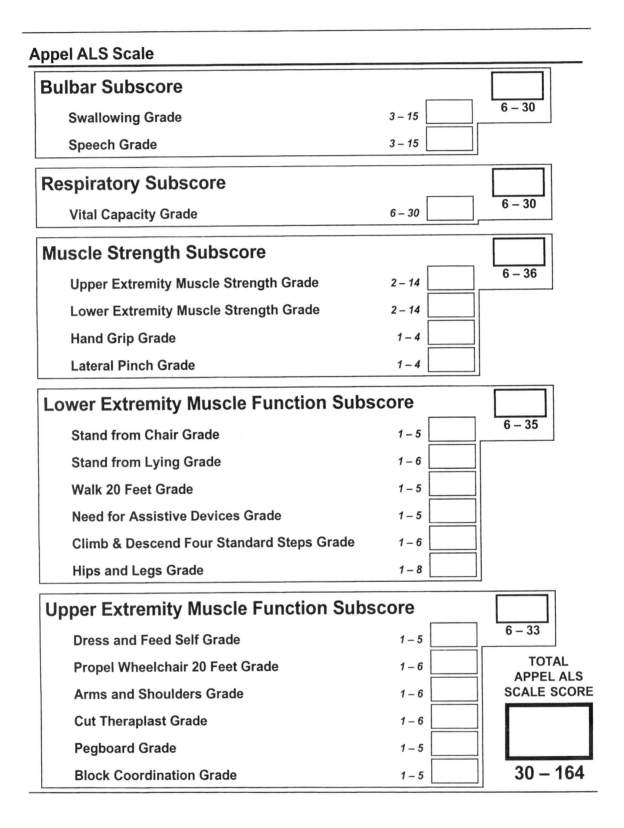

Figure 3-2. Appel ALS Scale rating form.

Table 3-4.   Guidelines for Administration/Scoring Appel ALS Scale

A. Bulbar Subscore (6–30 points)

1. *Swallowing Grade*

3 points	General Diet
6 points	Soft Diet [Soft, cooked; eliminates popcorn, crumbly foods, etc.]
9 points	Mechanical Soft Diet [Finely chopped or ground and thickened liquids]
12 points	Pudding Consistency Diet [Strained, pureed, blended, thickened liquids]

The score is determined by the nurse based on the recommendations given that clinic visit from either the neurologist or dietitian. For example, the patient may still say he/she is taking a general diet but if the team recommends that he/she should only have chopped or ground foods and thickened liquids, the patient receives a score of 9 points Please note that if the patient can take a General Diet or Soft Diet, he/she is taking regular liquids and has no need to use thickened liquids. If choking spells occur with regular liquids, thickened liquids should be recommended and the Bulbar Subscore should be designated as 9 points

2. *Speech Grade*

3 points	Clear
6 points	Slightly slurred
9 points	Slurred
12 points	Unintelligible
15 points	None

The score is determined by the nurse. If in doubt, other members of the ALS team should be consulted.

Bulbar Subscore (6–30 points)	**=**	***Swallowing Grade + Speech Grade***

B. Respiratory Subscore (6–30 points)

Vital Capacity Grade

6 points	Vital capacity within 80–100% of predicted value
12 points	Vital capacity within 60–79% of predicted value or incentive spirometry, medication or chest physical therapy
18 points	Vital capacity within 40–59% of predicted value or IPPB or suctioning
24 points	Vital capacity less than 39% of predicted value or tracheostomy being considered
30 points	Tracheostomy

Respiratory Subscore (6 –30 points)	**=**	***Vital Capacity Grade***

Table 3-4. *(continued)*

C. Muscle Strength Subscore (6–36 points)

1. *Upper Extremity Muscle Strength Grade* (Sum of right and left sides)

2 points	Sum of Muscle Strength is 70 (normal)
4 points	Sum of Muscle Strength is 62–69
6 points	Sum of Muscle Strength is 54–61
8 points	Sum of Muscle Strength is 46–53
10 points	Sum of Muscle Strength is 32–45
12 points	Sum of Muscle Strength is 18–31
14 points	Sum of Muscle Strength is ≤ 17

2. *Lower Extremity Muscle Strength Grade* (Sum of right and left sides)

2 points	Sum of Muscle Strength is 70 (normal)
4 points	Sum of Muscle Strength is 62–69
6 points	Sum of Muscle Strength is 54–61
8 points	Sum of Muscle Strength is 46–53
10 points	Sum of Muscle Strength is 32–45
12 points	Sum of Muscle Strength is 18–31
14 points	Sum of Muscle Strength is ≤ 17

3. *Hand Grip Grade* (Sum of right and left hand grips in pounds) divided by 2

1 points	Sum divided by 2 is ≥ 60
2 points	Sum divided by 2 is 46–59
3 points	Sum divided by 2 is 20–45
4 points	Sum divided by 2 is < 20

4. *Lateral Pinch Grade* (Sum of right and left lateral pinch in pounds) divided by 2

1 points	Sum divided by 2 is ≥ 14
2 points	Sum divided by 2 is 10–13
3 points	Sum divided by 2 is 5–9
4 points	Sum divided by 2 is < 5

Muscle Strength Subscore (6–36 points) = *Upper Extremity Grade + Lower Extremity Grade + Hand Grip Grade + Lateral Pinch Grade*

D. Lower Extremity Muscle Function Subscore (6–35 points)

1. *Standing from Chair Grade* (Best Time)

1 points	Standing time is 0.0–1.0 second
2 points	Standing time is 1.5–3.0 seconds

Table 3-4.   *(continued)*

3 points	Standing time is 3.5–5.0 seconds
4 points	Standing time is < 5.0 seconds
5 points	Unable to stand

2. *Standing from Lying Supine Grade* (Best Time)

1 points	Standing time is ≤ 2.0 seconds
2 points	Standing time is 2.5–4.0 seconds
3 points	Standing time is 4.5–6.0 seconds
4 points	Standing time is 6.5–10.0 seconds
5 points	Standing time is > 10.0 seconds
6 points	Unable to stand

3. *Walking 20 Feet Grade* (Best Time)

1 points	Walking time is ≤ 8.0 seconds
2 points	Walking time is 8.5–12.0 seconds
3 points	Walking time is 12.5–16.0 seconds
4 points	Walking time is > 16.0 seconds
5 points	Unable to stand

4. *Need for Assistive Devices Grade*

1 points	None
2 points	AFO / Cane / Boots
3 points	Walker, crutches and/or occasional wheelchair (for long trips, etc.)
4 points	Wheelchair bound or wheelchair most of the time
5 points	Bed confined

5. *Climbing and Descending Four Standard Steps Grade* (Best Time)

1 points	Climbing time is ≤ 5.0 seconds
2 points	Climbing time is 5.5–8.0 seconds
3 points	Climbing time is 8.5–12.0 seconds
4 points	Climbing time is 12.5–18.0 seconds
5 points	Climbing time is > 18.0 seconds
6 points	Unable to climb stairs

6. *Hips and Legs Grade*

1 points	Walks and climbs stairs without assistance
2 points	Walks and climbs stairs with aid of railing
3 points	Cannot climb stairs but walks unassisted and rises from chairs
4 points	Cannot climb stairs but walks unassisted with either ankle–foot orthosis or cane
5 points	Cannot climb stairs but walks with minimal assistance or walks unassisted with crutches or walker

Table 3-4.   *(continued)*

6 points	Cannot climb stairs but walks with crutches or walker with assistanc or walks with total support
7 points	Is in wheelchair
8 points	Confined to bed

Lower Extremity Function Subscore (6–35 points)	**=**	***Standing from Chair Grade*** *+ Standing from Lying Supine Grade* *+ Walking 20 Feet Grade* *+ Need for Assistive Devices Grade* *+ Climbing/Descending 4 Standard Steps Grade* *+ Hips and Legs Grade*

E. Upper Extremity Muscle Function Subscore (6–33 points)

1. *Dress and Feed Grade*

1 points	Independent
2 points	Independent with aids Button hooks, zipper pull, padded utensils, plate holder, etc. but patient does not need caretaker to assist
3 points	Minimal Assist Patient needs caretaker to assist (cutting meat, buttons, shifting clothing, etc.)
4 points	Major Assist Caretaker does majority of dressing and/or feeding
5 points	Dependent

The grade is based on questioning and the observed status.

2. *Propelling Wheelchair 20 Feet Grade* (Best Time)

1 points	Propelling time is ≤ 11.0 seconds
2 points	Propelling time is 11.5–20.0 seconds
3 points	Propelling time is 20.5–30.0 seconds
4 points	Propelling time is 30.5–40.0 seconds
5 points	Propelling time is > 40.0 seconds
6 points	Unable to stand

One trial is performed. No assistance can be given.

3. *Arms and Shoulders Grade* (Evaluate the most affected side)

1 points	Starting with arms at the sides, abducts the arms in a full circle until they touch above the head.
2 points	Raises arms above the head only by flexing at the elbow or using accessory muscles
3 points	Cannot raise hands above the head but raises glass of water to mouth
4 points	Raises hands to mouth but cannot raise glass of water to mouth
5 points	Cannot raise hands to mouth but can use hands to hold articles

Table 3-4. *(continued)*

6 points	Cannot raise hands to mouth and has no useful function of hands

The most affected side is graded. If a patient can raise one arm above his/her head but cannot raise the other arm above his/her head without flexing his/her arm at the elbow, then the weaker arm determines that the grade is 2 points.

4. *Cutting Theraplast Grade* (Time for Dominant Hand)

1 points	Cutting Time ≤ 5.0 seconds
2 points	Cutting Time 5.5–10.0 seconds
3 points	Cutting Time 10.5–15.0 seconds
4 points	Cutting Time 15.5–20.0 seconds
5 points	Cutting Time > 20.0 seconds
6 points	Unable

The patient cuts a 0.25" thick piece of theraplast that is set out on the board in the diameter of 4". Only the dominant hand is tested. The knife is positioned in the hand at the beginning of the timing.

5. *pegboard Grade*

(Sum of pegs constructed with right hand and left hand in 60 seconds) divided by 2

1 points	Sum divided by 2 is 27–36
2 points	Sum divided by 2 is 22–26
3 points	Sum divided by 2 is 18–21
4 points	Sum divided by 2 is 1–17
5 points	Unable

The Model 32030 Purdue Pegboard is 18″ × 11″ with two parallel rows of 25 hoses running vertically down the center of the board. The rows are 1″ apart, each hole is 1/3″ apart. The holes are 1/8″ diameter. At the base of the board are wells which hold the pegs that will be assembled. The fine motor test consists of forming the following construct of (1) a 1″ pin (1/8″ in diameter), (2) a washer (3/8″ in diameter) and (3) a collar (1/4″ long; 3/16″ in diameter). The patient is instructed to assemble the construct as follows:

> "Make as many constructs consisting of a pin, followed by a washer, followed by a collar as you can in 60 seconds with one hand."

The command is followed by a demonstration for the patient, then the command is repeated. The timing begins with the patient holding his hand above the tray containing the 1″ pins. There is no standard table height. Ideally, the table should be adjustable to allow the patient to easily rest his forearms on the table. The patient is given 60 seconds to assemble as many units as he/she can and is given credit for each component added to a construct. If the patient completes 2 units of pin, washer and collar plus one unit of pin and washer only, the score is 2 x 3 + 2 = 8 in 60 seconds.

6. *Block Coordination Grade*

(Sum of blocks turned with right hand and left hand in 60 seconds) divided by 2

1 points	Sum divided by 2 is 75–95
2 points	Sum divided by 2 is 62–74
3 points	Sum divided by 2 is 43–61

Table 3-4.   *(continued)*

4 points   Sum divided by 2 is 1–42

5 points   Unable

The Block Coordination Grade is part of the Gonzalez Evaluation of Coordination. This part is derived from the standardized test "Minnesota Rate of Manipulation." It may be administered by the occupational therapist. The board is 3´ long with 2 horizontal rows of 8 openings large enough to accommodate the round blocks (2.5˝ in diameter and 0.75˝ wide). Each hand is tested. The patient is instructed to turn as many blocks over as he/she can in one minute. When testing the right hand, the patient begins at the upper left hand corner of the board and goes clockwise. When testing the left hand, the patient begins at the upper right hand corner and goes counterclockwise.

Upper Extremity   =   *Dress and Feed Grade*
Function   *+ Propelling Wheelchair 20 feet Grade*
Subscore   *+ Arms and Shoulders Grade*
(6–33 points)   *+ Cutting Theraplast Grade*
                           + Pegboard Grade
                           + Block Coordination Grade

F. Total Appel ALS Score (30–164 points)

The grades for each subscore are determined. The subscores are then summed as described below to provide the Total Appel ALS Scale.

Total Appel   =   *Bulbar Subscore*
ALS Scale   *+ Respiratory Subscore*
(30–164 points)   *+ Muscle Strength Subscore*
                         + Lower Extremity Function Subscore
                         + Upper Extremity Function Subscore

Equipment List for Appel ALS Scale

Stopwatch	Pinch Dynamometer
Theraplast	Grip Dynamometer
Plastic Knife	Chair
Pegboard	Stairs
Wheelchair	Standard Examining Table
Board with Blocks	
Spirometer for Vital Capacity (see Table 3-5)	

Adapted with permission from ALS—Cyclosporine Treatment Study Principal Investigators Procedure Manual © 1987.

(muscle strength testing), the occupational therapist (blocks, pegboard, grip, lateral pinch), the respiratory therapist (vital capacity), and the research nurse (remainder of rating scale). The examination could easily be performed by a neurologist (muscle strength testing) and a nurse (remainder of the rating scale). The important principle is that parts of the test be performed by the same person at each subsequent visit.

The bulbar subscore is determined by the ALS clinic team based on the recommendations given at that clinic visit from either the neurologist or dietitian. The patient may say he or she is taking a general diet but if the ALS clinic team recommends that the patient should only have chopped or ground foods and thickened liquids, the patient should receive a grade of 9 points for swallowing. If choking spells occur with regular liquids, thickened liquids should be recommended and the grade will drop to 9 points.

The respiratory subscore is based on changes in the forced vital capacity (FVC) presented in terms of the predicted forced vital capacity for that patient based on gender, height, and age according to the Morris formula:

$$\text{Male predicted FVC} = [0.148 \times (\text{height in inches})] - [0.025 \times (\text{age})] - 4.241$$

$$\text{Female predicted FVC} = [0.115 \times (\text{height in inches})] - [0.024 \times (\text{age})] - 2.852$$

The FVC measurement should be performed with a nose clip and with the patient standing if possible. It is important to have masks available in case of poor lip seal. Each test should be performed at least twice to obtain a maximal effort. The best effort is recorded. If a patient with an FVC of 80% predicted receives respiratory medications, he or she should be recorded as 12 points (Fallat et al., 1979; Fallat, 1994; Glindmeyer et al., 1987; Norris & Fallat, 1998).

The muscle strength subscore consists of manual muscle testing according to the Medical Research Council grading system. Both the right and left deltoid, biceps, triceps, wrist extensors, wrist flexors, finger extensors, and finger flexors are tested. The sum of the right and left sides is determined and coded according to the algorithm in Table 3-4.

Hand grip is measured carefully. The handle of the Jamar dynamometer is adjusted to fit the subject's hand and allow metacarpophalangeal flexion. The subject rests his forearm on the desktop, but

the dynamometer is not rested on the desktop. Maximal hand grip is measured twice with a rest period between the two testing sessions (1–3 minutes). The sum of the right and left maximal hand grip is divided by two. The appropriate grade is assigned according to Table 3-4.

Lateral pinch is measured as the preceding with an Osco pinch gauge between the tip of the pad of the thumb and the lateral surface of the index finger. The right and left pinch is measured once, summed, and divided by two. The appropriate score is assigned according to Table 3-4.

The lower extremity function subscore involves timed functional tests. Standing from sitting in a chair is timed from the start of standing until the patient reaches the erect posture. The examiner is not allowed to assist. If assistance is required, the patient is graded as "unable" and receives a score of 5 points. Standing from lying supine is timed in arising from a supine position of a standard examining table height to a standing position. The examiner is not allowed to assist. If a patient requires assistance, he or she is graded as "unable" and given a score of 6 points. Timed walking 20 feet is timed from the first step through the first step across the finish line. The examiner is not allowed to assist, but should accompany the patient for safety. If assistance is needed, the patient is graded as "unable" and receives a grade of 5 points. Climbing and descending four standard stairs is timed. The examiner is not allowed to assist. If it is found that it would be unsafe to perform this task, the patient is scored "unable" and receives a grade of 6 points. The hips and legs portion is determined after the previous tests have been completed.

The upper extremity function subscore involves timed functional tests. Propelling wheelchair 20 feet with arms is timed from the initiation of wheelturning through the first point at which the bottom of the wheel of the wheelchair crosses the finish line. No assistance may be given. The arms and shoulders test should be graded according to the most affected side. A patient who can raise his or her right arm above the head with no problem but can only raise his or her left arm above the head by flexing the elbow is given a score of 2 points. Cutting theraplast requires the patient to employ the dominant hand to cut theraplast 0.25″ thick and 4″ in diameter. The knife is positioned in the hand at the beginning of the timing on the theraplast. Timing is measured from the initial cut until the entire theraplast is cut through. Pegboard testing requires the construction of peg units in sequence of a pin, followed by a washer, followed by a collar in 60 seconds by each hand. The construction of the peg unit should be demonstrated for the patient. The pegboard is placed on a table that will allow the patient to easily rest his or her forearms on the table. The Gonzalez Evaluation of Coordination subtest is derived from the standardized Minnesota Rate of Manipulation test. Each hand is tested. The patient is instructed to turn as many blocks over as he or she can in 60 seconds. When testing the right hand, the patient begins at the upper left hand corner of the board and goes clockwise. When testing the left hand, the patient begins at the upper right hand corner and goes counterclockwise.

Administration of ACTS ALS Evaluatilon

The Amyotrophic Lateral Sclerosis Ciliary Neurotrophic Factor Treatment Study (ACTS) ALS Evaluation evolved from previous standardized clinimetric scales developed by Munsat and collaborators (Andres et al., 1986; Munsat et al., 1988, 1989) as well as Ringel and collaborators (Ringel et al., 1993). The ACTS ALS Evaluation separately assesses impairments and disabilities. Impairments are measured by (1) quantitative function tests; (2) quantitative strength tests; and (3) spasticity, fasciculation, atrophy, and cramp scales. Disabilities are measured by the new ALS Functional Rating Scale, which was developed and then validated in three large multicenter clinical trials (ALS CNTF Treatment Study [ACTS] Phase I-II Study Group, 1995a, 1995b, 1996; ALS CNTF Treatment Study [ACTS] Phase II-III Study Group, 1996; Bradley et al., 1995).

The quantitative function tests include (1) speech diadochokinetic rates; (2) pulmonary function tests; (3) Purdue pegboard tests; and (4) the fifteen-foot walk. Standardized normalized age- and gender-controlled data are available for all these clinical measures (Guiloff & Goonetilleke, 1994; Tourtellotte et al., 1965).

The quantitative strength tests include isometric muscle strength measurements in five upper extremity muscles including hand grip and five lower extremity muscles including ankle dorsiflexion (Sanjak et al., 1996; Tourtellotte et al., 1965).

The spasticity, fasciculation, atrophy, and cramp scales measure with ordinal scales the status

of clinical features of the neurologic examination that relate to impairments specific to motor neuron diseases such as ALS (ALS CNTF Treatment Study [ACTS] Phase II-III Study Group, 1996; Ashworth, 1964; Tourtellotte et al., 1965).

These procedures and methods are described in Tables 3-5 and 3-6 with explanations and descriptions of equipment as necessary. All clinical evaluators should adhere to these procedures so that measurement errors are minimized. It is important to remember throughout this study that there are always three sources of error that will affect our measurements: (1) observer error (minimized by understanding what we are measuring and being consistent in our measurements); (2) patient error (minimized by explaining what is expected from them at the beginning of each test session; and (3) instrument error (minimized by regular calibration) (Hulley and Cummings, 1991).

Administration of ALS Functional Rating Scale (ALS FRS)

The ALS FRS (Figure 3-3) may be administered by the physician, nurse-coordinator, physical therapist, or a trained assistant to assess the patient's present ability to perform activities of daily living and functional improvement or decline at interval visits. The evaluator shall state to the patient (or spouse or other caregiver if the patient cannot communicate effectively):

"I now have a few questions I would like to ask you to help me better understand how you (or the patient) are functioning at home."

"Please answer each question to the best of your ability."

The evaluator then asks, "How are you doing at (. . .)?"

Record the patient's response, to the closest approximation available from the appropriate 5-point (0-4) list. If the patient is unable to volunteer a satisfactory response, the evaluator may prompt, using one of the available choices (e.g., asking, "Do you find that people are having trouble understanding your speech . . ." etc.). Record response on the case response form provided. Patients who become more independent because of the use of an assistive device, such as a wheelchair, walker, or elevator, cannot improve in their rating scores. The following examples elaborate on the scoring of

Table 3-5.   Guidelines for Administration/Scoring ACTS ALS Evaluation

A. Quantitative Function Tests

1. *Speech Diadochokinetic Rates*

   Equipment: Sony M-330 Pressman microcassette recorder/tape/Digital stopwatch

   The patient is seated and instructed to repeat the syllable "PaTa" as quickly and distinctly as possible, until told to stop.

   Start the recorder. Make sure the recorder is set to normal (2.4) speed.

   State the patient's name, date and trial number. Preset the timer at 5 seconds. Timing begins when the subject begins speaking (after you say "start") and ends after 5 seconds (when you say "stop"). The timer will beep after 5 seconds has expired.

   Perform two trials. Play back the tape and count the number of PaTas in each 5-second interval. Vary the speed as needed on playback, to slow (1.2) or fast (2.4), to determine the number of repetitions during each 5-second interval.

2. *Pulmonary Function Tests*

   Equipment: PB 100 Portable Spirometer (Puritan-Bennett Renaissance Spirometry System and PB110 Base Station/PB 130 Patient Data Memory Card/3-liter calibration syringe/BD250 Bi-Directional Flow Sensors (Pneumo Tach)/Nose clips and facemask (when indicated)/Printer

   Refer to Renaissance Spirometry System Operator's Guide for installation and calibration of equipment. Prior to initial use configure spirometer per operator's guide. Configuration will be retained in memory and should not have to be repeated until a protocol change.

   Turn on spirometer and printer; allow at least a 2-minute warm-up period prior to use.

   Spirometer should be calibrated each day prior to use with the 3-liter syringe provided. To calibrate, push the test button and then push button #4. Follow spirometer instructions. Repeat until error is less than 3%.

   Enter the new patient information data by pressing the new patient button. Follow spirometer instructions.

   Direct patient on how to perform the test. "The purpose of this test is to measure the biggest breath of air you can get in and out of your lungs on a single breath and also how fast you can get the air out of your lungs. The first thing I'll have you do is place your feet flat on the ground and sit up as straight as you can. "Next, I will place this mouthpiece in your mouth, between your lips and over your tongue (remove dentures if loose). Be sure your lips are sealed tightly around the outside of the mouthpiece—we don't want to lose any air."

   "I will close your nose with a noseclip. Hold your head up like your playing the trumpet. When I tell you, take a deep breath in and blow all of your air out of your lungs as fast as you possibly can; like blowing the birthday candles out on your birthday cake."

   REMEMBER: The object of this test is to measure how much air you are able to blow out along with how fast you can blow it out. From the very beginning, you'll want to use all the muscle groups you use to cough with, only don't cough, to try and get the air out as quickly as possible.

   "You can probably blow one continuous breath out for at least 8 seconds, but try and get most of the air out within the first second . . . like this (demonstrate). Remember, you have to keep pushing all of the air out of your lungs, even though you can't feel it coming out. You can only feel about the first 80% coming out of your lungs, and I'll keep coaching you to keep on pushing and squeezing with your chest and stomach muscles to get the last 15–20% out." Perform the test at least three good times but not more than eight trials.

   Print out the report as per manual instruction.

3. *Purdue Pegboard*

   Equipment: Purdue pegboard/Digital stopwatch

   The pegboard is placed directly in front of the patient, four inches (4") from the table's front edge, with at least 20 pegs in the exterior cup above the appropriate column. The pegboard may be moved closer or farther from the patient, but may not be moved or aligned diagonally.

Table 3-5.   *(continued)*

The patient is instructed to pick up one peg at a time from the cup and place it in order in the right hole column closest to the cup and tested side as quickly as possible. If the patient picks up 2 pegs, he/she must drop one of the pegs. When a peg is dropped intentionally or accidentally, the patient should not pick it up, but go on with another peg as quickly as possible.

Preset the timer at 30 seconds. Say "Ready . . . start." Timing begins when the patient touches the first peg and ends when 30 seconds has expired. The timer will beep. The number of pegs placed in the holes is recorded.

Perform the test on the right hand twice and then the left hand twice. The left column of holes and cup is used for the left hand. Record the number of pegs on the test report form provided.

4. *Fifteen-Foot Walk*

(This test should only be performed if the patient normally performs these tasks unassisted at home.

Equipment: Measuring tape (15 feet minimum)/Digital stopwatch

Fifteen feet (15′) walking distance should be marked in the room or hallway using two clearly visible tapes or other marking device. This is the start and finish distance. Two tapes similar in color and length are placed 3 feet exterior to the 15 feet tape. These are the target finish lines.

Instruct the patient to stand with feet touching the start line (the interior line) and to "walk as fast as you safely can to the target line," (but caution to not run or walk so fast as to risk falling). Clinical evaluator should walk slightly behind patient for safety.

Timing is started when the patient starts to move (not when you say to start) and ends as both feet cross the finish line.

Record the complete time to one decimal place (tenths of second) on scoring sheet.

B. Quantitative Strength Tests

1. *Isometric Muscle Strength Testing*

Equipment: Standard exam table (180 cm long, 60 cm wide, and 7.5 cm high)

Electronic strain gauge tensiometer (Interface and Advance Force Measurement—Scottsdale, AZ)/Aluminum upright and adjustable rings/Nylon straps

Macintosh Base Computerized Data Acquisition System and Printer

MacAdios II Jr. (Data acquisition A/D Board, GW Instruments)

MacAdios ABD Analog Breakout System (GW Instruments)

SuperScope for data acquisition

Excel for data management and final reports production

Maximal voluntary isometric force is measured with an electronic strain gauge connected to a Macintosh Data Acquisition System. The patient is tested in the supine position for the upper extremities and ankle dorsiflexors, sitting upright at the end of the table for lower extremities (knee extensor testing), and semi-reclined with a wedge for lower extremities (hip flexor testing).

After attaching the strap to the joint being measured, the patient is encouraged to "push" or "pull" against the strap as hard as he or she can "with all your strength." Contraction should be held for 3–4 seconds to assure maximal effort is reached. Encouragement needs to be consistent with all patients. A minimum of three (3) seconds should elapse between trials. Patients should not stabilize themselves by holding onto the table. The clinical examiner should be alert for any signs of respiratory distress when the patient is in the supine position.

To eliminate errors, the order of testing is always as follows:

1] Left Shoulder Extension	7] Left Knee Extension
2] Left Elbow Flexion	8] Right Knee Extension
3] Right Shoulder Extension	9] Right Hip Flexion
4] Right Elbow Flexion	10] Left Hip Flexion

Table 3-5.   *(continued)*

5] Right Ankle Dorsiflexion	11] Right Hand Grip
6] Left Ankle Dorsiflexion	12] Left Hand Grip

2. *Specific Muscle Testing Directions*

Shoulder Extension

Patient is supine with shoulder at 90 degrees of flexion, neutral rotation. Strap is placed just proximal to the elbow. Examiner supports the arm prior to the test (no tension on the strap). Stabilization is superior on the shoulder so that the shoulder does not elevate during the test, and the patient does not slide upward.

Elbow Flexion

Patient remains supine with arm resting on table. Elbow is positioned at 90 degrees, forearm in neutral rotation. The strap is placed just proximal to the styloid process. Examiner secures the elbow from an inferior position and holds the shoulder from protracting as well.

Foot Dorsiflexion

Patient is supine with hips and knees extended and ankle in slight plantarflexion. Strap placed across metatarsals. Heels are over the edge of the table. A towel roll is placed under the ankle. Patient attempts maximal dorsiflexion without pelvis elevation. Stabilization is downward over the proximal tibia. The ankle should be in slight plantarflexion initially so that with contraction it is a neutral ankle position (90 degrees). If the patient is unable to maintain a neutral ankle position (90 degrees) but is in some plantarflexion at the initiation of the trial, the clinical evaluator may "pinch" the strap manually around the patient's foot to prevent the strap from sliding off the foot.

Knee Extension

Patient is seated over the end of the table with knees at 90 degrees. Strap is placed just proximal to the malleoli. Femur is parallel to the table. Examiner provides stabilization by exerting downward force over the ipsilateral shoulder and contralateral hip or by exerting downward force over both shoulders if sitting behind the patient to prevent the hips from rising up off the table.

Hip Flexion

Patient is semi-reclined with head and shoulders supported by a wedge. A towel roll for increasing tension may be used and is placed under test leg which is at about 20 degrees of flexion at the hip. Knee is at 90 degrees of flexion. Strap is placed proximal to the knee joint. Strap not over patella or patient won't pull hard. The untested leg is supported by the tester with the hip and knee at 90 degrees of flexion to maintain pelvis in a posterior tilt. Patient attempts maximal hip flexion. Tension on the strain gauge should be enough at rest so that force is measured without actual elevation of the leg.

Hand Grip

Hand grip is measured manually with an adjustable hand grip dynamometer. The seated patient is positioned with wrist resting on lap and elbow flexed at approximately 110 degrees. The handle of the dynamometer should be adjusted to position 3. Place the dynamometer in the tested hand with dial facing toward the evaluator. Examiner supports the dynamometer from the side and should not pull on it. The wrist should not be supported. The patient is instructed to squeeze with his/her tested hand as hard as possible. Grip tests are performed twice on the right hand then twice on the left hand with dynamometer always set at 3. Measurements will be recorded in kilograms. Record score on test report form.

Equipment List for ACTS ALS Evaluation

PB100 Portable Spirometer
(Renaissance Spirometry System)
  PB110 Base Station
  PB130 Patient Data Memory Card
  3-Liter Calibration Syringe

Puritan-Bennett Corporation
265 Ballardvale Street
Wilmington MA 01887
(800) 842-8023

Table 3-5.   *(continued)*

Digital Thermometer BD250 Disposable Bi-Directional Flow Sensors	
Facemasks	Stuart Drug and Surgical Supply Anesthesia Inhalation Products Div. 4740 Moline Street Denver CO 80239 (303) 373-0530
Digital stopwatch with countdown timer capable of measuring to tenths of seconds	Radio Shack
Purdue Pegboard	Lafayette Instrument Company Box 5729 Lafayette IN 47903 (317) 423-1505
Eighteen inch (18″) high chair with arms	
Twenty-eight inch (28″) high desk or table	
Jamar Adjustable Hydraulic Hand Dynamometer (Model 2A)	Lafayette Instrument Company Box 5279 Lafayette IN 47903 (317) 423-1505
Sony M-330 Pressman Microcassette Recorder and Tape	

Isometric Strength Testing Table
   Standard treatment table
   Zimmer orthopedic bars
     and accessories
       18″ single clamp bar
       27″ plain bar
       66″ swivel clamp bar
       85″ plain bar
       96″ plain bar (heavy duty)
       cross clamp
       trapeze clamp w/D-ring and S-hook
   Connecting cables, straps
   S-hooks
   Calibration weights (25 kg)	

SM-250 Super Mini Load Cell
   20-foot cable
   Modular plug
   Two-28 thread eyebolts
	Interface and Advanced Force
	Measurement Corporation
	Scottsdale AZ
	(602) 948-5555

Macintosh Data Acquisition System Macintosh IIsi, 9 MB RAM, 80 MB hard drive, Nubus card, Monochrome monitor / Microsoft Excel software	

MacAdios Analog to Digital System
   MacAdios II Jr.
   12 mcs data acquisition board
	GW Instruments
	35 Medford Street
	Somerville MA 02143
	(617) 625-4096

MacAdios ABO (analog breakout system)
   modified to accommodate a modular jack
   34-wire cable (10 feet)
   SuperScope Software, version 1.6.3	

Printer	

Table 3-5. *(continued)*

C. Spasticity, Fasciculation, Atrophy and Cramp Scales

1. *Spasticity Scale:* Spasticity is assessed in the upper and lower extremities when the patients are seated. The grading is modified to be opposite to that previously reported (Ashworth, 1964).

Grading of Spasticity:

Modified Grade	Rating	Ashworth Grade
4	Normal	0
3	Slight catch; passive movement of limb, otherwise unimpeded	1
2	Definite resistance to passive movement	2
1	Increased tone sufficient to require effort on part of examiner to overcome resistance	3
0	Passive movement of joint impossible	4

Upper Extremities: Spasticity is assessed by passive range of motion on pronation and supination of the forearm and flexion and extension of the forearm at the elbow. Pronation and supination, flexion, and extension should be performed at less than one movement per second and then increased to a higher rate above 5 per second.

On the initial acceleration of the rate of movement above 3 cycles per second, if a single catch is felt with no passive movement of the limb impeded, then this is rated as a 3.

When the passive movement is restricted such that one or more catches are felt or the rate of movement cannot be increased as easily as in a limb without spasticity, then the limb is graded as 2.

In the forearm rapid-alternating movements occurring at rates below 3.0 Hz (not explained by muscular atrophy) are usually associated with grade 2 spasticity. Occasionally, there may be limitation of full supination in patients with grade 2 spasticity but this is usually limited to less than 160 degrees supination.

If passive range of motion at less than 1 cycle per second is inhibited and increasing the rate of supination-pronation or flexion-extension at the elbow limits the full range of motion of the muscle group being tested, then we give a rating of 1. Spasticity in the upper extremities associated with a rating of 1 usually is associated with a limitation of rapid-alternating movements to supination at an angle between 120–160 degrees.

If passive range of motion of the arm during supination-pronation or flexion-extension is limited at 1 cycle per second, then we give a grade of zero.

Lower Extremities: The limb is elevated and supported by the hand under the knee and the leg is moved in flexion-extension movement about the knee at less than 1 cycle per second, the movement is then accelerated to determine if there is any spastic catch. Spastic catches may be noted particularly in the quadriceps muscle group but occasionally can be felt in the hamstring muscle group.

When the acceleration is above 3 Hz, if one single catch is felt, then this would be given a grade of 3.

If the acceleration of the limb is above 3 cycles per second and one feels one or more catches where there is resistance to movement through the entire range of movement, then this is given a grade of 2.

If, with acceleration of flexion-extension of the leg at the knee, more than three catches or continuous resistance is felt but the leg can still be moved, this is given the score of 1.

If on passive movement at less than 1 cycle per second there is minimal movement or if on acceleration full movement cannot be completed, then a score of zero is given.

Flexion and extension of the foot at the ankle may also be used to assess spasticity. If there is one spastic catch on accelerating the dorsiflexion-plantar flexion movement of the foot to greater than 3 cycles per second, then a rating of 3 will be given to that limb.

If on accelerating the rate of flexion-extension of the ankle on dorsiflexion there is more than one catch or increased resistance of forced dorsiflexion, then this will be rated as 2.

Table 3-5. *(continued)*

If on accelerating the passive range of motion to above 3 cycles per second there is continuous resistance of movement, then this is given a rating of 1.

If the forced dorsiflexion creates clonus, then the rating is given as zero.

In the lower extremity, contractures are much more common in the hamstrings and the posterior leg compartment muscles. This may limit passive range of motion. The distinction between spasticity and contracture is determined by the lack of full range of motion at low frequency passive range of motion.

2. *Fasciculation Scale:* Fasciculations should be evaluated by both inspection and palpation.

Grading of Fasciculations:

Grade	Rating	Explanation
4	Absent	____
3	Rare	Felt only once during examination or reported by patient
2	Evident on inspection	Consistently seen after exercise
1	Obvious	Consistently seen before exercise
0	Continuous	____

The patient should be graded as no fasciculations if there is no report of fasciculations and there are no fasciculations observed on examination.

Continuous fasciculations are present regardless of activity and are graded zero. The rate of fasciculation is unimportant; whether they completely go away is the crucial determinant.

Bulbar Muscles: The tongue should be observed in repose and on protrusion.

If fasciculations occur after protrusion when the tongue is at rest, fasciculations should be graded as 2 (evident on inspection).

Fasciculations noted at rest without protrusion of the tongue would be graded as 1 (obvious).

Submentalis fasciculations are graded as 2 (evident on inspection after contraction) if they occur after facial testing with grimacing or blowing out the cheeks.

Submentalis fasciculations should be graded as 1 (obvious) if they occur spontaneously without exercise-induced production of fasciculation.

Arm and Hand Muscles:

If active or passive range of motion induced fasciculations are palpated or observed, this is a 2 (evident on inspection after contraction).

If the fasciculations are present without active or passive range of motion of the arm, this would be graded as 1 (obvious).

Trunk Muscles: The trunk, shoulder, chest, abdomen and rhomboids should be observed or palpated for fasciculations.

In the trunk region, rare fasciculations are those reported by the patient that may or may not be felt or observed once during the examination.

If only one fasciculation is noted, it should be graded as 3.

Leg and Foot Muscles: Fasciculation should be observed or palpated in the quadriceps, hamstrings, and posterior calf muscles and anterior compartment muscles.

Fasciculations are noted as 1 (obvious) if they are observed or palpated on examination before active or passive range of motion of the muscle.

Fasciculations are noted as 2 (evident on inspection) if they are present only after active or passive range of motion of the muscle.

3. *Atrophy Scale:* Atropy should be evaluated by both inspection and palpation.

Table 3-5. *(continued)*

Grading of Atrophy:

Grade	Rating	Explanation
4	None	___
3	Mild	Loss of normal muscle contour
2	Moderate	Shallowing of muscle belly in anatomical compartment
1	Severe, but without complete loss of muscle bulk	Bony limits of muscle in anatomical compartment easily palpated
0	Complete loss of muscle bulk	No muscle palpated

Bulbar Muscles: Atrophy is graded in the muscles innervated by the hypoglossal and facial cranial motor nerves.

Tongue atrophy is graded mild as 3 if there is only lateral furrowing.

Tongue atrophy is graded moderate as 2 if there is lateral furrowing and dimpling throughout the muscle mass.

Tongue atrophy is graded severe as 1 if there is extreme deepening of the central ridge and lateral furrowing.

Tongue atrophy is graded severe as 0 if there is marked dimpling and lateral furrowing with loss of bulk evident on attempted protrusion.

Tongue muscle bulk is graded as complete loss of muscle bulk when there is very little muscle mass usually smaller than the thumb of the patient with lateral furrowing, dimpling and, in a late stage, even loss of fasciculation.

Facial atrophy is graded mild as 3 when the orbicularis oris cannot purse with lip protrusion.

Facial atrophy is graded moderate as 2 when there is loss of muscle mass such that zygomatic dysfunction is lost with no elevation of the corners of the mouth and the smile is not made as a flat smile over the entire breadth of the face but is only an oval smile.

Facial atrophy is graded severe as 1 when there is decreased elevation of the forehead, poor closure of the eyes, or incomplete closure of the eyes with poor burying of the eyelashes and loss of facial expression.

Facial atrophy is graded complete as 0 when muscle bulk is such that the lips cannot approximate and no facial expression is possible.

Arm and Hand Muscles:

Arm atrophy is noted as mild when the biceps or first dorsal interosseus has lost its normal contour.

Arm atrophy is noted as moderate when there is flattening of either of these muscles.

Arm atrophy is noted as severe when there is severe hollowing of the first dorsal interossei and the interosseus muscle or loss of the normal curvature of the biceps muscle.

Triceps muscle should not be assessed for atrophy. Forearm muscles may be assessed if the biceps and first dorsal interosseus cannot be assessed.

Trunk Muscles:

Trunk atrophy is graded as mild when there is some decrease in the deltoid bulk bilaterally.

Trunk atrophy is graded as moderate when deltoid bulk is lost anteriorly but present laterally.

Trunk atrophy is graded as severe when there is easy palpation of the shoulder joint

Trunk atrophy is graded as zero with complete loss of muscle bulk when the shoulders are ptotic and the shoulder joint is visually apparent.

Spine extensor atrophy is graded as mild when muscle bulk is asymmetrically lost in a focal manner.

Spine extensor atrophy is graded as moderate when extensor muscles of the back are lost to palpation.

Spine extensor atrophy is graded as severe when there is marked bony prominence.

Table 3-5. *(continued)*

> Spine extensor atrophy is graded as zero when there is complete loss of muscle bulk, associated with extreme extensor weakness of the back
>
> ***Leg and Foot Muscles:***
>
> Lower extremity atrophy is graded as mild if there is flattening of the anterior compartment muscles.
>
> Lower extremity atrophy is graded as moderate if there is shallowing of the anterior compartment muscles.
>
> Lower extremity atrophy is graded as severe if there is easily apparent bony ridging of the anterior compartment.
>
> Lower extremity atrophy is graded as zero when there is complete loss of muscle bulk and is usually associated with complete foot drop and easy palpation of the ridge of the tibia with no apparent muscle (Saber shins).
>
> Posterior compartment muscles are most difficult to evaluate from the point of view of atrophy but may be affected. Mild atrophy is loss of the medial head of the gastrocnemius, moderate atrophy is decreased bulk in both heads, severe atrophy is flattening of the posterior compartment muscle.
>
> It is rare to see complete loss of posterior compartment muscle bulk.
>
> 4. *Cramp Scale:* The patient should be asked if he has any cramps described as pain with contraction or tightness of muscle group either occurring spontaneously or brought on by exercise, which causes the patient to want to lengthen the muscle to relieve the pain or contraction.
>
> Patients sometimes confuse spasms due to spasticity with cramps and that has to be sorted out by history and topography. Patients may have cramps when they are stretching their legs at night or when they are getting up. They may have spasms, however, shortly after going to bed with extensor or flexor spasms. These spasms may or may not be painful. The cramps usually are painful. There is a diurnal variation in cramping with cramping being primarily in the supine position in some patients at night. Tongue cramps are very unusual in ALS.
>
> **Grading of Cramps:**
>
> | Grade | Rating | Explanation |
> |:---:|:---|:---|
> | 4 | None | —— |
> | 3 | Rare cramps, related to voluntary muscle activity | Induced by stretching or brisk stiff contractions or < 1 cramp/week |
> | 2 | Spontaneous cramps 1-7 times weekly | Occur with or without movement but strong contractions not required to cause cramp |
> | 1 | > 1 cramp/day, or 7/week | Occur with or without movement but strong contractions not required to cause cramp |
> | 0 | Activity interrupted by severe cramps on multiple occasions daily | —— |
>
> ***Bulbar and Neck Muscles:*** The patient may describe that his tongue gets stuck but it is not truly a cramp.
>
> Neck cramps may be common particularly on extension but occasionally on flexion or rotation. These are usually induced by activity.
>
> If they occur with every activity, they are graded as 0 (activity interrupted by severe cramps on multiple occasions daily). Most patients, however, have these cramps with some maneuvers and not with others. Temporal mandibular joint dislocation with or without forced yawning is not a cramp.
>
> ***Arm and Hand Muscles:*** Upper extremity cramps are more common in the fingers of the hand and the forearm. Flexor cramps are much more common than extensor cramps. Biceps cramps occur commonly on lifting; triceps cramps are extremely rare.

Table 3-5.   *(continued)*

> ***Trunk Muscles:*** Back or flank cramps are occasionally present on extension when yawning. The patient occasionally has abdominal cramps on sneezing or coughing. Chest wall cramps are unusual.
>
> ***Leg and Foot Muscles:*** In the lower extremity, foot cramps are common at night when small intrinsic muscles of the foot with contract with curling of the toes. There are also posterior compartment cramps that involve extension of the leg. It is rare to have anterior compartment cramps except on repetitive activity.

Anterior thigh compartment cramps are much less common than posterior compartment cramps but they may occur. The grading of cramps is done by history and rarely by examination. A patient will usually report that there are no cramps but sometimes further questioning is required to ascertain specifically in anatomical areas where there may be cramping when there is activity that the patient does not interpret as cramps.

Cramps may be rare, less than one per week, and occur only on voluntary muscle activity. These are rated as 3.

Spontaneous cramps that occur without voluntary activity are rated as 2. Sometimes it is difficult to sort out whether voluntary activity activates cramps. If the cramping is very frequent (1–7 times weekly) and it is unclear whether it is voluntary muscle activity-induced cramping or spontaneous cramping, rate it as a 2 nevertheless.

If there is greater than one cramp per day or greater than seven cramps per week due to voluntary or spontaneous activity about specific muscle groups, grade these cramps as 1.

Adapted with permission from ACTS Group Principal Investigator and Procedure Manuals © 1993

Table 3-6. Guidelines for Administration/Scoring ALS Functional Rating Scale (ALS FRS)

Item	Description	Grade
1.	SPEECH	
	Normal speech processes	4
	Detectable speech disturbance	3
	Intelligible with repeating	2
	Speech combined with nonvocal communication	1
	Loss of useful speech	0
2.	SALIVATION	
	Normal	4
	Slight but definite excess of saliva in mouth; may have nighttime drooling	3
	Moderately excessive saliva; may have minimal drooling	2
	Marked excess of saliva with some drooling	1
	Marked drooling; requires constant tissue or handkerchief	0
3.	SWALLOWING	
	Normal eating habits	4
	Early eating problems—occasional choking	3
	Dietary consistency changes	2
	Needs supplemental tube feeding	1
	NPO (exclusively parenteral or enteral feeding)	0
4.	HANDWRITING (with dominant hand prior to ALS onset)	
	Normal	4
	Slow or sloppy: all words are legible	3
	Not all words are legible	2
	Able to grip pen but unable to write	1
	Unable to grip pen	0
5a.	CUTTING FOOD AND HANDLING UTENSILS (patients without gastrostomy)	
	Normal	4
	Somewhat slow and clumsy, but no help needed	3
	Can cut most foods, although clumsy and slow; some help needed	2
	Food must be cut by someone, but can still feed slowly	1
	Needs to be fed	0
5b.	CUTTING FOOD AND HANDLING UTENSILS (patients with gastrostomy)	
	Normal	4
	Clumsy but able to perform all manipulations independently	3
	Some help needed with closures and fasteners	2
	Provides minimal assistance to caregiver	1
	Unable to perform any aspect of task	0
6.	DRESSING & HYGIENE	
	Normal function	4
	Independent and complete self-care with effort or decreased efficiency	3
	Intermittent assistance or substitute methods	2
	Needs attendant for self-care	1
	Total dependence	0

Table 3-6. *(continued)*

Item	Description	Grade
7.	TURNING IN BED AND ADJUSTING BED CLOTHES	
	Normal	4
	Somewhat slow and clumsy, but no help needed	3
	Can turn alone or adjust sheets, but with great difficulty	2
	Can initiate, but not turn or adjust sheets alone	1
	Helpless	0
8.	WALKING	
	Normal	4
	Early ambulation difficulties	3
	Walks with assistance (any assistive device including AFOs)	2
	Nonambulatory functional movement only	1
	No purposeful leg movement	0
9.	CLIMBING STAIRS	
	Normal	4
	Slow	3
	Mild unsteadiness or fatigue	2
	Needs assistance (including handrail)	1
	Cannot do	0
10.	BREATHING	
	Normal	4
	Shortness of breath with minimal exertion (e.g., walking, talking)	3
	Shortness of breath at rest	2
	Intermittent (e.g., nocturnal) ventilatory assistance	1
	Ventilator dependent	0

ALS Functional Rating Scale

1). SPEECH
4 Normal speech processes.
3 Detectable speech disturbance.
2 Intelligible with repeating.
1 Speech combined with nonvocal communication.
0 Loss of useful speech.

2). SALIVATION
4 Normal.
3 Slight but definite excess of saliva in mouth; may have nighttime drooling.
2 Moderately excessive saliva; may have minimal drooling.
1 Marked excess of saliva with some drooling.
0 Marked drooling; requires constant use of tissue or handkerchief.

3). SWALLOWING
4 Normal eating habits.
3 Early eating problems — Occasional choking.
2 Dietary consistency changes.
1 Needs supplemental tube feeding.
0 NPO (exclusively parenteral or enteral feeding).

4). HANDWRITING
4 Normal.
3 Slow or sloppy; all words are legible.
2 Not all words are legible.
1 Able to grip pen but unable to write.
0 Unable to grip pen.

5a). CUTTING FOOD & HANDLING UTENSILS (w/o gastrostomy)
4 Normal.
3 Somewhat slow and clumsy, but no help needed.
2 Can cut most foods, although clumsy and slow; no help needed.
1 Food must be cut by someone, but can still feed self slowly.
0 Needs to be fed.

5b). CUTTING FOOD & HANDLING UTENSILS (with gastrostomy)
4 Normal.
3 Clumsy but able to perform all manipulations independently.
2 Some help needed with closures and fasteners.
1 Provides minimal assistance to caregiver.
0 Unable to perform any aspect of task.

6). DRESSING & HYGIENE
4 Normal function.
3 Independent and complete self-care with effort or decreased efficiency.
2 Intermittent assistance or substitute methods.
1 Needs attendant for self-care.
0 Total dependence.

7). TURNING IN BED & ADJUSTING BED CLOTHES
4 Normal.
3 Somewhat slow and clumsy, but no help needed.
2 Can turn alone or adjust sheets, but with great difficulty.
1 Can initiate, but not turn or adjust sheets alone.
0 Helpless.

8). WALKING
4 Normal.
3 Early ambulation difficulties.
2 Walks with assistance (any assistive device including ankle foot orthosis).
1 Nonambulatory functional movement only.
0 No purposeful leg movement.

9). CLIMBING STAIRS
4 Normal.
3 Slow.
2 Mild unsteadiness or fatigue.
1 Needs assistance (including handrail).
0 Cannot do.

10). BREATHING
4 Normal.
3 Shortness of breath with minimal exertion (e.g., walking, talking).
2 Shortness of breath at rest.
1 Intermittent (e.g., nocturnal) ventilator dependence.
0 Ventilator dependent.

☐ Speech

☐ Salivation

☐ Swallowing

☐ Handwriting

☐ Cutting Food & Handling Utensils   Gastrostomy ☐

☐ Dressing & Hygiene

☐ Turning in Bed & Adjusting Bed Clothes

☐ Walking

☐ Climbing Stairs

☐ Breathing

Total Score
☐

Figure 3-3. ALS Functional Rating Scale form.

patients who require assistance or assistive devices for ambulation: (1) walking score as "walks with assistance" or worse; (2) climbing stairs score as "needs assistance" or worse (requiring use of handrail equates to "needs assistance").

Comparison of ALS Clinimetric Scales

The clinical usefulness and robustness of clinimetric scales for ALS depend on their accuracy, sensitivity, reproducibility, and validity (Hulley & Cummings, 1988). The clinimetric scales described in this chapter vary in their accuracy, sensitivity, reproducibility, and validity. Moreover, practical issues are important in the choice of particular clinimetric scales. The Norris scale has historical precedence. The Appel scale has been used in fewer clinical trials, but it is the only clinimetric scale to date that has been instrumental in demonstrating a potential treatment effect of a neurotrophic factor in ALS (Lai et al., 1996; Lange et al., 1996). The ACTS ALS Evaluation consists of quantitative functional tests, quantitative strength tests, and associated spasticity, fasciculation, atrophy, and cramp ordinal scales that measure impairment. These measures of impairment are kept separate from measures of disability, evaluated by the ALS Functional Rating Scale (ALS FRS), which has been validated by other standard techniques. The ALS FRS is a simple, accurate, sensitive, reproducible measure of disability resulting from ALS-related impairments that is validated and may be used easily in the primary physician's office, the consulting neurologist's office, the ALS multidisciplinary clinic, or clinical trials.

The Norris ALS Scale has been used in many studies from 1974 through 1993. Its properties have been well described (Brooks, 1994). It has many difficulties, including the mixing of impairments and disabilities in the same scale (Feinstein, 1987; Louwerse et al., 1990). The total Norris ALS score for the individual patient may have a variable course over time but it generally shows stability or a linear decline. Similar behavior is noted for the Norris ALS score for groups of patients (Figure 3-4).

The Appel ALS Scale has been used in fewer studies from 1984 to the present. Its properties are less well described (Brooks et al., 1991; Lai et al., 1996; Haverkamp et al., 1995). In order to understand the properties of this scale, we have provided a summary of the changes in Appel subscores over time in 18 ALS patients who also had isometric

muscle strength testing with the ACTS ALS Evaluation. We employed time to failure analysis to permit comparison among the different subscores (Figure 3-5). It is clear that muscle strength testing, lower extremity muscle function, and upper extremity muscle function change more dramatically over time than the bulbar function or respiratory function subscores. It is clear, however, that isometric strength testing is much more sensitive than manual muscle testing that is used in the Appel ALS Scale (Figure 3-6). The functional scores for this group of ALS patients followed for up to 12 months demonstrate changes in upper extremity function by 3 months of follow-up compared with delayed changes in lower extremity function after 6 months of follow-up (Figure 3-7). These properties of the subscores of the Appel scale will be instrumental in allowing the scale to demonstrate clinically significant changes that may occur in the active treatment arms of clinical trial. More importantly, however, is the fact that the Appel ALS Scale still mixes impairments and disabilities in attempting to define a single score for the ALS patient. This problem makes interpretation of Appel scale score changes difficult. In the individual patient, the Appel ALS Scale provides sufficient follow-up information that is useful for clinical management. Its use in clinical trials has been demonstrated, but the interpretation of clinically significant improvement or stabilization is fraught by the difficulty in mixing impairments and disabilities.

The ACTS ALS Evaluation is based on Airlie House Guidelines prepared by the Subcommittee on Motor Neuron Diseases of the World Federation of Neurology Research Group on Neuromuscular Diseases (Subcommittee on Motor Neuron Diseases, 1995). It is divided into quantitative function tests, quantitative strength tests and ordinal scales of impairments, and a clinimetric disability scale (ALS CNTF Treatment Study [ACTS] Phase I-II Study Group, 1995a, 1995b, 1996). The impairments measured by quantitative functional tests are specifically related to disability measured by the ALS FRS (Figure 3-8). Additionally, the impairments measured by quantitative strength tests are specifically related to disability measured by the ALS FRS (Figure 3-9). The change over time in the isometric strength of specific muscles in ALS patients is a function of the anatomical location of the muscles tested (Figure 3-10). Proximal muscles are stronger overall as a percent of the normal predicted value for each patient. Distal muscles are weaker. These individual differences among mus-

Norris Scale

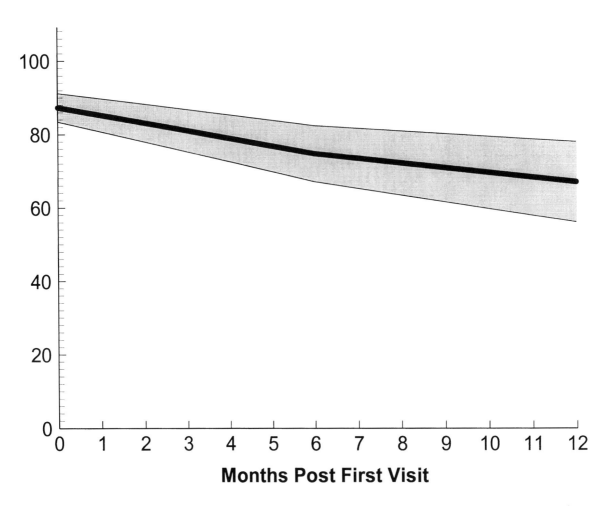

Figure 3-4. Norris ALS Scale changes over 12 months. Mean ± 95% confidence limits of total Norris ALS Scale score in 18 ALS patients.

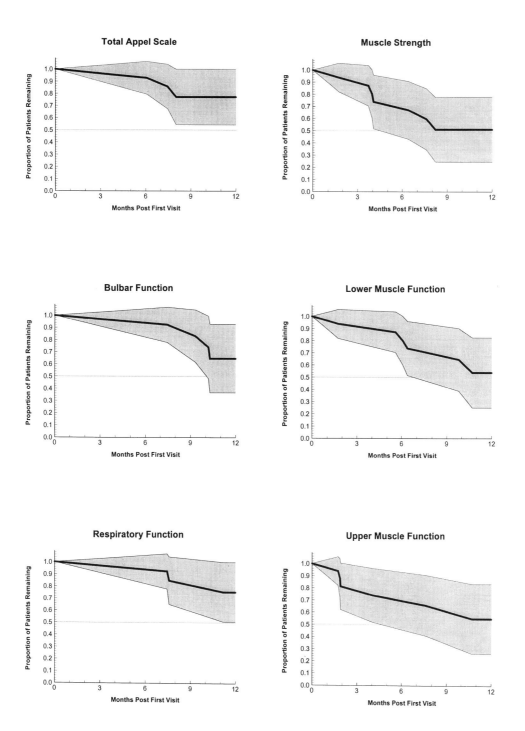

Figure 3-5. Time to failure for total Appel ALS Scale score and subscores over 12 months.

A. Proportion ± 95% confidence limits of 18 ALS patients maintaining total Appel ALS Scale Score < 103 points.

B. Proportion ± 95% confidence limits of 18 ALS patients maintaining muscle strength Appel ALS Scale subscore < 22 points.

C. Proportion ± 95% confidence limits of 18 ALS patients maintaining bulbar Appel ALS Scale subscore < 17 points.

D. Proportion ± 95% confidence limits of 18 ALS patients maintaining lower extremity function Appel ALS Scale subscore < 21 points.

E. Proportion ± 95% confidence limits of 18 ALS patients maintaining respiratory Appel ALS Scale subscore < 24 points.

F. Proportion ± 95% confidence limits of 18 ALS patients maintaining upper extremity function Appel ALS Scale subscore < 19 points.

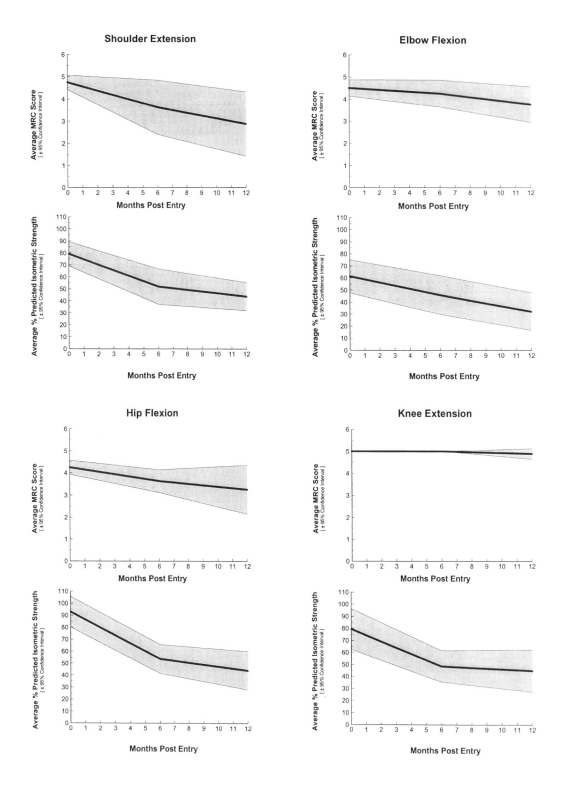

Figure 3-6. Comparison of change in MRC score with change in isometric strength in ALS patients. The average MRC score ± 95% confidence limits was compared over 12 months with the average percent predicted isometric muscle strength ± 95% confidence limits for the following right and left muscle groups of 18 ALS patients

    A. Shoulder extension.

    B. Elbow flexion.

    C. Hip flexion.

    D. Knee extension.

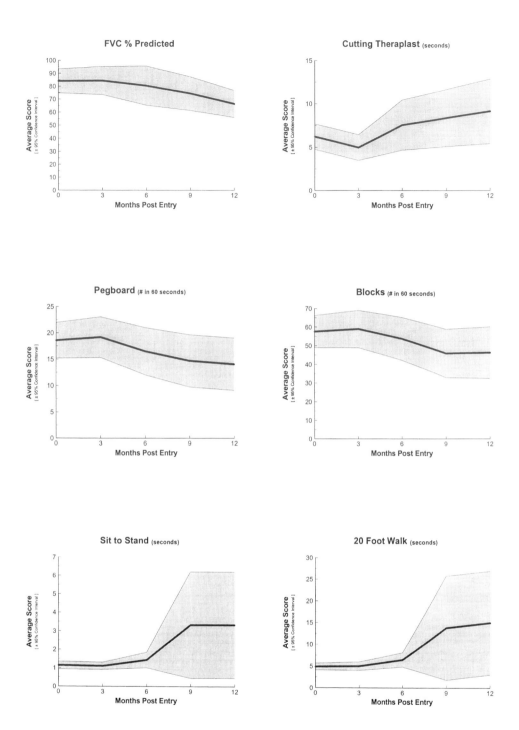

Figure 3-7. Average score for functional measurements in Appel ALS subscores. The average score ± 95% confidence limits for 18 ALS patients followed 12 months by the Appel ALS Scale was determined for the following respiratory, upper extremity and lower extremity functions:

A. Forced vital capacity percent predicted.
B. Cutting theraplast time.
C. Pegboard constructs in time interval.
D. Block turning in time interval.
E. Standing from chair tIme.
F. Twenty foot walk time.

Missing data imputed by the last value carried forward technique.

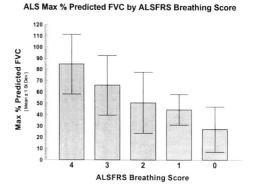

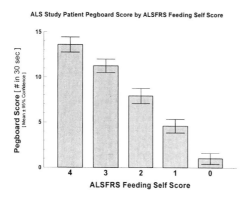

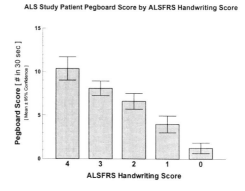

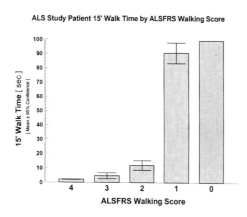

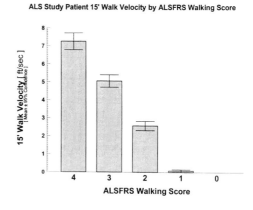

Figure 3-8. Comparison of functional measurements in ACTS ALS Evaluation with ALS FRS subscores. The average value ± 95% confidence limits for functional measurements in the ACTS ALS Evaluation of 132 ALS patients was compared with the ALS FRS subscore for the following functional measurements:

A. Bulbar diadochokinetic [PaTa] score with ALS FRS summed bulbar subscore.
B. Forced vital capacity percent predicted with ALS FRS breathing subscore.
C. Pegboard constructs in time tnterval with ALS FRS feeding subscore.
D. Pegboard constructs in time interval with ALS FRS handwriting subscore.
E. Walking time with ALS FRS walking subscore.
F. Walking velocity with ALS FRS walking subscore.

Elbow Flexion % Pred Isometric Strength by Mean Arm FRS

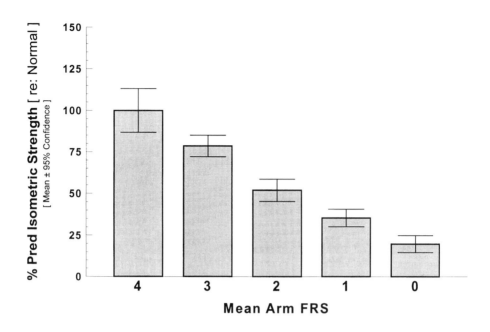

Ankle Dorsiflexion % Pred Isometric Strength by Mean Leg FRS

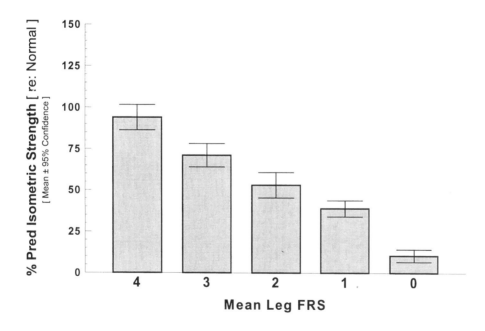

Figure 3-9. Comparison of isometric strength measurements in ACTS ALS Evaluation with ALS FRS subscores. The average value ± 95% confidence limits for right and left isometric strength (as percent predicted relative to normal) measurements in the ACTS ALS Evaluation of 132 ALS patients was compared with the ALS FRS subscore for the following muscle groups:

A. Elbow flexion.
B. Ankle dorsiflexion.

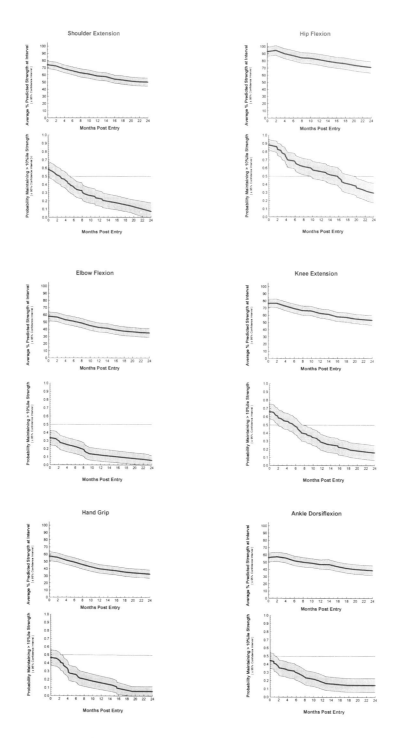

Figure 3-10. Isometric muscle strength changes over time in ACTS ALS Evaluation. The average value ± 95% confidence limits for right and left isometric strength (as percent predicted relative to normal) measurements over time in the ACTS ALS Evaluation of 132 ALS patients was compared with time to failure (< 10% predicted normal strength) for the following muscle groups:

   A. Shoulder extension.
   B. Hip flexion.
   C. Elbow flexion.
   D. Knee extension.
   E. Hand grip.
   F. Ankle dorsiflexion.

cles make it difficult to form a composite score of muscle strength since some muscles are further along in the disease process than others. Isometric strength measurements are crucial in the individual patient to identify significant changes in clinical strength not measurable by manual muscle testing (Figure 3-6). This change over time will be instrumental in providing information of progression required to increase the certainty of the diagnosis of ALS according to the El Escorial criteria (Subcommittee on Motor Neuron Diseases/Amyotrophic Lateral Sclerosis, 1994). Early diagnosis is enhanced by the employment of isometric muscle strength changes over time in addition to other neurodiagnostic techniques. Isometric strength measurements are also important in determining treatment effects in short-term studies where survival or other clinimetric scales do not show changes during the shorter time period (ALS CNTF Treatment Study [ACTS] Phase II-III Study Group, 1996; Bradley, et al., 1995; Miller et al., 1996a, 1996b).

The ALS FRS is a measure of disability in ALS patients. It has been validated against other quantitative measures of function and strength changes resulting from impairments caused by ALS. It is a sensitive, accurate, and reproducible measure of the clinical course of ALS. Its properties have been described in some detail (Brooks et al., 1995; Brooks, 1996). In this chapter, we present the course of disability due to ALS measured by ALS FRS subscores in a large group of ALS patients described in two different ways. The average score over time is contrasted with the probability of maintaining a specific ALS FRS subscore over time (Figure 3-11). In this manner, different disability states may be seen in a population of ALS patients. There is a 1-point drop from normal in the dressing and hygiene subscore in nearly all patients by 12 months while handwriting and feeding subscores

drop 1 point from normal between 12 and 24 months after entry. Climbing stairs and walking subscores drop 1 point from normal in this same time period, but the drop from grade 2 to grade 1 occurs in a shorter time span. Bulbar subscore measures do not drop 1 point from normal in the majority of patients until after 24 months from entry. The speech subscore changes in the majority of patients occur earlier than the salivation or swallowing subscores.

The ALS FRS permits a definition of the time spent in different disability states as a function of the time spent following entry before a 1-point drop from normal (4 to 3), from mildly affected (3 to 2), from moderately affected (2 to 1), and from severely effected to moribund (1 to 0) (Figure 3-12). The range of the time spent in these different states is broad (Table 3-7). Nevertheless, this new means of describing disability due to ALS will permit a simple mode for obtaining clinical information that will allow follow-up of individual patients in different clinical settings, as well as application of sophisticated biomedical statistical methods for efficient and economical future clinical trials.

Acknowledgments. The information provided in this chapter derives from a cooperative effort of many collaborators at the ALS Clinical Research Center (Daryn Belden, Mohammed Sanjak, Jennifer Parnell, Christy Dewitt, John Wheat, Kelly Wheat), the ALS Clinic (Kathryn Roelke, Andrew Waclawik, Barend Lotz, Bradley Beinlich), and the Wisconsin Chapter of the Muscular Dystrophy Association (Paula McGuire).

Information obtained for this review was obtained during studies that were supported in part by the Muscular Dystrophy Association, Department of Veterans Affairs, Regeneron Pharmaceuticals, Amgen-Regeneron Partners, and Rhone-Poulenc Rorer Pharmaceuticals.

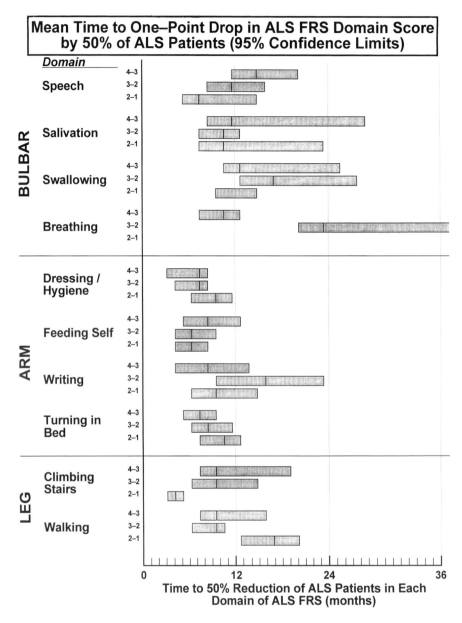

Figure 3-11. ALS FRS subscore changes over time in ACTS ALS Evaluation. The average value ± 95% confidence limits for individual subscore measurements over time in the ACTS ALS Evaluation of 132 ALS patients was compared with time to failure (by 1-point drop to lower score: 4 to 3 (solid black line), 3 to 2 (thick horizontal dashed black line), 2 to 1 (thin vertical dashed line)] for the following ALS FRS subscores:

Bulbar
Speech
Salivation
Swallowing
Arm
Dressing and hygiene
Feeding self
Writing
Turning in bed
Leg
Climbing stairs
Walking

Speech

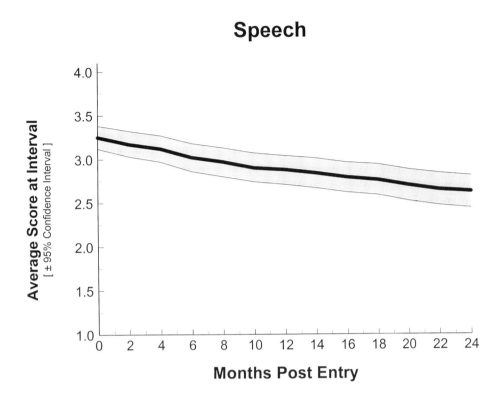

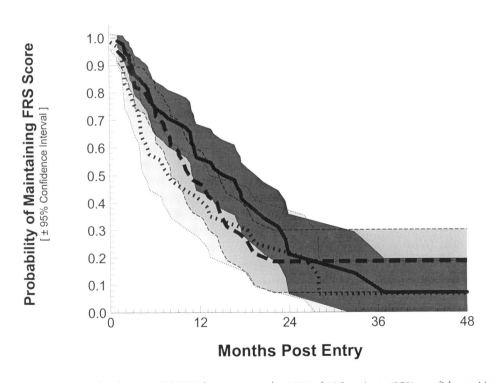

Figure 3-11a. Mean time to 1-point drop in ALS FRS domain score by 50% of ALS patients (95% confidence Limits). The mean time in months ± 95% confidence limits for 1-point drop to lower score: 4 to 3 (solid line), 3 to 2 (horizontal dash), 2 to 1 (diagonal dash) for ALS FRS subscores.

Salivation

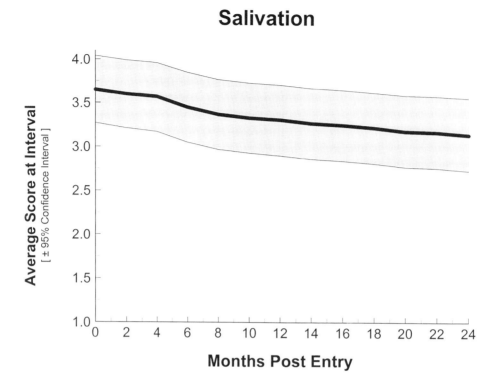

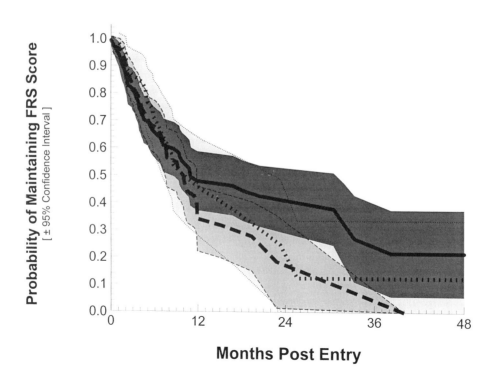

Figure 3-11b.

Swallowing

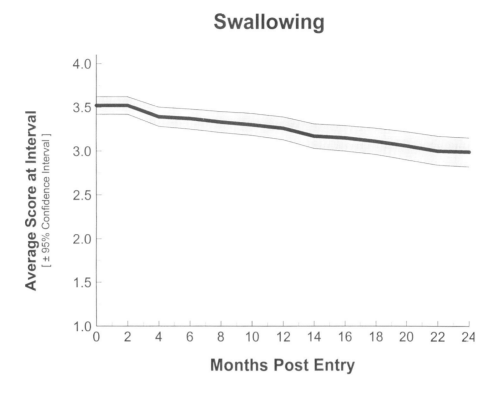

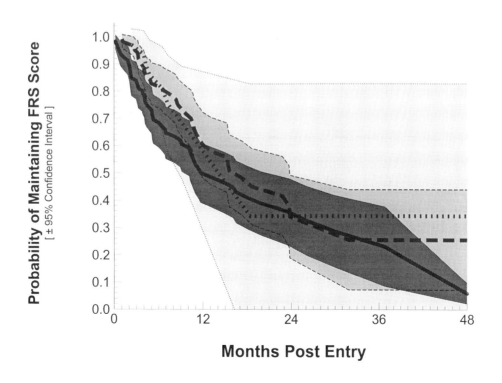

Figure 3-11c.

Handwriting

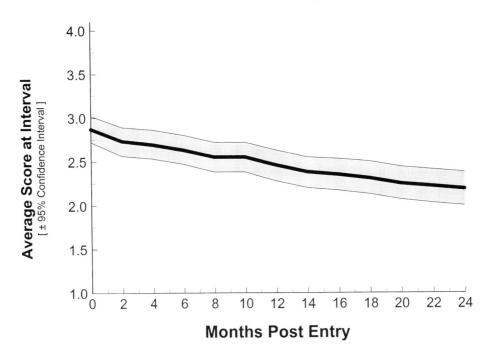

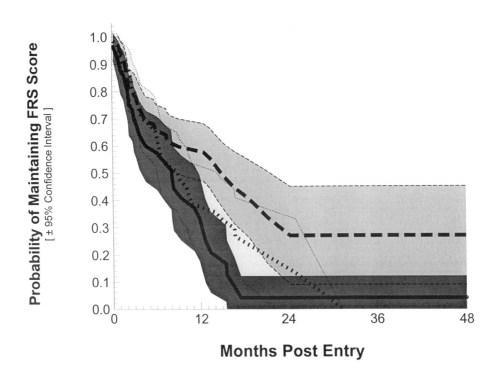

Figure 3-11d.

Feeding Self

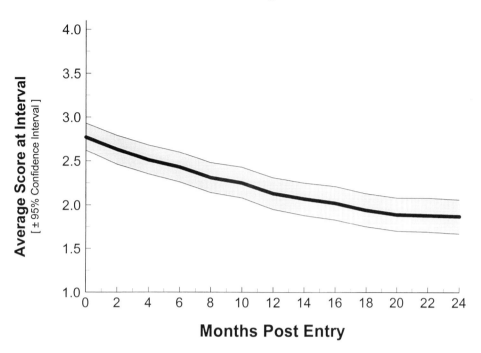

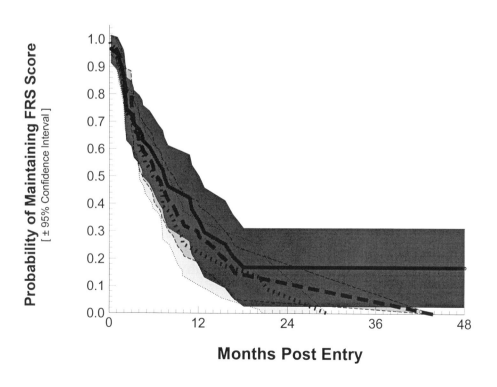

Figure 3-11e.

Dressing & Hygiene

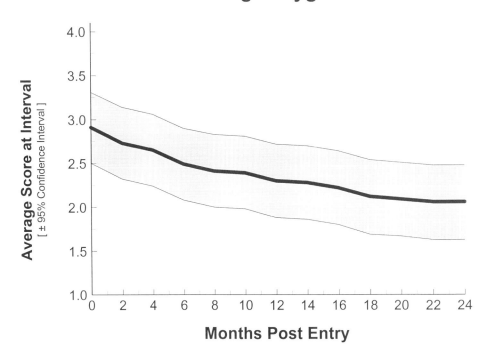

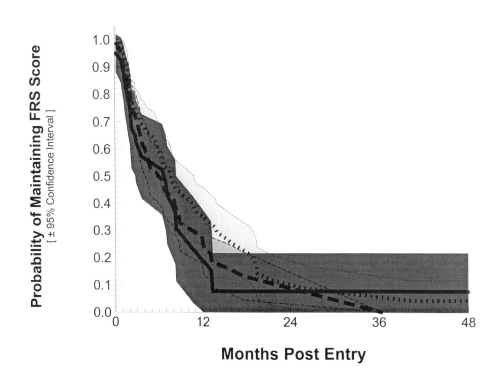

Figure 3-11f.

Turning in Bed

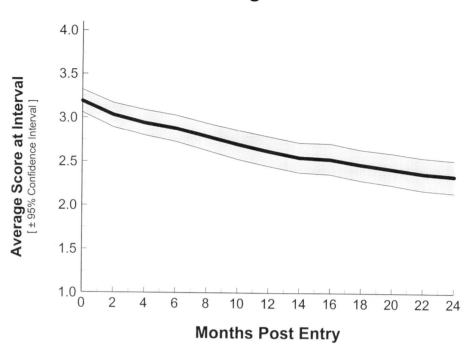

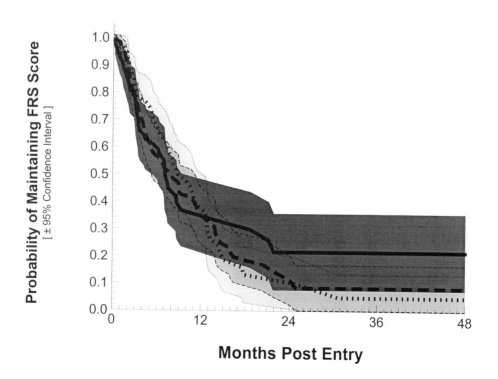

Figure 3-11g.

Walking

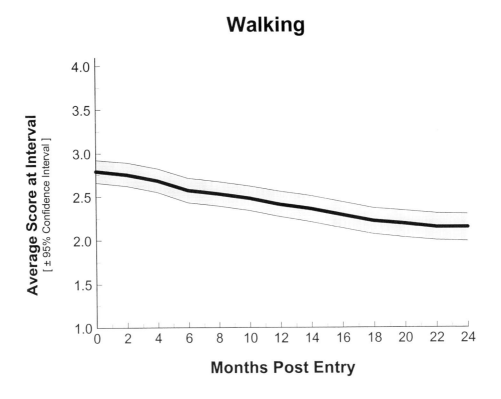

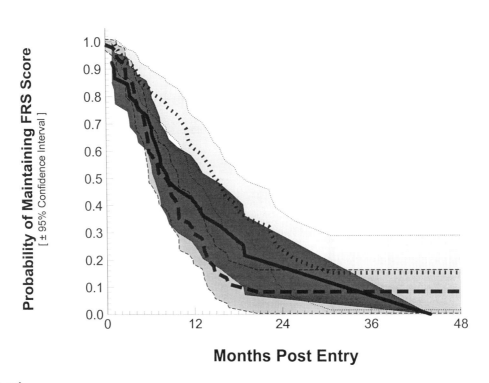

Figure 3-11h.

Climbing Stairs

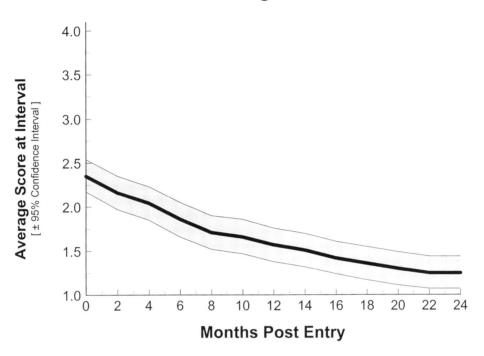

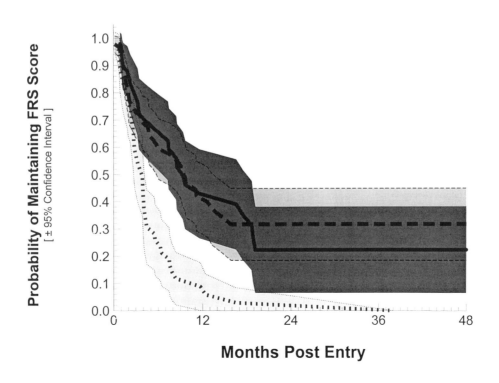

Figure 3-11i.

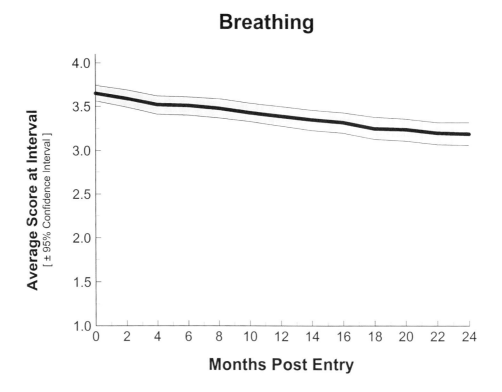

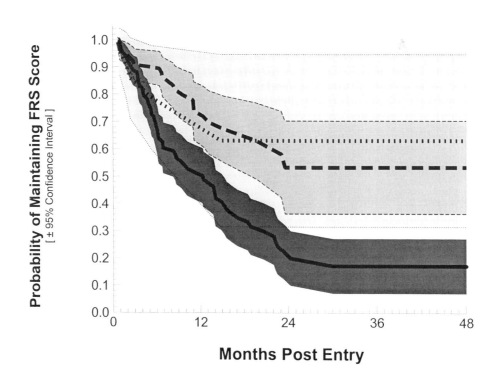

Figure 3-11j.

Table 3-7.   Mean Time to One-Point Drop in ALS FRS Domain Score by 50% of ALS Patients

Time to 50% Reduction of ALS Patients in each Domain of ALS FRS (95% Confidence Limits)

Score Change *Domain*	*4 → 3*	*3 → 2*	*2 → 1*
Bulbar			
Speech	14 mo detectable (11–19)	11 mo repeating required (8–15)	7 mo nonverbal aids used (5–14)
Salivation	11 mo nocturnal drooling (8–27)	10 mo mild saliva during day (7–12)	10 mo moderate saliva (7–22)

Swallow	12 mo
	detectable, occasional
	  choking
	(10–24)
		16 mo
		soft diet
		(8–15)
			14 mo
			supplemental
			  tube feedings
			(9–Indeterminate)

Respiratory			
Breathing	10 mo SOB exertion (7–12)	22 mo SOB at rest (19–40)	indeterminate BiPAP/CPAP (–)
Arm			
Dressing/Hygiene	7 mo decreased efficiency (3–8)	7 mo intermittent assistance (7–12)	9 mo with full assistance (7–22)
Feeding/Cutting	8 mo slow but full turn, unaided (5–12)	6 mo clumsy, occasionally aided (4–9)	6 mo cutting by aide (4–8)
Writing	8 mo slow, legible (4–13)	15 mo illegible (9–22)	9 mo hold pen, not write (6–14)
Trunk			

Turning in Bed	7 mo
	slow, unaided
	(10–24)
		8 mo
		worse but full turn,
		  unaided
		(8–15)
			10 mo
			can initiate but not turn
			  fully without aide
			(9–10)

Leg			
Climbing Stairs	9 mo slow, unaided (7–18)	9 mo unsteady, unaided (6–14)	4 mo with hand rail or assistance (3–5)
Walking	9 mo slow, unaided (7–15)	9 mo requires assistive device, including APO (6–10)	16 mo nonambulatory (12–19)

References

ALS CNTF Treatment Study (ACTS) Phase I-II Study Group. The pharmacokinetics of subcutaneously administered recombinant human ciliary neurotrophic factor (RHCNTF) in patients with amyotrophic lateral sclerosis—Relation to parameters of the acute-phase response. *Clin Neuropharmacol* 1995;18:500–14.

ALS CNTF Treatment Study (ACTS) Phase I-II Study Group. A phase I study of recombinant human ciliary neurotrophic factor (RHCNTF) in patients with amyotrophic lateral sclerosis. *Clin Neuropharmacol* 1995;18:515–32.

ALS CNTF Treatment Study (ACTS) Phase I-II Study Group. The amyotrophic lateral sclerosis functional rating scale—Assessment of activities of daily living in patients with amyotrophic lateral sclerosis. *Arch Neurol* 1996;53:141–47.

ALS CNTF Treatment Study (ACTS) Phase II-III Study Group. A double-blind placebo-controlled clinical trial of subcutaneous recombinant human ciliary neurotrophic factor (RHCNTF) in amyotrophic lateral sclerosis. *Neurology* 1996;46:1244–49.

Andres PL, Hedlund W, Finison L, Conlon T, Felmus M, Munsat TL. Quantitative motor assessment in amyotrophic lateral sclerosis. *Neurology* 1986;36:937–41.

Appel V, Stewart SS, Smith G, Appel SH. A rating scale for amyotrophic lateral sclerosis: description and preliminary experience. *Ann Neurol* 1987;22:328–33.

Ashworth B. Preliminary trial of carisoprodol in multiple sclerosis. *Practitioner* 1964;192:540–42.

Bradley WG and the BDNF Study Group. A phase I/II of recombinant human brain derived neurotrophic factor in amyotrophic lateral sclerosis [Works in Progress Abst 1]. *Ann Neurol* 1995;38:971.

Bromberg MB, Brooks BR. Issues in clinical trial design II: selection of end point measures. *Neurology* 1996;47(Suppl 2):S100–S102.

Brooks BR. Natural history of ALS: Symptoms, strength, pulmonary function and disability. *Neurology* 1996;47(Suppl 2):S71–S82.

Brooks BR, DePaul R, Tan YD, Sanjak M, Sufit RL, Robbins JE. Motor neuron disease. In: Porter RJ, Schoenberg BS (eds.). *Controlled clinical trials in neurological disease.* Boston: Kluwer Academic, 1990:249–81.

Brooks BR, Lewis D, Rawling J, et al. The natural history of amyotrophic lateral sclerosis. In: William AC (ed.). *Motor neuron disease.* London: Chapman & Hall, 1994:131–69.

Brooks BR, Sufit RL, Clough JA, Conrad J, Sanjak M, Schram M, Erickson LM. Isokinetic and functional evaluation of muscle strength over time in amyotrophic lateral sclerosis. In: Munsat TL (ed.). *Quantification of neurologic deficit.* Boston: Butterworths, 1989:143–54.

Brooks BR, Sufit RL, DePaul R, Tan YD, Sanjak M, Robbins J. Design of clinical therapeutic trials in amyotrophic lateral sclerosis. In: Rowland LP (ed.). *Amyotrophic lateral sclerosis and other motor neuron diseases.* New York: Raven, 1991:521–46.

Brooks BR. Test protocol development: further preliminary experience with the effects of TRH in ALS. *Muscle Nerve* 1985;8:460–65.

Brooks BR. The Norris ALS score: insight into the natural history of amyotrophic lateral sclerosis provided by Forbes Norris. In: Rose FC (ed.). *ALS—From Charcot to the present and into the future—The Forbes H. Norris (1928-1993) Memorial Volume.* London: Smith-Gordon, 1994:21–29. [Advances in ALS/MND, Vol. 3].

Caroscio JT, Mulvihill MN, Sterling R, Abrams B. Amyotrophic lateral sclerosis—Its natural history. *Neurol Clinics* 1987;1–8.

Fallat RJ, Jewitt B, Bass M, Kamm B, Norris FH. Spirometry in amyotrophic lateral sclerosis. *Arch Neurol* 1979;36:74–80.

Fallat RJ. Pulmonary function in amyotrophic lateral sclerosis: caveats and value in clinical management and future clinical trials. In: Rose FC (ed.). *ALS—From Charcot to the present and into the future—The Forbes H. Norris (1928-1993) Memorial Volume.* London, Smith-Gordon, 1994:309–313. [Advances in ALS/MND, Vol. 3].

Feinstein AR. *Clinimetrics.* London: Yale University Press, 1987.

Guiloff RJ, Goonetilleke A. Longitudinal clinical assessments in motor neurone disease. Relevance to clinical trials. In: Rose FC (ed.). *ALS—From Charcot to the present and into the future—The Forbes H. Norris (1928–1993) Memorial Volume.* London: Smith-Gordon, 1994:73-82. [Advances in ALS/MND, Vol. 3].

Haverkamp LJ, Appel V, Appel SH. Natural history of amyotrophic lateral sclerosis in a database population—Validation of a scoring system and a model for survival prediction. *Brain* 1995;118:707-19.

Glindmeyer HW, Jones RN, Barkman HW, Weill H. Spirometry: quantitative test criteria and test acceptability. *Am Rev Respir Dis* 1987;136:449-52.

Hillel AD, Miller RM, Yorkston K, McDonald E, Norris FH, Konifow N. Amyotrophic lateral sclerosis severity scale. In: Rose FC (ed.). *Amyotrophic lateral sclerosis.* New York: Demos, 1990:93-97.

Hillel AD, Miller RM, Yorkston K, McDonald E, Norris FH, Konikow N. Amyotrophic lateral sclerosis severity scale. *Neuroepidemiology* 1989:8:142-50.

Hulley S, Cummings R. *Designing clinical research.* Baltimore: Williams & Wilkins, 1988.

Italian ALS Study Group. Branched-chain amino acids and amyotrophic lateral sclerosis: a treatment failure. *Neurology* 1993;43:2466–70.

Lai EC, Felice K, Gawel M, Gelinas D, Kratz R, Lange DJ, Natter HM, Rudnicki SA, Miller K, Murphy MF and the ALS/North American IGF-1 Study Group, Appel V, Haverkamp LJ, Appel SH. Amyotrophic lateral sclerosis disease progression in a historical database group accurately reflects the rate of decline of placebo controls in a phase III clinical trial for insulin-like growth factor [Abst S64.003]. *Neurology* 1996;46(Suppl 2):A469–A470.

Lange DJ, Felice KJ, Festoff BW, Gawel MJ, Gelinas DF, Kratz R, Lai EC, Murphy MF, Natter HM, Norris FH, Rudnicki S and the North American ALS/IGF-1 Study Group. Recombinant human insulin-like growth factor-I in ALS: description of a double-blind, placebo-controlled study. *Neurology* 1996;47 (Suppl 2):S93–S95.

Louwerse ES, de Jong JMBV, Kuether G. Critique of assessment methodology in amyotrophic lateral sclerosis. In: Rose FC (ed.). *Amyotrophic lateral sclerosis.* New York: Demos, 1990:151–79.

McGuire D, Garrison L, Armon C, et al. Relationship of the Tufts quantitative neuromuscular exam (TQNE) and the Sickness Impact Profile (SIP) in measuring progression of ALS. *Neurology* 1996;46:1442–44.

Miller RG, Gelinas D, Moore M, et al. A placebo-controlled trial of gabapentin in amyotrophic lateral sclerosis [Abst S64.002]. *Neurology* 1996a;46(Suppl 2):A469.

Miller RG, Petajan JH, Byan WW, et al. A placebo-controlled trial of recombinant human ciliary neurotrophic (RHCNTF) factor in amyotrophic lateral sclerosis. *Ann Neurol* 1996b;39:256–60.

Munsat TL, Andres PL, Finison L, Conlon T, Thiodeau L. The natural history of motoneuron loss in amyotrophic lateral sclerosis. *Neurology* 1988;38:409–13.

Munsat TL, Andres PL, Skerry LM. The use of quantitative techniques to define amyotrophic lateral sclerosis. In: Munsat TL (ed.). *Quantification of neurologic deficit.* Boston: Butterworths, 1989:129–42.

Norris FH, Calanchini PR, Fallat R, Panchri S, Jewett BJ. The administration of guanidine in amyotrophic lateral sclerosis. *Neurology* 1974;24:721–28.

Norris FH, Fallat RJ. Staging respiratory failure in ALS. In: Tsubaki T, Yase Y (eds.). *Amyotrophic lateral sclerosis.* Amsterdam: Elsevier Excerpta Medica, 1988:217–22.

Ottenbacher KJ. *Evaluating clinical change—Strategies for occupational and physical therapists.* Baltimore: Williams & Wilkins, 1986.

Ringel SP, Murphy JR, Alderson MK, et al. The natural history of amyotrophic lateral sclerosis. *Neurology* 1993;43:1316–22.

Sanjak M, Belden D, Cook T, Brooks BR. Muscle strength measurement. In: Lane RJM (eds). *Handbook of muscle disease.* New York: Marcel Dekker, 1996:19–34.

Smith RA, Melmed S, Sherman B, Frane J, Munsat TL, Festoff BW. Recombinant growth hormone treatment of amyotrophic lateral sclerosis. *Muscle Nerve* 1993;16:624–33.

Streiner DL, Norman GR. *Health measurement scales—A practical guide to their development and use.* Oxford: Oxford University Press, 1989.

Subcommittee on Motor Neuron Diseases/Amyotrophic Lateral Sclerosis of the World Federation of Neurology Research Group on Neuromuscular Disease and the El Escorial "Clinical Limits Amyotrophic Lateral Sclerosis" Workshop Contributors. El Escorial World Federation of Neurology Criteria for the Diagnosis of Amyotrophic Lateral Sclerosis. *J Neurol Sci* 1994;124(Suppl):96–107.

Subcommittee on Motor Neuron Diseases of the World Federation of Neurology Research Group on Neuromuscular Disease and the Airlie House "Therapeutic Trials in ALS" Workshop Contributors. Airlie House Guidelines—Therapeutic Trials in Amyotrophic Lateral Sclerosis. *J Neurol Sci* 1995; 129(Suppl):1–10.

Tourtellotte WW, Haerer AF, Simpson JF, et al. Quantitative clinical neurological testing 1. A study of a battery of tests designed to evaluate in part the neurological function of patients with multiple sclerosis and its use in a therapeutic trial. *Ann NY Acad Sci* 1965;122:480–505.

Wade DT. Pathology, impairment, disability, handicap: a useful model. *Measurement in neurologic rehabilitation.* Oxford: Oxford University Press, 1992.

CHAPTER 4 Scales for the Assessment of Movement Disorders

Stephen T. Gancher, MD

A variety of scales have been developed during the last several decades for measurement of the severity of various movement disorders. They vary from simple, limited assessments that are easily performed to comprehensive scales that may be time-consuming and take practice to administer.

One common feature of these scales is an emphasis on motor signs. Depending on the disease, various symptoms associated with the condition have also been used for rating, and some scales or portions of scales use descriptions of functional status and ability to perform self-care activities as a basis for rating disease. This chapter reviews the most widely used scales for Parkinson's disease, dystonia, tic disorders, and tardive dyskinesias.

Parkinson's Disease

Introduction

Prior to the development of levodopa treatment of Parkinson's disease, studies describing the efficacy of drug treatment or surgical therapy largely relied on an overall subjective impression of disease severity rather than formal ratings. With the advent of levodopa therapy, many drug trials were conducted and created a need to rate the severity of parkinsonism in a more standardized fashion.

One of the first widely used scales is a single-item assessment, reported by Drs. Margaret Hoehn and Melvin Yahr in a study of the natural history of Parkinson's disease (Hoehn et al., 1967). Although this scale is mainly useful for broad classification of patients and is not sufficiently detailed to follow patients who exhibit motor fluctuations, it is easily administered and still widely used. Other early scales, such as the Northwestern University Disability Scale (Canter et al., 1961), evaluated functional status and both functional and objective tests (Webster, 1968; Schwab, 1960), and a scale developed at Columbia University (Yahr et al., 1969) was extensively used. These scales, as well as others, are comprehensively reviewed by Martinez-Martin (1993).

Because of the marked variability between scales and differences in weighting signs and symptoms, a committee chaired by Stanley Fahn, M.D., was created in 1984 to develop a standardized scale. This scale, the Unified Parkinson's Disease Rating Scale (UPDRS) (Fahn et al., 1987), is a composite of various previous scales and its use in the United States has largely supplanted other scales.

The Unified Parkinson's Disease Rating Scale

Description

The UPDRS (Table 4-1) is a composite scale consisting of six sections. Unless indicated otherwise, all items are rated from 0 (normal) to 4 (severely affected); each item is defined by a short sentence.

Part I of the UPDRS consists of four items that assess mentation, behavior, and mood. Although helpful as a general screen, these items are inadequate for measurement of dementia or depression, so other instruments should be used for their assessment.

Part II consists of 13 items and assesses the performance of activities of daily living. Items include assessment of difficulty with speech and swallowing, self-care, speaking, turning over in bed, and walking.

Two limitations should be mentioned in the use of this subscale. First, as it is based on symptoms, there may be disagreement between items that reflect bradykinesia and objective estimates of bradykinesia in the physical examination portion of the scale (Part III). Also, since patients may perceive symptoms differently despite similar signs, it is possible for them to have different scores despite a similar degree of bradykinesia or tremor.

A second difficulty with this subscale relates to its use in comparing "on" and "off" states. Because many items are based on specific activities such as dressing or eating, in patients who time these activities to coincide with "on" states, a rating of functional difficulties performing these activities during "off" states may be artificial and difficult to interpret.

Part III is a 14-item rating of motor signs that is based on items in the Columbia disability scale. In addition to ratings of tremor and an assessment of facial and generalized bradykinesia, performance on several tasks is used to rate disease severity, including any difficulty noted while repeatedly tapping the index finger against the thumb, clenching and unclenching a fist, and arising from a chair. The definitions of difficulties with each task are straightforward, and the scale is reproducible. However, this motor scale does not take into account interference from dyskinesias or dystonias, which may present difficulty in motor performance in some patients.

Part IV rates complications of therapy. It includes several questions that attempt to quantify the duration and severity of dyskinesias and motor fluctuations and a 3-item section concerning anorexia, sleep disturbance, and orthostatic hypotension. Unlike the previous sections, some items in this section are not graded, and it may be difficult to consistently rate patients who describe minor difficulties with sleep or minimal orthostatic dizziness.

Part V is a modified version of the Hoehn and Yahr staging system; overall disease severity is divided into unilateral (stage I), bilateral but without a gait or balance disorder (stage II), and bilateral disease with progressively more difficulty with mobility and balance (stage III–V); half points are allowed between stages I–II and II–III.

Part VI is a disability scale based on a scale reported by Schwab & England (Martinez-Martin, 1993). It is an estimation of the degree of interference with normal functioning and dependency due to parkinsonism; like other symptom-based scales, it reflects subjective perception, and patients with similar motor difficulties may sometimes report discrepant scores.

The CAPIT Rating Scale

This scale, an acronym for the Core Assessment Program for Intracerebral Transplantation, was devised in an attempt to standardize the ratings obtained in studies of transplantation in Parkinson's disease. In addition to utilizing the UPDRS, the CAPIT protocol also includes 0–5 scales for both the duration and the severity of dyskinesias. Other items include diary information, timed motor tasks, and evaluation both before and after an oral dose of L-dopa (Langston et al., 1992)

Diary Ratings

Another popular instrument for the assessment of motor fluctuations involves self-reporting of hourly status by patients. The patient is instructed to rate motor symptoms, averaging performance over each hour. In some centers, this information is visually conveyed by constructing a table such that each horizontal line represents a different day and each vertical line a block of time; blacking in the individual squares during either "on" or "off" states graphically conveys patterns that may be unapparent on a single day but may become obvi-

Table 4-1. Unified Parkinson's Disease Rating Scale (UPDRS)

I. Mentation, Behavior and Mood

1. Intellectual Impairment:

0—None.

1—Mild. Consistent forgetfulness with partial recollection of events and no other difficulties.

2—Moderate memory loss, with disorientation and moderate difficulty handling complex problems. Mild but definite impairment of function at home with need of occasional prompting.

3—Severe memory loss with disorientation for time and often to place. Severe impairment in handling problems.

4—Severe memory loss with orientation preserved to person only. Unable to make judgments or solve problems. Requires much help with personal care. Cannot be left alone at all.

2. Thought Disorder: (Due to dementia or drug intoxication)

0—None.

1—Vivid dreaming.

2—"Benign" hallucinations with insight retained.

3—Occasional to frequent hallucinations or delusions; without insight; could interfere with daily activities.

4—Persistent hallucinations, delusions, or florid psychosis. Not able to care for self.

3. Depression:

0—Not present.

1—Periods of sadness or guilt greater than normal, never sustained for day or weeks.

2—Sustained depression (1 week or more).

3—Sustained depression with vegetative symptoms (insomnia, anorexia, weight loss, loss of interest).

4—Sustained depression with vegetative symptoms and suicidal thoughts or intent.

4. Motivation/Initiative:

0—Normal.

1—Less assertive than usual; more passive.

2—Loss of initiative or disinterest in elective (non-routine) activities.

3—Loss of initiative or disinterest in day to day (routine) activities.

4—Withdrawn, complete loss of motivation.

II. Activities of Daily Living (Determine for "on/off")

5. Speech:

0—Normal.

1—Mildly affected. No difficulty being understood.

2—Moderately affected. Sometimes asked to repeat statements.

3—Severely affected. Frequently asked to repeat statements.

4—Unintelligible most of the time.

6. Salivation:

0—Normal.

1—Slight but definite excess of saliva in mouth; may have nighttime drooling.

2—Moderately excessive saliva; may have minimal drooling.

3—Marked excess of saliva with some drooling.

4—Marked drooling, requires constant tissue or handkerchief.

Table 4-1. *(continued)*

7. Swallowing:

   0—Normal.
   1—Rare choking.
   2—Occasional choking.
   3—Requires soft food.
   4—Requires NG tube or gastrotomy feeding.

8. Handwriting:

   0—Normal.
   1—Slightly slow or small.
   2—Moderately slow or small; all words are legible.
   3—Severely affected; not all words are legible.
   4—The majority of words are not legible.

9. Cutting Food and Handling Utensils:

   0—Normal.
   1—Somewhat slow and clumsy, but no help needed.
   2—Can cut most foods, although clumsy and slow; some help needed.
   3—Food must be cut by someone, but can still feed slowly.
   4—Needs to be fed.

10. Dressing:

    0—Normal.
    1—Somewhat slow, but no help needed.
    2—Occasional assistance with buttoning, getting arms in sleeves.
    3—Considerable help required, but can do some things alone.
    4—Helpless.

11. Hygiene:

    0—Normal.
    1—Somewhat slow, but no help needed.
    2—Needs help to shower or bathe, or very slow in hygienic care.
    3—Requires assistance for washing, brushing teeth, combing hair, going to bathroom.
    4—Foley catheter or other mechanical aids.

12. Turning in Bed and Adjusting Bed Clothes:

    0—Normal.
    1—Somewhat slow and clumsy, but no help needed.
    2—Can turn alone or adjust sheets, but with great difficulty.
    3—Can initiate, but not turn or adjust sheets alone.
    4—Helpless.

13. Falling (unrelated to freezing):

    0—None.
    1—Rare falling.
    2—Occasionally falls, less than once per day.
    3—Falls an average of once daily.
    4—Falls more than once daily.

Table 4-1.   *(continued)*

14. Freezing When Walking:

0—None.

1—Rare freezing when walking; may have start-hesitation.

2—Occasional freezing when walking.

3—Frequent freezing. Occasionally falls from freezing.

4—Frequent falls from freezing.

15. Walking:

0—Normal.

1—Mild difficulty. May not swing arms or may tend to drag leg.

2—Moderate difficulty, but requires little or no assistance.

3—Severe disturbance of walking, requiring assistance.

4—Cannot walk at all, even with assistance.

16. Tremor:

0—Absent.

1—Slight and infrequently present.

2—Moderate; bothersome to patient.

3—Severe; interferes with many activities.

4—Marked; interferes with most activities.

17. Sensory Complaints Related to Parkinsonism:

0—None

1—Occasionally has numbness, tingling, or mild aching.

2—Frequently has numbness, tingling, or aching; not distressing.

3—Frequent painful sensations.

4—Excruciating pain.

III. Motor Examinations:

18. Speech:

0—Normal.

1—Slight loss of expression, diction, and/or volume.

2—Monotone, slurred but understandable; moderately impaired.

3—Marked impairment, difficult to understand.

4—Unintelligible.

19. Facial Expression:

0—Normal.

1—Minimal hypomimia, could be normal "poker face."

2—Slight but definitely abnormal diminution of facial expression.

3—Moderate hypomimia; lips parted some of the time.

4—Masked or fixed facies with severe of complete loss of facial expression; lips parted 1/4 inch or more.

20. Tremor at Rest:

0—Absent.

1—Slight and infrequently present.

2—Mild in amplitude and persistent. Or moderate in amplitude, but only intermittently present.

3—Moderate in amplitude and present most of the time.

4—Marked in amplitude and present most of the time.

Table 4-1. *(continued)*

21. Action or Postural Tremor of Hands:

    0—Absent.
    1—Slight; present with action.
    2—Moderate in amplitude, present with action.
    3—Moderate in amplitude with posture holding as well as action.
    4—Marked in amplitude; interferes with feeding.

22. Rigidity: (Judged on passive movement of major joints with patient relaxed in sitting position. Cogwheeling to be ignored.)

    0—Absent.
    1—Slight or detectable only when activated by mirror or other movements.
    2—Mild to moderate.
    3—Marked, but full range of motion easily achieved.
    4—Severe, range of motion achieved with difficulty.

23. Finger Taps: (Patient taps thumb with index finger in rapid succession with widest amplitude possible, each hand separately.)

    0—Normal.
    1—Mild slowing and/or reduction in amplitude.
    2—Moderately impaired. Definite and early fatiguing. May have occasional arrests in movement.
    3—Severely impaired. Frequent hesitation in initiating movements or arrests in ongoing movement.
    4—Can barely perform the task.

24. Hand Movements: (Patient opens and closes hand in rapid succession with widest amplitude possible, each hand separately.)

    0—Normal.
    1—Mild slowing and/or reduction in amplitude.
    2—Moderately impaired. Definite and early fatiguing. May have occasional arrests in movement.
    3—Severely impaired. Frequent hesitation in initiating movements or arrests in ongoing movement.
    4—Can barely perform the task.

25. Rapid Alternating Movements of Hands: (Pronation-supination movements of hands, vertically or horizontally, with as large an amplitude as possible, both hands simultaneously.)

    0—Normal.
    1—Mild slowing and/or reduction in amplitude.
    2—Moderately impaired. Definite and early fatiguing. May have occasional arrests in movement.
    3—Severely impaired. Frequent hesitation in initiating movements or arrests in ongoing movement.
    4—Can barely perform the task.

26. Foot Agility: (Patient taps heel on ground in rapid succession, picking up entire foot. Amplitude should be about 3 inches.

    0—Normal.
    1—Mild slowing and/or reduction in amplitude.
    2—Moderately impaired. Definite and early fatiguing. May have occasional arrests in movement.
    3—Severely impaired. Frequent hesitation in initiating movements or arrests in ongoing movement.
    4—Can barely perform the task.

Table 4-1.   *(continued)*

27. Arising from Chair: (Patient attempts to arise from a straight-back wood or metal chair with arms folded across chest.)

   0—Normal.
   1—Slow; or may need more than one attempt.
   2—Pushes self up from arms of seat.
   3—Tends to fall back and may have to try more than one time, but can get up without help.
   4—Unable to arise without help.

28. Posture:

   0—Normal erect.
   1—Not quite erect, slightly stooped posture; could be normal for older person.
   2—Moderately stooped posture, definitely abnormal; can be slightly leaning to one side.
   3—Severely stooped posture with kyphosis; can be moderately leaning to one side.
   4—Marked flexion with extreme abnormality of posture.

29. Gait:

   0—Normal
   1—Walks slowly, may shuffle with short steps, but no festination or propulsion.
   2—Walks with difficulty, but requires little or no assistance; may have some festination, short steps, or propulsion.
   3—Severe disturbance of gait, requiring assistance.
   4—Cannot walk at all, even with assistance.

30. Postural Stability: (Response to sudden posterior displacement produced by pull on shoulders while patient erect with eyes open and feet slightly apart. Patient is prepared.)

   0—Normal.
   1—Retropulsion, but recovers unaided.
   2—Absence of postural response; would fall if not caught by examiner.
   3—Very unstable, tends to lose balance spontaneously.
   4—Unable to stand without assistance.

31. Body Bradykinesia and Hypokinesia: (Combining slowness, hesitancy, decreased arm swing, small amplitude, and poverty of movement in general.)

   0—None.
   1—Minimal slowness, giving movement a deliberate character; could be normal for some persons. Possibly reduced amplitude.
   2—Mild degree of slowness and poverty of movement which is definitely abnormal. Alternatively, some reduced amplitude.
   3—Moderate slowness, poverty or small amplitude of movement.
   4—Marked slowness, poverty or small amplitude of movement.

IV. Complications of Therapy (in the past week)

   A. *Dyskinesias*

32. Duration: What proportion of the waking day are dyskinesias present? (Historical information)

   0—None
   1—1–25% of day
   2—26–50% of day
   3—51–75% of day
   4—76–100% of day

Table 4-1.   *(continued)*

33. Disability: How disabling are the dyskinesias? (Historical information; may be modified by office examination.)

    0—Not disabling
    1—Mildly disabling
    2—Moderately disabling
    3—Severely disabling
    4—Completely disabling

34. Painful Dyskinesias: How painful are the dyskinesias?

    0—No painful dyskinesias
    1—Slight
    2—Moderate
    3—Severe
    4—Marked

35. Presence of Early Morning Dystonia: (Historical information)

    0—No
    1—Yes

B.   *Clinical Fluctuations*

36. Are any "off" periods predictable as to timing after a dose of medication?

    0—No
    1—Yes

37. Are any "off" periods unpredictable as to timing after a dose of medication?

    0—No
    1—Yes

38. Do any of the "off" periods come on suddenly, e.g., over a few seconds?

    0—No
    1—Yes

39. What proportion of the waking day is patient "off" on average?

    0—None
    1—1–25% of day
    2—26–50% of day
    3—51–75% of day
    4—76–100% of day

C.   *Other Complications*

40. Does the patient have anorexia, nausea, or vomiting?

    0—No
    1—Yes

41. Does the patient have any sleep disturbances, e.g., insomnia or hypersomnolence?

    0—No
    1—Yes

Table 4-1. *(continued)*

42. Does the patient have symptomatic orthostasis?

    0—No

    1—Yes

V. Modified Hoehn and Yahr Staging

Stage 0—No signs of disease.

Stage 1—Unilateral disease.

Stage 1.5—Unilateral plus axial involvement.

Stage 2—Bilateral disease, without impairment of balance.

Stage 2.5—Mild bilateral disease with recovery on pull test.

Stage 3—Mild to moderate bilateral disease; some postural instability; physically independent.

Stage 4—Severe disability; still able to walk or stand unassisted.

Stage 5—Wheelchair bound or bedridden unless aided.

VI. Modified Schwab and England Activities of Daily Living Scale

100%—Completely independent. Able to do all chores without slowness, difficulty, or impairment. Essentially normal. Unaware of any difficulty.

90%—Completely independent. Able to do all chores with some degree of slowness, difficulty, and impairment. Might take twice as long. Beginning to be aware of difficulty.

80%—Completely independent in most chores. Takes twice as long. Conscious of difficulty and slowness.

70%—Not completely independent. More difficulty with some chores. Three to four times as long in some. Must spend a large part of the day with chores.

60%—Some dependency. Can do most chores, but exceedingly slowly and with much effort. Errors; some impossible.

50%—More dependent. Help with half, slower, etc. Difficulty with everything.

40%—Very dependent. Can assist with all chores, but few alone.

30%—With effort, now and then does a few chores alone or begins alone. Much help needed.

20%—Nothing alone. Can be a slight help with some chores. Severe invalid.

10%—Total dependent, helpless. Complete invalid.

  0%—Vegetative functions such as swallowing, bladder and bowel functions are not functioning. Bedridden.

ous over three to five days of assessment. In some versions, the patient is asked to distinguish between "on" and "on with dyskinesias."

Although patient diaries can be helpful, a number of problems are encountered with diary information. The major one is that in some patients a poor correlation may be noted between their self-reports and objective assessment of parkinsonism. This may be due to several factors. First, in patients with diphasic or peak-dose dyskinesias, motor functioning may be impaired by dyskinesias and it may be difficult for patients to reliably distinguish between "on" and "off" states. An additional problem is compliance; patients may fill out diaries retrospectively, and their recall of performance may be inaccurate; our group has noted a relatively poor correlation between nursing rating of parkinsonism under controlled conditions in a research ward and patient self-reports. Although these problems represent a serious limitation in their usefulness, patient diaries may be a simple and effective way of reporting a number of symptoms, including prolonged "off" periods, levodopa dose failures, and severe dyskinesias that otherwise may prove difficult to quantify and can be useful in both patient care and drug studies.

Validation

Until recently, little effort was made to estimate the variability either in the assessments between individual raters (interrater reliability) or in the reproducibility of scales over time. In recent years, several studies have validated scales in Parkinson's disease using a variety of methods.

In a study by Richards and colleagues (Richards et al., 1994), 24 patients with Parkinson's disease were rated by two of three neurologists with experience in the use of this scale. Overall, ratings agreed between raters (the correlation coefficient, r, was 0.8), suggesting good interrater reliability. Selected items such as speech ($r = 0.29$) and facial akinesia ($r = 0.07$) were less reliable. One potential cause for the latter is that a score of 1 is assigned to patients with equivocal impairment. For example, a facial hypokinesia score of 1 reflects an appearance "possibly within normal limits for an older person," and the authors suggested that this ambiguity hinders agreement between different raters.

A second study assessed reproducibility of a modification of the Columbia rating scale by comparison with a second scale (Hely et al., 1993). From videotaped exams of 41 patients, five neurologists rated parkinsonism on both scales; some patients were also assessed at the time of video recording. A close correlation was found between the live and videotaped ratings ($r = 0.97$ and 0.95); repeated assessment of videotapes was also reproducible within an individual rater ($r = 0.86$). Although good, the concordance rates between different raters was less close; a correlation of 0.71 was found for the Columbia scale overall. Facial expression and seborrhea (an item not in the UPDRS) had poor reliability.

A third study assessed 111 patients with Parkinson's disease using the UPDRS and the Hoehn and Yahr staging system, using a single rating physician (van Hilten et al.,1994). This study found a close correlation between the two measures, but found that some items in the UPDRS dealing with activities of daily living correlated poorly; it also found that some items appeared to be redundant and could be omitted without adverse effects on the overall scale.

A fourth study validated the UPDRS by assessing 40 patients with multiple raters and by a single neurologist's assessment of 127 patients over four hospitals in different regions (Martinez-Martin et al., 1994). They found good agreement between different raters (overall $r = 0.98$). The least reliable items were facial expression, estimating the severity of sensory symptoms, and estimating overall bradykinesia. Using the Hoehn and Yahr stage as an independent variable, this study found a significant correlation ($r = 0.71$) between the UPDRS and the Hoehn and Yahr stage, also noting that six items in the UPDRS accounted for most of the correlation.

Finally, good correlation was recently reported between Hoehn and Yahr stage and the striatal uptake of 18-F-labeled deoxyglucose (Eidelberg et al., 1995).

Taken together, these studies demonstrate that motor ratings of parkinsonism have good interrater reliability and reproducibility, and reflect disease severity as measured by an independent, metabolic marker.

Administration

The UPDRS is administered by a combination of patient interview and physical examination. It can be administered by a physician, a nurse experienced in Parkinson's disease, or a trained technician. Depending on the skill of the rater and interactions with the patient, the UPDRS requires approximately 20 to 30 minutes to administer; in one of the previous studies, the UPDRS took an average of 17 minutes to administer. In practice, the motor portion of the UPDRS is the briefest to administer, particularly in mildly affected patients.

Dyskinesia

Description

A dyskinesia scale appropriate for Parkinson's disease was reported by Goetz and colleagues (1994) using a scale based on videotaped ratings of performance of motor tasks (Table 4-2). Patients are videotaped performing four tasks (walking, drinking from a cup, putting on a coat, and buttoning), and an overall severity score is assigned (0–5). The different types and most severe dyskinesias are also identified.

Validation

The description of the scale also included validation measures. Videotapes of 20 patients were reviewed on two occasions by multiple raters, including physicians and study coordinators. Agreement between raters on the severity, type of dyskinesia, and severity of dyskinesia was good for both groups of raters (r = 0.8–0.9). Ratings were also reproducible within individual raters.

Administration

The dyskinesia scale is easily performed by either a physician or a trained technician and may be used either during an interview or from a videotape. One advantage of this scale is that the rating is clearly defined relative to physical appearance and by performance of a motor task, features that reduce subjectivity.

Although it is useful, there are some limitations to this scale. First, it does not assess the distribution or amplitude of movements and may not be appropriate for some studies or uses. Second, many dyskinesias only occur at specific times of the day and may not be readily observed during office evaluations. Finally, the intensity of pain or other symptoms is not estimated on this scale. Nonetheless, the scale can be performed reasonably quickly and may be useful as an adjunct to the UPDRS.

Dystonia

Introduction

A number of scales have been developed for dystonia, including scales for assessment of generalized dystonia and torticollis. Separate scales for craniocervical dystonia and writer's cramp have also been devised (Weiner et al., 1989).

Description

A scale for generalized dystonia was devised by Fahn and Marsden in 1981, originally for use in a therapeutic trial of trihexyphenidyl. It has been subsequently used in a variety of genetic and pharmacologic studies (Burke et al., 1985). The scale rates the severity of movements affecting different body parts, each on a 5-point scale. The appearance of dystonic movements in each body part is also rated in relationship to the amount of activity required to produce the movements; while 1 represents dystonia appearing only with action, 4 is assigned to persistent dystonia at rest. Truncal and limb movements are assigned a weight of 1, and cranial or cervical movements are assigned a weight of 0.5, for a maximal total score of 120 (Table 4-3).

A similar process is used in a scale described by Tsui and colleagues for evaluation of the effects of botulinum injections for spasmodic torticollis (Tsui et al., 1986). The amplitude of rotation, tilt, and either antecollis or retrocollis are each assigned a rating of 0–3; these scores are added (maximum of 9), and this rating is then multiplied by a value assigned for either 1 for intermittent or 2 for constant movements. Second, tremulous movements are rated as either absent to severe (0–2), and multiplied by 1 (intermittent) or 2 (constant). Third, shoulder elevation is rated on a scale of 0–3. These three ratings are then added, for a maximal score of 27 (Table 4-4).

A second scale for torticollis was described by Fahn and colleagues (see Weiner et al., 1989) (Table 4-5). This scale rates turn and tilt, each on a scale from 0 to 6, and sagittal movements (antecollis or retrocollis) from 0 to 3. These are added (maximal score of 15), and multiplied by a severity factor, ranging from 0 (none) to 4 (maximal movements present 75% or more of the time), for a maximal score of 60. Other more limited scales have been used in pharmacologic trials of botulinum toxin and were able to demonstrate beneficial effects of

Table 4-2. Dyskinesia Rating Scale

Directions:

1. View the patient walk, drink from a cup, put on a coat, and button clothing.
2. Rate the severity of dyskinesias. These may include chorea, dystonia, and other dyskinetic movements in combination. Rate the patient's worst function.
3. Check which dyskinesias are observed (more than one response possible).
4. Check the type of dyskinesia that is causing the most disability on the tasks seen on the tape (only one response is permitted).

Severity rating code:

0	absent;
1	minimal severity, no interference with voluntary motor acts
2	dyskinesias may impair voluntary movements but patient is normally capable of undertaking most motor acts
3	intense interference with movement control and daily life activities are greatly limited
4	violent dyskinesias, incompatible with any normal motor task

Dyskinesias Present
(more than one choice possible)

	Chorea (C)	Dystonia (D)	Other (list)	Most disabling dyskinesia (choose one)		
Severity of worst dyskinesia observed	(0–4)	(0–4)	(0–4)	C	D	Other

Table 4-3. Dystonia Movement Scale

Region Product	Provoking Factor		Severity Factor	Weight
Eyes 0–8	0–4	X	0–4	0.5
Mouth 0–8	0–4	X	0–4	0.5
Speech/swallowing 0–16	0–4	X	0–4	1.0
Neck 0–8	0–4	X	0–4	0.5
R arm 0–16	0–4	X	0–4	1.0
L arm 0–16	0–4	X	0–4	1.0
Trunk 0–16	0–4	X	0–4	1.0
R leg 0–16	0–4	X	0–4	1.0
L leg 0–16	0–4	X	0–4	1.0

Sum: (Maximum = 120)

I. Provoking Factor

    A. General

        0—No dystonia at rest or with action

        1—Dystonia on particular action

        2—Dystonia on many actions

        3—Dystonia on action of distant part of body or intermittently at rest

        4—Dystonia present at rest

    B. Speech and swallowing

        1—Occasional, either or both

        2—Frequent either

        3—Frequent one and occasional other

        4—Frequent both

II. Severity Factors

    Eyes

        0—No dystonia present

        1—Slight. Occasional blinking

        2—Mild. Frequent blinking without prolonged spasms of eye closure

        3—Moderate. Prolonged spasms of eyelid closure, but eyes open most of the time

        4—Severe. Prolonged spasms of eyelid closure, with eyes closed at least 30% of the time

Table 4-3. *(continued)*

Mouth

0—No dystonia present
1—Slight. Occasional grimacing or other mouth movements (e.g., jaw open or clenched; tongue movements)
2—Mild. Movement present less than 50% of the time
3—Moderate dystonic movements or contractions present most of the time
4—Severe dystonic movements or contractions present most of the time

Speech and Swallowing

0—Normal
1—Slightly involved; speech easily understood or occasional choking
2—Some difficulty in understanding speech or frequent choking
3—Marked difficulty in understanding speech or inability to swallow firm foods
4—Complete or almost complete anarthria, or marked difficulty swallowing soft foods and liquids

Neck

0—No dystonia present
1—Slight. Occasional pulling
2—Obvious torticollis, but mild
3—Moderate pulling
4—Extreme pulling

Arm

0—No dystonia present
1—Slight dystonia. Clinically insignificant
2—Mild. Obvious dystonia, but not disabling
3—Moderate. Able to grasp, with some manual function
4—Severe. No useful grasp

Trunk

0—No dystonia present
1—Slight bending, clinically insignificant
2—Definite bending, but not interfering with standing or walking
3—Moderate bending, interfering with standing or walking
4—Extreme bending of trunk preventing standing or walking

Leg

0—No dystonia present
1—Slight dystonia, but not causing impairment; clinically insignificant
2—Mild dystonia. Walks briskly and unaided
3—Moderate dystonia. Severely impaired walking or requires assistance
4—Severe. Unable to stand or walk on involved leg

2. Disability Scale

Function	Score
Speech	0–4
Writing	0–4
Feeding	0–4
Eating	0–4
Hygiene	0–4
Dressing	0–4
Walking	0–6

Sum: (Maximum = 30)

Table 4-3.   *(continued)*

Disability Scale

A. *Speech*

   0—Normal
   1—Slightly involved; easily understood
   2—Some difficulty in understanding
   3—Marked difficulty in understanding
   4—Complete or almost complete anarthria

B. *Handwriting (tremor or dystonia)*

   0—Normal
   1—Slight difficulty; legible
   2—Almost illegible
   3—Illegible
   4—Unable to grasp to maintain hold on pen

C. *Feeding*

   0—Normal
   1—Uses "tricks"; independent
   2—Can feed, but not cut
   3—Finger food only
   4—Completely dependent

D. *Eating/swallowing*

   0—Normal
   1—Occasional choking
   2—Chokes frequently; difficulty swallowing
   3—Unable to swallow firm foods
   4—Marked difficulty swallowing soft foods and liquids

E. *Hygiene*

   0—Normal
   1—Clumsy; independent
   2—Needs help with some activities
   3—Needs help with most activities
   4—Needs help with all activities

F. *Dressing*

   0—Normal
   1—Clumsy, independent
   2—Needs help with some activities
   3—Needs help with most activities
   4—Helpless

G. *Walking*

   0—Normal
   1—Slightly abnormal; hardly noticeable
   2—Moderately abnormal; obvious to naive observer
   3—Considerably abnormal
   4—Needs assistance to walk
   6—Wheelchair-bound

Table 4-4. Spasmodic Torticollis Rating Scale*

A. *Turn/Tilt + Sagittal*

Rate degrees of turn (chin to side of turn) plus degrees of tilt (ear down toward shoulder)

    0—0°
    1—1–15°
    2—15–30°
    3—30–45°
    4—45–60°
    5—60–75°
    6—75–90

Add rating for sagittal deviation (antecollis/retrocollis)

    0—Absent
    1—Mild
    2—Moderate
    3—Severe

	Left	*Right*
Turn		
Tilt		
Sagittal		
Total		

B. *Severity factor*

    0—None
    1—Occasional deviation only
    2—Mild. Deviation present < 50% of time
    3—Moderate. Excursions to maximal deviation present 50–75% of time

OR

    Deviation present most of the time but excursions largely submaximal

        4—Severe. Excursions to maximal deviation present 75–100% of time

Score (A) Turn/Tilt + Sagittal X (B) Severity Factor = Total Score
    Add rating for dystonia elsewhere (Fahn-Marsden Scale)
    Also record duration able to hold head in fixed central position; taken to first twitch of movement in direction of torticollis: maximum = 60 sec (mean of two trials).

* Some torticollis rating scales include a separate score for shoulder elevation.

Table 4-5.   Torticollis Severity Scale

(A)   Amplitude of sustained movements:

    1.   Rotation: 0 = absent, 1= < 15°, 2 = 15–30°, 3 = > 30°

    2.   Tilt: 0 = absent, 1 = < 15°, 2 = 15–30°, 3 = > 30°

    3.   Anterograde/retrograde: 0 = absent, 1 = mild, 2 = moderate, 3 = severe

Combined A score—

(B)   Duration of sustained movements: 1 = intermittent, 2 = constant

(C)   Shoulder elevation: 0 = absent, 1 = mild and intermittent, 2 = mild and constant or severe and intermittent, 3 = severe and constant

(D)   Tremor severity: 1 = mild, 2 = severe

Duration:

1 = occasional, 2 = continuous

Severity + duration = D score

Total score = (A + B) + C + D

injections (Jankovic et al., 1990). More recently, other composite scales are under development for the comprehensive assessment of patient outcomes with cervical dystonia. Like the UPDRS in Parkinson's disease, these newer scales include patient and physician assessment of functional disability, pain, and interference with daily activities.

Validation

The scale for evaluation of primary torsion dystonia has been validated by assessment of videotapes. In this evaluation (Burke et al., 1985), ten patients were rated on a simple global evaluation scale (0–5) and by the Dystonia Movement Scale; additionally, patients were rated twice by two examiners. A close correlation ($r = 0.9$) was found in ratings between different raters, and an almost 100% correlation between repeated ratings, demonstrating both good interrater and intrarater reliability; both trained and untrained raters performed consistently.

Administration

The scales for both generalized dystonia and torticollis can be administered by either a physician or a technician trained in evaluation and recognition of dystonia. Both scales are brief and quick to administer.

Special Considerations

One feature of dystonia is that in some patients a variety of sensory "tricks" (*geste antagoniste)*, such as touching the chin or talking, may partially or completely suppress the dystonic movements, and patients should be instructed to not use such maneuvers while they are being evaluated. Other patients with task-specific dystonias may only exhibit involuntary movements under specific situations, such as writing; such triggering factors should be used for rating these patients.

Tourette's Syndrome

Introduction

Among the movement disorders, tic disorders can be the most difficult to evaluate and assess quantitatively. Patients may exhibit a large variety of simple and complex motor and phonic tics that may appear and disappear over time.

Many patients also experience psychological symptoms such as obsessions, and many complex motor tics may blend into compulsive behaviors and make distinction between tics and compulsions arbitrary.

Several scales have been devised in an effort to quantify tics and associated behaviors. These include rating instruments based on a symptom checklist, an objective tic rating, or both. One symptom checklist that has been extensively used is the Tourette Syndrome Symptom List (TSSL), which was developed at Yale to assist parents in assessing tic behaviors (Cohen et al., 1984); similar scales have been described by other investigators, ranging from simple, such as the Hopkins Motor/Vocal Tic Scale (see Walkup et al., 1992), to complex, such as the Tourette's Syndrome Global Scale (TSGS).

Objective tic ratings are included in several scales. A scale described by Goetz and colleagues in 1987 is based on tic counts from a short videotaped protocol. Other tic ratings are included in composite scales; these include the Tourette's Syndrome Global Scale (TSGS) described by Harcherik and colleagues in 1984 (Harcherik et al., 1984) and the Shapiro TS Severity Scale (TSSS) (Leckman et al., 1988). Many of these investigators also participated on a committee to develop a standardized scale, the Unified Tic Rating Scale, which is under development.

Description

The Tourette's Syndrome Global Scale (TSGS) (Table 4-6) is a composite scale, roughly divided into two sections. The first section rates the frequency of simple motor tics, complex motor tics, simple phonic tics, and complex phonic tics on a scale of 1–5 (1 is 1 or fewer tics in 5 minutes, 5 is virtually uncountable), and the degree of disruption is graded on a scale of 1–5 (1 is easy to camouflage, 5 is disruptive to the point of making it impossible to otherwise function); each of these is multiplied, and is added and averaged. A second section uses a simple 0–25 scale for behavior, motor restlessness, school/learning or work/occupational problems, and these three items are also averaged; they are then weighted for a composite total score.

A second scale is described by Goetz and colleagues and utilizes videotape ratings. The patient is recorded for two minutes, seated at rest, without the examiner present; segments taped at near and at far are obtained. They are scored on a 5-point motor tic and vocal tic scale, identifying tics in 11

Table 4-6. Tourette's Syndrome Global Scale (TSGS)

Name _____   Date_____   Rater_____

Code for Frequency	*Frequency (F)*	*Disruption (D)*
1 = 1 or less in 5 min		
2 = 1 in 2–4.9 min		
3 = from 1 in 1.9 min to 4 in 1 min		
4 = 5 or more in 1 min		
5 = virtually uncountable		
SIMPLE MOTOR (SM): Nonpurposeful tics, jerks and/or movements	0 1 2 3 4 5	1 2 3 4 5 FXD =
COMPLEX MOTOR (CM): Purposeful, thoughtful actions (systematic actions), rituals, touching self, others, or objects	0 1 2 3 4 5	1 2 3 4 5 FXD =
SIMPLE PHONIC (SP): Nonpurposeful noises, throat clearing, coughing	0 1 2 3 4 5	1 2 3 4 5 FXD =
COMPLEX PHONIC (CP): Purposeful, insults, coprolalia, words, distinguishable speech	0 1 2 3 4 5	1 2 3 4 5 FXD =

BEHAVIOR (B) (conduct)

0	No problem
5	Subtle problems normal peer, school, and family relations
10	Some problems, at least one relationship area impaired
15	Clear impairment in more than one area
20	Serious impairment, affects all areas
25	Unacceptable social behavior, constant supervision

SCHOOL AND LEARNING PROBLEMS

0	No problem
5	Low grades
10	Should be or in some special classes, or repeated
15	All special classes
20	Special school
25	Unable to remain in school, homebound

MOTOR RESTLESSNESS (MR)

0	Normal movement
5	Adventitial movements, visible, no problem

WORK AND OCCUPATION PROBLEMS

0	No problem
5	Stable job, some difficulty

Table 4-6.   *(continued)*

10	Increased motor restlessness, clearly visible, some problem	10	Serious problems
15	Clear motor restlessness, moderate problem	15	Lost lots of jobs
20	Mostly in motion but occasionally stops, impaired functioning	20	Almost never employed
25	Nonstop motion, clearly cannot function	25	Unemployed

((SM + CM)/2) = ((SP + CP)/2) + ((B + MR + school or work problems) x 2/3) = Global Score

Severity Rating Scales

Motor tics

  0—Absent

  1—Minimal; could be normal

  2—Mild; limited to a single muscle group

  3—Moderate; limited to a single body part

  4—Severe; involving more than one body part

  5—Extreme; complex behavior

Vocalizations

  0—Absent

  1—Minimal; could be normal

  2—Mild; single words or sounds, separated by at least one breath or 4 seconds.

  3—Moderate; words or sounds repeated two or three times in series or single obscenities separated by at least one breath or 4 seconds

  4—Severe; words or sounds repeated four or more times in series or obscenities repeated two or three times in series

  5—Extreme; obscenities repeated four or more times in series

different body parts. Tics are counted for one minute.

Validation

Twenty patients with Tourette's syndrome were compared using the TSGS, TSSS, the Hopkins Motor/Vocal Scale, the Clinical Global Impression (reviewed in Leckman et al., 1988), and the Child Behavior Checklist, using three raters and an hour-long, structured interview. This study found excellent interrater reliability for all scales, as well as good reliability between tests. The study found that the ratings of tics did not correlate with the presence of ADHD or obsessive-compulsive symptoms (Walkup et al.,1992). Similar results were obtained in a separate study of the TSGS (see Leckman et al., 1988).

The videotape protocol was also validated (Goetz et al., 1987). Thirty patients were evaluated at 3-week intervals while taking placebo tablets as part of a controlled trial of clonidine. The scale was found to be highly reliable between raters (Pearson's ranged from $r = 0.8$ to $r = 0.98$ for evaluation of motor and vocal tic frequency and severity, and $r = 0.6$ for tic distribution). A moderate agreement ($r = 0.5–0.6$) was found following repeated evaluations, suggesting some waxing and waning of tic severity. This study also found that although rating of motor tic severity and frequency correlated with each other closely ($r = 0.8$), as did vocal tics ($r = 0.9$), there was a poor correlation between these two different tic types ($r = 0.4$), suggesting that a single summary measure is inadequate. A second portion of the study compared the tic counts to the TSGS in 12 patients and found a moderate correlation (motor tics, $r = 0.5$, vocal tics, $r = 0.6$). Finally, 9 patients given neuroleptics for tics demonstrated a significant improvement in videotape tic counts.

Administration

Although portions of these scales may be administered by a trained technician, assessment and distinction between tics and other movements or sounds is difficult and requires special expertise and training; it is best performed by a physician or an experienced research nurse. Many items are rated by answers to structured interviews, also requiring internal consistency in quantifying answers.

A quiet room is required for video recording; if more than one assessment is obtained, it is best to standardize the conditions under which video recordings are obtained.

Time to Administer

Unlike other movement disorders, the assessment of Tourette's syndrome is time-consuming. Even the simpler scales may take 30 to 45 minutes to administer, and evaluation by the Unified Rating Scale may take over an hour. This scale also requires special training; many items are obtained by structured interview, and interpretation of answers to questions by patient, spouse, or parents at times may be subjective.

Although the previously described scales have been validated and appear to be integrally reliable and consistent, the evaluation of Tourette's syndrome is difficult and is affected by a variety of factors. These include waxing and waning of signs, a poor correlation between symptoms and motor signs, and a poor correlation between psychological and physical symptoms, and the overall clinical utility of ratings in a clinic setting is uncertain. If a rating is used, a simple rating of motor and vocal tic frequency and severity, such as the TSGS, is more quickly performed and therefore may be of greater practical utility than more comprehensive scales.

Tardive Dyskinesia

A number of scales have been developed to evaluate extrapyramidal side effects seen in patients treated with dopaminergic antagonists. Of these, the Abnormal Involuntary Movement Scale (AIMS), described in the 1970s, is the most widely used and has been used to assess choreic movements in other disorders, including Parkinson's and Huntington's diseases (Guy, 1976). A second scale, the St. Hans Rating Scale for extrapyramidal syndromes, was also developed in the 1970s and has been widely applied (Gerlach et al., 1993).

Description

The Abnormal Involuntary Movement Scale (AIMS) (Table 4-7) consists of rating the severity of movements in 7 regions, each on a 5-point scale, ranging from 0 = none to 4 = severe, and a separate rating of the overall severity of the abnormal movements, judged on the amplitude of movements, incapacitation, and patient awareness of movements. Specific postures and positions, including

Table 4-7. Abnormal Involuntary Movement Scale (AIMS)

Definitions of 0–4 Scale

Rate highest severity observed. Rate movements that occur upon activation one less than those observed spontaneously. Use the following scale:

0 = None
1 = Minimal
2 = Mild
3 = Moderate
4 = Severe

Movement Ratings

Muscles of Facial Expression

Examples: Movements of forehead, eyebrows, periorbital area, cheeks; include frowning, blinking, smiling, grimacing.

Lips and Periorbital Area

Examples: Puckering, pouting, smacking.

Jaw

Examples: Biting, clenching, chewing, mouth opening, lateral movement.

Tongue

Examples: Rate only increase in movements, both in and out of mouth, NOT inability to sustain movement.

Upper Extremities

Include choreic movements (i.e., rapid, objectively, purposeless, irregular, spontaneous), athetoid movements (i.e., slow, irregular, complex, serpentine). Do NOT include tremor (i.e., repetitive, regular, rhythmic).

Lower Extremities

Examples: Lateral knee movement, foot tapping, heel dropping, foot squirming, inversion and eversion of foot.

Trunk

Examples: Rocking, twisting, squirming, pelvic gyrations.

Global Judgment

Patient's Awareness of Abnormal Movements

0 = None
1 = Aware, no distress
2 = Aware, mild distress
3 = Aware, moderate distress
4 = Aware, severe distress

Either before or after completing the examination procedure, observe the patient unobtrusively at rest (e.g., in waiting room). The chair to be used in this examination should be a hard, firm one without arms.

1. Ask patient whether there is anything in his/her mouth (i.e., gum, candy, etc.) and if there is to remove it.
2. Ask patient about the current condition of his/her teeth. Ask patient if he/she wears dentures.
3. Ask patient whether he/she notices any movements in mouth, face, hands, or feet. If yes, ask to describe and to what extent they currently bother patient or interfere with his/her activities.

Table 4-7.   *(continued)*

4. Have patient sit in chair with hands on knees, legs slightly apart, and feet flat on floor. (Look at entire body for movements while in this position.)

5. Ask patient to sit with hands hanging unsupported. If male, between legs, and if female and wearing a dress, hanging over knees. (Observe hands and other body areas.)

6. Ask patient to open mouth. (Observe tongue at rest within mouth.) Do this twice.

7. Ask patient to protrude tongue. (Observe similarities of tongue movement.) Do this twice.

8. Ask patient to tap thumb with each finger, as rapidly as possible for 10–15 seconds; separately with right hand, then with left hand. (Observe facial and leg movements.)

9. Flex and extend patient's left and right arm (one at a time).

10. Ask patient to stand up. (Observe in profile. Observe all body parts again, hips included.)

11. Ask patient to extend both arms outstretched in front with palms down. (Observe trunk, legs, and mouth.)

12. Have patient walk a few paces, turn and walk back to chair. (Observe hands and gait.) Do this twice.

Scoring System Instructions

Complete examination procedure before making ratings.

Movement ratings: Rate highest severity noted. Rate movements that occur upon activation one less than those observed spontaneously.

Code: 0 = none; 1 = minimal may be extreme normal; 2 = mild; 3 = moderate; 4 = severe
(Circle one)

FACIAL AND ORAL MOVEMENTS

1.	Muscles of facial expression, e.g., movements of forehead, eyebrows, periorbital area, cheeks; include frowning, blinking, smiling, grimacing	0	1	2	3	4
2.	Lips and periorbital area, e.g., puckering, pouting, smacking	0	1	2	3	4
3.	Jaw, e.g., biting, clenching, chewing, mouth opening, lateral movement	0	1	2	3	4
4.	Tongue. Rate only increase in movement both in and out of mouth, *not* inability to sustain movement	0	1	2	3	4

EXTREMITY MOVEMENTS

5.	Upper (arms, wrist, hands, fingers). Include choreic movements (i.e., rapid, objectively, purposeless, irregular, spontaneous), athetoid movements (slow, irregular, complex, serpentine). Do *not* include tremor (i.e., repetitive, regular, rhythmic)	0	1	2	3	4
6.	Lower (legs, knees, ankles, toes), e.g., lateral knee movement, foot tapping, heel dropping, foot squirming, inversion and eversion of foot	0	1	2	3	4

Table 4-7.   *(continued)*

TRUNK MOVEMENTS					
7. Neck, shoulders, hips, e.g., rocking, twisting, squirming, pelvic gyrations	0	1	2	3	4
GLOBAL JUDGEMENTS					
8. Severity of abnormal movements	0	1	2	3	4
9. Incapacitation due to abnormal movements					
10. Patient's awareness of abnormal movements					
DENTAL STATUS					
11. Current problems with teeth and/or dentures	No 0 Yes 1				
12. Does patient usually wear dentures?	No 0 Yes 1				

sitting in the chair, opening the mouth, tapping the thumb against each finger, holding the hands outstretched, and standing and walking, are included. Dental status is also rated, as the presence or absence of problems with teeth or dentures (this latter assessment is included because edentulous individuals may sometimes exhibit involuntary movements without exposure to drugs).

Validation

Thirty-three patients were rated by two experienced and two inexperienced psychiatrists on at least two occasions. Significant correlations of moderate degree were found between raters (r ranged from 0.5 to 0.8, depending on body region). In general, the experienced raters were more consistent over time and had greater agreement (Lane et al., 1985).

A second study compared the AIMS to the St. Hans Rating Scale for the assessment of tardive dyskinesia (Gerlach et al., 1993). In this study, 30 patients were evaluated three times, once from a live exam, and two additional times from review of a videotape from the same examination. Seven raters (2 experienced, 2 with less experience, 3 naive) performed the examinations and ratings. Intrarater reliability was generally good; correlations ranged from 0.7 to 0.9 and did not differ between experienced and inexperienced raters. Interrater reliability also was good, with the experienced raters showing slightly greater agreement. There was good agreement between the two scales

Administration

The AIMS is simple to administer, taking 10 minutes or less to perform. It may be performed by either a physician or a nurse trained in evaluation of involuntary movements

Summary

A number of scales for the assessment of movement disorders are presented in this chapter. Most have been demonstrated to be reasonably reproducible and to correlate well with each other. In the case of the UPDRS, a good correlation has been seen between the extent of loss of dopaminergic nerve terminals and the motor score, suggesting that for this scale (and presumably others), the disease severity score does reflect the pathological abnormalities seen in the disease.

Practical issues, such as the ease of use and availability of the scale, should be emphasized in selecting a scale. For patient care, these scales sometimes add little and their routine use should not be viewed as mandatory; for example, the appearance of tics may not correlate well with the patient's perception of interference with daily activities, and quantification of these diseases may not be helpful. However, quantitative assessment of other diseases, such as Parkinson's disease or dystonia, may allow comparison of different patients and may reveal trends in symptom patterns which may otherwise not be apparent. For Parkinson's disease, the motor section of the UPDRS is quickly performed, and its inclusion in a patient clinic visit may be useful. Similarly, one of the brief assessments of dystonia may be useful in a variety of settings; assessment of torticollis by a brief scale, for example, may aid not only in the overall assessment of disease severity but also in the selection of different muscles for injection

References

Burke RE, Fahn S, Marsden CD, Bressman SB, Moskowitz C, Friedman J. Validity and reliability of a rating scale for the primary torsion dystonias. *Neurology* 1985;35:73–77.

Canter CJ, de la Torre R, Mier M. A method of evaluating disability in patients with Parkinson's disease. *J Nerv Ment Dis* 1961;133:143–47.

Cohen DJ, Leckman JF, Shaywitz BA. The Tourette syndrome and other tics. In: Shaffer D, Ehrhardt AA, Greenwill L (eds.). *The clinical guide to child psychiatry.* New York: Free Press, 1984,

Eidelberg D, Moeller JR, Ishikawa T, et al. Assessment of disease severity in parkinsonism with fluorine-18-fluorodeoxyglucose and PET. *J Nucl Med* 1995;36:378–83.

Fahn S, Elton RL, Members of the UPDRS Development Committee. In: Fahn S, Marsden CD, Calne DB, Goldstein M (eds.). *Recent developments in Parkinson's disease, Vol. 2.* Florham Park, NJ: Macmillan Health Care Information, 1987:153–64.

Gerlach J, Korsgaard S, Clemmensen P, et al. The St. Hans rating scale for extrapyramidal syndromes: reliability and validity. *Acta Psychiatr Scand* 1993;87:244–52.

Goetz CG, Stebbins GT, Shale HM, et al. Utility of an objective dyskinesia rating scale for Parkinson's disease: inter- and intrarater reliability assessment. *Mov Disord* 1994;9:390–94.

Goetz CG, Tanner CM, Wilson RS, Shannon KM. A rating scale for Gilles de la Tourette's syndrome: description, reliability, and validity data. *Neurology* 1987;37:1542–44.

Guy, W. *ECDEU assessment manual for psychopharmacology*. DHEW publication, No. 76–338. Washington, DC: U.S. Government Printing Office, 1976:534–37.

Harcherik DF, Leckman JF, Detlor J, Cohen DJ. A new instrument for clinical studies of Tourette's syndrome. *J Am Acad Child Adolesc Psychiatry* 1984;23:153–60.

Hely MA, Chey T, Wilson A, Williamson PM, O'Sullivan DJ, Rail D, Morris JGL. Reliability of the Columbia scale for assessing signs of Parkinson's disease. *Mov Disord* 1993;8:466–72.

Hoehn MM, Yahr MD. Parkinsonism: onset, progression, and mortality. *Neurology* 1967;17:427–42.

Jankovic J, Schwartz K. Botulinum toxin injections for cervical dystonia. *Neurology* 1990;40:277–80.

Lane RD, Glazer WM, Hansen TE, Berman WH, Kramer SI. Assessment of tardive dyskinesia using the abnormal involuntary movement scale. *J Nerv Ment Dis* 1985;173:353–57.

Langston JW, Widner H, Goetz CG, Brooks D, Fahn S, Freeman T, Watts R. Core Assessment Program for Intracerebral Transplantations (CAPIT). *Mov Disord* 1992;7:2–13.

Leckman JF, Towbin KE, Ort SI, Cohen DJ. Clinical assessment of tic disorder severity. In: Cohen DJ, Bruun RD, Leckman JF (eds.). *Tourette's syndrome and tic disorders*. New York: John Wiley, 1988:55–78.

Martinez-Martin P. Rating scales in Parkinson's disease. In: Jankovic J, Tolosa E (eds.). *Parkinson's disease and movement disorders*. Baltimore: Williams & Wilkins, 1993:281–92.

Martinez-Martin P, Gil-Nagel A, Gracia LM, Gomez JB, Martinez-Sarries J, Bermejo F, The Cooperative Multicentric Group. Unified Parkinson's Disease Rating Scale characteristics and structure. *Mov Disord* 1994;9:76–83.

Richards M, Marder K, Cote L, Mayeux R. Interrater reliability of the Unified Parkinson's Disease Rating Scale Motor Examination. *Mov Disord* 1994;9:89–91.

Schwab RS. Progression and prognosis in Parkinson's disease. *J Nerv Ment Dis* 1960;130:556–66.

Tsui JK, Calne DB. Botulinum toxin in cervical dystonia. *Adv Neurol* 1988;49:473–78.

Tsui JK, Eisen A, Mak E, Carruthers J, Scott AB, Calne DB. Double-blind study of botulinum toxin in spasmodic torticollis. *Lancet* 1986;2:245–47.

van Hilten JJ, van der Zwan AD, Zwinderman AH, Roos RAC. Rating impairment and disability in Parkinson's disease: evaluation of the Unified Parkinson's Disease Rating Scale. *Mov Disord* 1994;9:84–88.

Walkup JT, Rosenberg LA, Brown J, Singer HS. The validity of instruments measuring tic severity in Tourette's syndrome. *J Am Acad Child Adolesc Psychiatry* 1992;30:472–77.

Webster DD. Critical analysis of the disability in Parkinson's disease. *Mod Treatment* 1968;5:257–282.

Weiner WJ, Lang, AE. *Movement disorders: a comprehensive survey*. Mount Kisco, NY: Futura, 1989.

Yahr MD, Duvoisin RC, Schear MJ, Barrett RE, Hoehn MM. Treatment of parkinsonism with levodopa. *Arch Neurol* 1969;21:343–54.

5 Multiple Sclerosis
and Demyelinating
Diseases

Robert M. Herndon, M.D.,
and Donald Goodkin, M.D.

Diagnostic Criteria for Multiple Sclerosis

Accurate diagnosis is critical for understanding the natural history of multiple sclerosis (MS) and for interpreting the results of clinical trials of promising therapies. Unfortunately, despite the newer imaging techniques and the availability of more sensitive and reliable spinal fluid and evoked potential testing, misdiagnosis remains a problem that must be dealt with in clinical trials (Rudick et al., 1986; Herndon, 1994). The earliest known diagnostic criteria for MS, intended for use in clinical practice, were proposed by Charcot (1877). In the 1950s, it became evident that better diagnostic criteria were needed for clinical trials and a committee chaired by Dr. George Schumacher was convened to develop the new criteria. Subsequently, as new diagnostic tools developed, it became necessary to revise these criteria and Dr. Charles Poser convened a panel for this purpose.

Schumacher Committee Criteria

The Schumacher Committee diagnostic criteria (Table 5-1) were designed to provide a clear defini-

tion of clinically definite multiple sclerosis for use in evaluating patients for clinical trials using agreed upon diagnostic criteria. The purpose was, in so far as possible, to establish uniform diagnostic criteria for individuals to be included in therapeutic trials.

Validation

In the only available validation study of the Schumacher Criteria, neuropathological examination of 518 consecutive patients with clinically definite MS revealed a correct diagnosis in 485 cases (94%) (Engell, 1988). The same authors were only able to obtain postmortem confirmation of MS in 66% of 33 patients with clinically probable MS.

Administration

The evaluation of the patient requires a competent clinical neurologist and depends on a mixture of history and neurologic findings obtained in a standard neurologic evaluation.

Time to Administer

It usually requires 45 to 60 minutes to obtain a history and examination adequate to see if a patient meets these criteria. For established patients, one

Table 5-1. Schumacher Committee Criteria

The following six criteria are deemed essential to characterize the disease state as clinically "definite multiple sclerosis" (Schumacher et al., 1965).

a. There must be objective abnormalities on neurologic examinations attributable to dysfunction of the central nervous system. Symptoms alone, no matter how suggestive, cannot be accepted as diagnostic of multiple sclerosis.

b. On neurologic examination or by history there must be evidence of involvement of two or more separate parts of the central nervous system.

c. The objective neurologic evidence of central nervous system disease must reflect predominantly white matter involvement, i.e., fiber tract damage. Thus, signs must consist mainly of optic nerve, cerebral subcortical, corticobulbar, corticospinal, medial longitudinal fasciculus, cerebellar subcortical, spinocerebellar, and long sensory tract (especially posterior column dysfunction. More than a minor proportion of signs of lower motor neuron (brainstem, spinal nuclear gray matter, or peripheral nerve) dysfunction will disqualify a subject as having multiple sclerosis for purposes of an experimental trial of therapy.

d. The involvement of the neuraxis must have occurred temporally in one or the other of the following patterns:

  (1) In two or more episodes of worsening, separated by a period of one month or more, each episode lasting at least 24 hours.

  (2) Slow or step-wise progression of signs and symptoms, over a period of at least six months. These arbitrary time limits are necessary to exclude: (1) fluctuation or transitory neurologic impairment due to other causes (e.g., vascular); and (2) acute disseminated neurologic disease which is short-lived and non-recurrent (such as encephalomyelitis).

e. The ages of the patient at the onset of the disease must fall within the range of 10 to 50 years, inclusive.

f. The patient's signs and symptoms cannot be explained better by some other disease process, a decision which must be made by a physician competent in clinical neurology.

can usually determine whether or not an individual meets criteria from the record in a few minutes.

Special Considerations

The Schumacher Criteria are mainly of historical interest but were widely used prior to publication of the Washington Conference Criteria in 1983. They may still have limited use in situations in which one is evaluating a diagnostic test such as MRI against another test, particularly if spinal fluid results are not available in the cohort.

Advantages

The criteria are strictly clinical with no requirement for MRI or CSF examination and therefore can be used in areas with limited medical resources.

Disadvantages

The Schumacher Committee Criteria have been superseded for most purposes by the Washington Conference (Poser) Criteria.

Summary

Once useful and widely used formal diagnostic criteria, now of mainly historical interest.

Washington Conference (Poser) Criteria

Description

These criteria, known as the Washington Conference or Poser Criteria (Table 5-2), are the current standard diagnostic criteria for inclusion in MS clinical trials. They include clinical, paraclinical (i.e., magnetic resonance imaging, evoked responses), and laboratory tests (e.g., measures of intrathecal cerebrospinal fluid immunoglobulin G production) to minimize diagnostic errors. To a considerable extent, they are an expansion and refinement of the Schumacher Criteria, incorporating the newer laboratory and imaging tests. Using these criteria, only cases with clinically definite MS or laboratory supported definite MS should be included in clinical trials.

Validation

The criteria have obvious face validity since they formalize common clinical diagnostic criteria. No clinico-pathoanatomical validation study of

these criteria has been reported. It should be recognized that the Washington Conference Criteria, in contrast to the Schumacher Criteria, will exclude many cases that are progressive from onset or cases of progressive myelopathy with normal spinal fluid and no paraclinical evidence of disease outside the spinal cord.

Administration

Determination of which criteria an individual meets is accomplished by the neurologist's history and examination or chart review in conjunction with review of any diagnostic procedures that have been carried out.

Time to Administer

For new patients, 45 to 60 minutes of history, neurologic exam, and record review. For established patients, it may require as little as 5 to 10 minutes to determine which diagnostic level the individual meets.

Advantages

The Washington Conference or Poser Criteria are useful criteria that utilize modern imaging and modern laboratory testing to add to the certainty of diagnosis. They have become the standard criteria used to establish diagnosis for clinical trials.

Disadvantages

These criteria will exclude many cases of MS that are progressive from onset and cases of progressive myelopathy with normal spinal fluid and no paraclinical evidence of disease outside the spinal cord. While some investigators believe that these cases represent a different disease process and should be treated separately, other investigators consider it to be simply a different disease pattern.

Summary

The Washington Conference or Poser Criteria are the *de facto* standard for MS diagnosis for clinical trials. They are relatively straightforward and will result in inclusion of very few incorrectly diagnosed patients while excluding only a small number who do have the disease. In general, except in special purpose trials, only clinically or laboratory definite patients are suitable for inclusion in a clinical trial.

Table 5-2. Washington Conference Criteria

Category	Clinical Attacks	Clinical Evidence	Paraclinical Evidence	CSF OB/Ig
Clinically definite				
CDMS A1	2	2		
CDMS A2	2	1 and	1	
Laboratory supported definite				
LSDMS B1	2	1 or	1	+
LSDMS B2	1	2		+
LSDMS B3	1	1 and	1	+
Clinically probable				
CPMS C1	2	1		
CPMS C2	1	2		
CPMS C3	1	1 and	1	
Laboratory supported probable				
LSPMS D1	2			+

Definitions related to the criteria:

Attack (bout, episode, exacerbation): The occurrence of a symptom or symptoms of neurological dysfunction, with or without objective confirmation, lasting more than 24 hours.

Historical information: The description of symptoms by the patient.

Clinical evidence of a lesion: Signs of neurologic dysfunction demonstrable by neurologic examination. This includes signs no longer present if they were previously found on examination by a competent examiner.

Paraclinical evidence of a lesion: This includes such items as high signal areas on MRI, abnormal evoked responses, and other tests that establish the presence of a lesion in the central nervous system.

Separate lesions: Separate signs or symptoms that cannot be explained on the basis of a single lesion.

Laboratory Support: For purposes of these criteria includes evidence of elevated IgG synthesis on CSF examination and oligoclonal bands.

Rating Scales to Measure the Consequences of MS-Related Pathology

The consequences of MS-related pathology are classified by the World Health Organization as *impairment, disability,* and *handicap.* Impairment is caused by underlying pathology that produces abnormalities on the neurologic examination. The earliest published attempts to develop rating scales for MS-related impairment appear to be those of Arkin et al. (1950) and Alexander (1951). The Kurtzke Disability Status Scale (DSS), published in 1955, appears to be an outgrowth of these earlier scales. The DSS was revised and expanded as the Expanded Disability Status Scale (EDSS) in 1983. Although other scales, including the Scripps Neurologic Rating Scale (NRS) (Sipe et al., 1984), the Troiano Scale (TS) (Cook et al., 1986), Quantitative Examination of Neurological Function (QENF) (Syndulko et al., 1983), and the Hauser Ambulation Index (Hauser et al., 1983), have been proposed as alternative approaches to measure impairment, the EDSS is currently the only widely accepted standard for providing validated measures of impairment in the context of MS clinical research.

Disability reflects the impact of neurologic impairment on activities of daily living. Although measures focused on disability are not widely used in the context of MS clinical trials, disability resulting from MS-related impairment may be measured by the Incapacity Status Scale (ISS) (Haber & LaRocca, 1985) or the Functional Independence Measure (FIM) (Granger et al., 1986).

Handicaps are the vocational or social role limitations resulting from the interaction between disability and the environment. Although measures focused on handicap are not widely used in the context of MS clinical trials, handicap may be measured by the Environmental Status Scale (ESS) or the Minimal Record of Disability (MRD) (Haber & LaRocca, 1985) or by various patient-based reports of quality of life. These are discussed further in Chapter 10.

In this chapter we first review the characteristics of an ideal outcome measure for use in MS clinical trials. We critically review the EDSS, the standard measure of impairment in MS clinical trials, to see how it compares to an ideal outcome measure. We then briefly review other measures of impair-

ment, disability, and handicap, including the NRS, TS, AI, quantified tests of upper extremity function, ISS, FIM, and ESS. Proposed measures of quality of life are currently not validated or generally accepted for use in MS clinical trials and are therefore beyond the scope of this chapter.

Measuring change in clinical status in patients with MS is problematic because clinical manifestations vary widely between patients and within patients. The course of the disease may be characterized by unpredictable recurring attacks of symptoms that may not be accompanied by neurologic impairment, gradual accumulation of neurologic disability, or periods of clinical stability. Optimally, any instrument designed to assess change in clinical status should (1) reflect disease-specific activity; (2) be sensitive to the full range of clinically significant changes that may occur over a short time interval; (3) possess high intra- and interrater reliability; (4) be quantitative with defined distance between points of the scale; (5) be easy to administer; (6) be acceptable to patients and those administering the instruments; and (7) be cost-effective.

Instruments to Measure Neurologic Impairment

The Expanded Disability Status Scale (EDSS)

Although it is the most widely accepted measure of neurologic impairment in MS clinical trials, the EDSS (Table 5-3) fails to satisfy several characteristics of an ideal outcome measure reviewed by Goodkin (1993). There are at least five categories of difficulty with the EDSS. These include (1) imprecise levels of measurement; (2) suboptimal reliability; (3) unequal levels of sensitivity for detecting change in impairment across the range of the scale; (4) limited validity; and, (5) problems with administration.

Precision may be optimized with interval scales. Interval scales are characterized by equal distance between ordered points on the scale (i.e., age, weight). Change on interval scales is easily interpreted with straightforward arithmetic operations (i.e., "you are 5 years older"). Ordinal scales may be derived from interval scales by creating less precise categories to define measures of interest (i.e., < 15 years = "youthful," 16–21 years = "ado-

Table 5-3. Kurtzke Extended Disability Status Scale (EDSS)

0.0—Normal neurologic exam [all grade 0 in all Functional System (FS) scores].

1.0—No disability, minimal signs in one FS (i.e., grade 1).

1.5—No disability, minimal signs in more than one FS (more than 1 grade 1).

2.0—Minimal disability in one FS (one FS grade 2, others 0 or 1).

2.5—Minimal disability in two FS (two FS grade 2, others 0 or 1).

3.0—Moderate disability in one FS (one FS grade 3, others 0 or 1) or mild disability in three or four FS (three or four FS grade 2 others 0 or 1) though fully ambulatory.

3.5—Fully ambulatory but with moderate disability in one FS (one grade 3) and one or two FS grade 2; or two grade 3 (others 0 or 1) or 5 grade 2 (others 0 or 1).

4.0—Fully ambulatory without aid, self-sufficient, up and about some 12 hours a day despite relatively severe disability consisting of one FS grade 4 (others 0 or 1), or combination of lesser grades exceeding limits of previous steps and the patient should be able to walk > 500 m without assist or rest.

4.5—Fully ambulatory without aid, up and about much of the day, may otherwise require minimal assistance; characterized by relatively severe disability usually consisting of one FS grade 4 (others or 1) or combinations of lesser grades exceeding limits of previous steps and walks > 300 m without assist or rest.

5.0—Ambulatory without aid for at least 50 meters; disability severe enough to impair full daily activities (e.g., to work a full day without special provision). (Usual FS equivalents are one grade 5 alone, others 0 or 1; or combinations of lesser grades). Patient walks > 200 m without aid or rest.

5.5—Ambulatory without aid for at least 100 meters; disability severe enough to preclude full daily activities. (Usual FS equivalents are one grade 5 alone, others 0 or 1; or combinations of lesser grades). Enough to preclude full daily activities. (Usual FS equivalents are one grade 5 alone, others 0 or 1; or combinations of lesser grades).

6.0—Intermittent or unilateral constant assistance (cane, crutch, brace) required to walk at least 100 meters. (Usual FS equivalents are combinations with more than one FS grade 3).

6.5—Constant bilateral assistance (canes, crutches, braces) required to walk at least 20 meters. (Usual FS equivalents are combinations with more than one FS grade 3).

7.0—Unable to walk at least 5 meters even with aid, essentially restricted to wheelchair; wheels self and transfers alone; up and about in wheelchair some 12 hours a day. (Usual FS equivalents are combinations with more than one FS grade 4+; very rarely pyramidal grade 5 alone).

7.5—Unable to take more than a few steps; restricted to wheelchair; may need aid in transfer; wheels self but cannot carry on in wheelchair a full day. (Usual FS equivalents are combinations with more than one FS grade 4+; very rarely pyramidal grade 5 alone.)

8.0—Essentially restricted to chair or perambulated in wheelchair, but out of bed most of day; retains many self-care functions; generally has effective use of arms. (Usual FS equivalents are combinations, generally grade 4+ in several systems).

8.5—Essentially restricted to bed most of day; has some effective use of arm(s) ; retains some self-care functions. (Usual FS equivalents are combinations, generally 4 in several systems).

9.0—Helpless bed patient; can communicate and eat. (Usual FS equivalents are combinations, mostly grade 4+).

9.5—Totally helpless bed patient; unable to communicate effectively or eat or swallow. (Usual FS equivalents are combinations, almost all grade 4+).

10.0—Death due to MS.

lescent," 22–45 years = "young adult," 45–65 years = "middle-aged," > 65 years = "senior citizen"). Ordinal scales may also be used when interval scales cannot be used readily to measure a parameter of interest (i.e., "mild, moderate, or severe" loss of vibratory sensation in the legs). As such, change measured by ordinal scales must be determined with nonparametric methods and may be more difficult to interpret (i.e., "progression from a mild to a moderate loss of vibratory sensation"). The EDSS is an ordinal scale that is characterized by imprecise categorical distinctions of impairment (i.e., mild, moderate, severe).

Reliability refers to the reproducibility of an outcome measure. The EDSS is characterized by limited intra- and interrater reliability. This limitation is in part due to imprecise definitions of ordered categorizations of impairment (i.e., mild, moderate, severe) and may also reflect a tendency for certain aspects of neurologic impairment to fluctuate during the day because of fatigue or issues related to patient motivation. Additionally, intra- and interrater scoring reproducibility are not constant across the full range of scores of the EDSS. Scoring reproducibility is poorest in the 1.0–3.5 EDSS point range, where the EDSS score is determined entirely by scores on each of the functional systems. Scoring reproducibility appears to be greater in the 4.0–7.0 range, where the EDSS score is determined by the distance a patient walks and whether ambulation is performed independently or with assistive devices such as a cane or walker. Scoring reproducibility in the 7.5–9.5 point range of the EDSS has not been rigorously assessed.

Sensitivity refers to the ability of an instrument to detect change when change is observed. The EDSS is insensitive to detecting change in functional status reported by patients and their family members and is also insensitive to detecting gadolinium-enhanced brain MRI activity. Poor sensitivity is related in part to the characteristics of the EDSS scale. A change in the score of one of the functional systems (FSS) (Table 5-4) may result in a change in the EDSS score within the 1.0–3.5 point range but may not result in a change in EDSS score above that range. For example, it is possible for a patient's EDSS score to change from 2.0 to 3.5 if the visual FS score changes from 0 to 3. However, the same change in the visual FS score will not change the EDSS score of a patient whose EDSS score was greater than 3.5.

Validity is defined as measuring what is intended to be measured. The face validity of the EDSS may be compromised because change in the EDSS score may not reflect disease-specific change (i.e., motivational issues or weakness that may worsen as a result of fever or an asymptomatic urinary tract infection). Construct validity is limited because the EDSS is not equally sensitive to change across its full range of points. Criterion validity is limited because change in the EDSS correlates poorly (r = 0.22) with change in MRI activity (The IFNB Study Group and the University of British Columbia MS/MRI Analysis Group, 1995). Content validity is compromised because the EDSS is heavily weighted to ambulatory status and fails to provide an adequate assessment of upper extremity function. Predictive validity is limited because cross-sectional EDSS scores do not reliably predict future EDSS scores in individual patients.

Ease of administration of the EDSS is also problematic. Acceptable intrarater reproducibility using the EDSS is only achieved after formal training sessions. As a result, the EDSS is rarely used in clinical practice. In one clinical trial, a 15-page manual was required to address questions related to administration and scoring of the EDSS.

The Scripps Neurologic Rating Scale (NRS)

Description

The Scripps Neurologic Rating Scale (NRS) (Table 5-5) translates the neurologic examination into a standardized impairment scale. It provides scores for mentation and mood (10 points), visual cranial nerves (21 points), other cranial nerves (5 points), strength for limbs (20 points), deep tendon reflexes (8 points), Babinski sign (4 points), sensory function for limbs (12 points), cerebellar function for limbs (10 points), and gait and balance (10 points). The maximum score for a normal subject is 100 points. As many as 10 points can be deducted for bladder, bowel, or sexual dysfunction. The NRS differs conceptually from the EDSS in that it scores motor, sensory, and cerebellar functions separately for each limb. It is not known if this improves sensitivity for detecting change in longitudinal studies. The weighting of scores is arbitrary and the scale is characterized by imprecise terms such as mild, moderate, and severe. This is problematic since a change from mild to moderate in deficits in the motor and cerebellar scores of this scale could result in an overall scoring change of 12 points.

Table 5-4. Functional System Scores (FSS)

Note: Clarifications for imprecise FSS terms appear in parentheses. These clarifications were validated by Goodkin et al. for use in a phase III clinical trial of interferon beta-1a in relapsing MS in the EDSS 1.0–3.5 point range (Goodkin et al., 1992) and were used in a phase II clinical trial of methotrexate in chronic progressive MS in the EDSS 3.0–6.5 point range (low-dose oral methotrexate for the treatment of chronic progressive multiple sclerosis. (Goodkin DE, Rudick RA. In: Goodkin DE, Rudick RA (eds.).*Treatment of multiple sclerosis: advances in trial design, results and future perspectives.* In press.

Pyramidal Functions

0. Normal
1. Abnormal signs without weakness
2. Mild weakness (4/5 in one extremity or 4+/5 in more than one extremity)
3. Moderate paraparesis or hemiparesis (4/5 or 4–/5); or severe monoparesis (≤ 3/5)
4. Severe triparesis, paraparesis or hemiparesis (≤ 3/5); moderate quadriparesis (4/5 or 4–/5); or monoplegia
5. Paraplegia, hemiplegia, or severe quadriparesis (≤ 3/5)
6. Quadriplegia
7. (Untestable)
8. (Unknown)

Cerebellar Functions

(Note: Test finger to nose, heel/knee/shin, rapid alternating movements, and gait. This is a test of cerebellar function and not of weakness. If one or more limbs cannot be tested for any reason, score only the remaining limbs.)

0. Normal. (No evidence of cerebellar dysfunction. This score may be used if one or more limbs are uncoordinated due to weakness, apraxia, or sensory loss.)
1. Abnormal signs without disability (Interference in routine function)
2. Mild ataxia. (Limb ataxia in any or all limbs or gait ataxia that is adequate to interfere with routine function.)
3. Moderate ataxia. (Moderate ataxia of one or more limbs or gait that requires some physical or mechanical adaptation to complete a targeted activity. Examples include the requirement to hold a wall or a companion's arm to hop or tandem walk, or to use a buttonhole device to fasten buttons. The adaptation permits the activity to be completed.)
4. Severe ataxia, all limbs. (This score is applied when there is ataxia of one or more limbs or gait. Patients with a severe ataxia cannot complete a targeted activity even with mechanical or human assistance even though the activity may be initiated).
5. Unable to perform coordinated movements due to ataxia. (This score is only used when routine activities in one or more limbs or gait cannot even be initiated because ataxia is so severe that injury will result.)
6. (Untestable. This score will be applied most commonly when motor strength is 3/5 or less in all four limbs.)
7. (Unknown)

Brain Stem Functions

0. Normal
1. Signs only. (There is no interference with function. Use this score for unsustained nystagmus.)
2. Moderate impairment. (Use this score for sustained conjugate nystagmus, dysconjugate eye movements without associated nystagmus (incomplete INO), or paresis of one or more extraocular muscles innervated by neurons originating in the brainstem.)

Table 5-4.   *(continued)*

3. Severe nystagmus, marked extraocular weakness, or moderate disability of other cranial nerves. (Use this score for dysconjugate nystagmus (complete INO), paralysis of one or more extraocular muscles innervated by neurons originating in the brainstem, or when speech is affected due to brainstem dysfunction but remains intelligible.)

4. Marked dysarthria or other marked disability. (Use this score when speech is impaired by brainstem dysfunction and is marginally intelligible.)

5. Inability to swallow or speak (due to brainstem dysfunction)

6. (Untestable)

7. (Unknown)

Sensory Function

0. Normal

1. Vibration or figure-writing decrease only, in one or two limbs. (There is a loss of vibration, pain or temperature, or position sense involving the toes or fingers of one or more limb.)

2. Mild decrease in touch or pain or position sense, and moderate decrease in vibration on one or two limbs; or vibratory decrease alone in three or four limbs. (There is a loss of vibration, pain or temperature, or position sense up to the ankle or wrist in one or more limbs.)

3. Moderate decrease in touch or pain or position sense, and essentially lost vibration in one or two limbs; or mild decrease in touch or pain, or moderate decrease in touch or pain or severe proprioceptive decrease in more than two limbs. (Severe impairment. There is a loss of vibration, pain or temperature, or position sense up to the knee or elbow in one or more limbs.)

4. Marked decrease in touch or pain or loss of proprioception alone or combined, in one or two limbs; or moderate decrease in touch or pain or severe proprioceptive decrease in more than two limbs. (Loss of above described sensory function(s) proximal to the knee or elbow in one limb.)

5. Loss of sensation in one or two limbs; or moderate decrease in touch or pain or loss of proprioception for most of the body below the head. (Loss of above described sensory function(s) in more than one limb.)

6. Sensation lost below the head. (Untestable)

7. (Unknown)

Bowel and Bladder Function

(Ask about both bladder and bowel function during the past two weeks. Score the worst as follows. Place an "X" after bladder score if the patient performs intermittent self-catheterization).

Bladder

0. Normal

1. Mild urinary hesitance, urgency, or retention. (Bladder symptoms but not incontinence)

2. Moderate hesitance, urgency, retention of bowel or bladder, or rare urinary incontinence. (Incontinence less than twice per week)

3. Frequent urinary incontinence. (Incontinence two or more times per week but not daily)

4. In need of almost constant catheterization. (Daily incontinence)

5. Loss of bladder function. (Indwelling catheter)

6. Loss of bowel and bladder function. (Grade 5 bladder function plus grade 5 bowel function)

7. (Untestable). (Use this score if change in function is due to change in medication or presence of infection.)

8. (Unknown)

Table 5-4. *(continued)*

Bowel

0. Normal
1. Mild or intermittent constipation but no incontinence
2. Severe and continuous constipation but no incontinence
3. Incontinence less than twice per week
4. Incontinence two or more times per week but not daily
5. Daily incontinence
6. Grade 5 bowel function plus grade 5 bladder function
7. (Untestable: use this score if change in function is appears to be due to change in medication or presence of infection)
8. (Undetermined)

Visual Function

[Note: All visual acuities (VA) are best corrected.]

0. Normal. (VA better than 20/30 and no sign of optic nerve disease)
1. Scotoma with visual acuity better than 20/30. [VA equal to or better than 20/30 with signs of optic nerve disease (e.g. afferent pupil defect)].
2. Worse eye with scotoma with maximal visual acuity of 20/30–20/59. (Worst eye with maximal corrected VA 20/40–20/50).
3. Worse eye with large scotoma, or moderate decrease in visual fields but with maximal visual acuity of 20/60–20/99. (Worst eye with maximal corrected VA 20/70).
4. Worse eye with marked decrease of fields and maximal visual acuity of 20/100–20/200; grade 3 plus maximal acuity of better eye of 20/60 or less. (Worst eye with maximal corrected VA 20/100–20/200).
5. Worse eye with maximal visual acuity less than 20/200; grade 4 plus maximal acuity of better eye of 20/60 or less. (Worst eye with maximal corrected VA worse than 20/200 and maximal VA of better eye better than 20/60).
6. Grade 5 plus maximal VA in better eye worse than 20/60.
7. (Untestable)
8. (Unknown)

Mental Functions

(Note: This score is not used in calculation of EDSS scores when neuropsychological testing is performed as part of a controlled clinical trial).

0. Normal
1. Mood alteration only (does not affect EDSS score)
2. Mild decrease in mentation
3. Moderate decrease in mentation
4. Marked decrease in mentation
5. Dementia or chronic brain syndrome
6. (Untestable)
7. (Unknown)

Table 5-5. Scripps Neurologic Rating Scale (NRS

System Examined	Maximum Points	Normal	Degree of Impairment		
			Mild	Moderate	Severe
Mentation and Mood	10	10	7	4	0
Cranial Nerves	21				
Visual Acuity		5	3	1	0
Fields, Discs, Pupils		6	4	2	0
Eye Movements		5	3	1	0
Nystagmus		5	3	1	0
Lower Cranial Nerves	5	5	3	1	0
Motor	20				
RU		5	3	1	0
LU		5	3	1	0
RL		5	3	1	0
LL		5	3	1	0
DTRS	8				
UE		4	3	1	0
LE		4	3	1	0
Babinski R/L (2 ea)	4	4	0	0	0
Sensory	12				
RU		3	2	1	0
LU		3	2	1	0
RL		3	2	1	0
LL		3	2	1	0
Cerebellar	10				
UE		5	3	1	0
LE		5	3	1	0
Gait, Trunk, Balance	10	10	7	4	0
Special Category					
Bladder/Bowel/Sexual					
Dysfunction	0	0	−3	−7	−10
Totals	100				

Validation

The NRS has not been widely validated. The group most familiar with the scale report an interrater agreement of 85% when agreement is defined as a difference of no more than 10 points and a weighted kappa coefficient for intrarater scoring agreement of 2 NRS scores of 0.978–0.998 (Sipe et al., 1994). The NRS and EDSS evidenced similar sensitivity for detecting change in neurologic impairment in a clinical trial of interferon beta-1b. (The IFNB Multiple Sclerosis Study Group, 1993.

Administration

The scale is based on the neurologic examination, which is a requirement. Time required for examination and scoring is 15 to 25 minutes.

Advantages

Since it tests and scores individual limbs separately, the Scripps scale may be more sensitive to change than the EDSS, although this has not been demonstrated. Since it is based on the neurologic examination and scoring from the examination is straightforward, it is probably slightly more efficient than the EDSS, which often requires walking the patient for a substantial distance in addition to the neurologic examination.

Disadvantages

The NRS requires a neurologist to administer, uses nonquantifiable values such as mild, moderate, and severe, which increase intra- and interobserver variability, and has not been adequately validated.

Summary

The NRS shares most of the limitations of the EDSS, has not been widely validated, and has received limited use in MS clinical trials.

The Ambulation Index (AI)

Description

The AI (Table 5-6) provides a focused assessment of timed walking and ability to transfer. Like the EDSS, it is an ordinal scale. The scores range from 0 (normal gait) to 9 (unable to ambulate or transfer independently).

Validation

The test has face validity as a direct measure of mobility but has not undergone formal validation. Although the AI provides a measure of mobility, it fails to account for the broader range of impairments experienced by patients with MS. It has been suggested that the AI may be more sensitive than the EDSS in detecting a change of neurologic impairment but this has not been borne out in controlled clinical trials (Goodkin et al., 1995). The correlation between EDSS and AI scores appears to be very high (Beatty W, Goodkin DE. Screening for cognitive impairment in multiple sclerosis: an evaluation of the Mini-Mental State Exam. *Arch Neurol* 1990;3:297–304).

Administration

Perhaps the most appealing feature of the AI is that the test can be administered by a nurse or family member in less than one minute.

Summary

A rapid and easily performed test of mobility; it is both simple and useful.

The Troiano Scale (TS)

Description

The Troiano Scale (Table 5-7) derives an ordinal measure of impairment and disability from an assessment of gait (5 points), activities of daily living (4 points), and ability to perform transfers (3 points). Although the points on the scale are well defined and the instrument is easy to administer, the TS provides no assessment of vision, sphincter function, brainstem, or cognitive functions; the weighting of scores appears to be arbitrary.

Validation

The TS has not been formally validated and has not gained widespread acceptance for use in MS clinical trials.

Administration

The scale can be administered by a nurse or technician in a few minutes.

Table 5-6. Hauser Ambulation Index

0. Asymptomatic; fully active.

1. Walks normally, but reports fatigue that interferes with athletic or other demanding activities.

2. Abnormal gait or episodic imbalance; gait disorder is noticed by family and friends; able to walk 25 ft. in 10 sec. or less.

3. Walks independently; able to walk 25 ft. in 20 sec. or less.

4. Requires unilateral support (cane or single crutch) to walk; walks 25 ft. in 20 sec. or less.

5. Requires bilateral support (canes, crutches, or walker) and walks 25 ft. in 25 sec. or less; or requires unilateral support but needs more than 20 sec. to walk 25 ft.

6. Requires bilateral support and more than 20 sec. to walk 25 ft., may use wheelchair on occasion.

7. Walking limited to several steps with bilateral support; unable to walk 25 ft., may use wheelchair for most activities.

8. Restricted to wheelchair; able to transfer self independently.

9. Restricted to wheelchair; unable to transfer self independently.

Table 5-7. Troiano Functional Scale

Gait

0. Normal.
1. Abnormal, independent.
2. Uses unilateral assistance device.
3. Uses bilateral assistance device; may use wheelchair for longer mobility; walking is sufficient to serve various routine daily activities.
4. Depends mainly on wheelchair for mobility; may stand and take some steps with bilateral assistance; walking not very useful for practical purposes, done largely for short transfers and exercise activity, preferably with supervision.
5. No standing or steps excluding active human support or rigid support such as Kim stander.

Activities of Daily Living

0. Normal.
1. Independent with minimum dysfunction; may choose to use assistance or device for speed and efficiency.
2. Routinely uses partial human assistance for some dexterity functions (writing, managing utensils, buttons, etc.) and dressing and bathing of lower body.
3. Uses substantial human assistance for most activities, including bathing and dressing lower and upper body actively participates.
4. Dependent for all activities; passive with no effective participation.

Transfers

0. Slight or no difficulty.
1. Uses arms to shift weight, sitting to standing, or sitting to sitting, from a straight chair or wheelchair; transfers are independent.
2. Routinely uses assistance for most transfers; actively participates.
3. Dependent for all transfers; passive with no effective participation.

Summary

A very simple scale that has not been formally validated and has not gained wide acceptance.

Quantified Tests of Upper Extremity Function

The 9-Hole Peg Test (9HPT) and Box and Block Test (BBT) are standardized tests of upper extremity function (Goodkin et al., 1988). Both tests are commercially available [Craftsman Carpentry, Moorhead Minnesota, (218) 233-8162] and can be easily administered by a nurse in less than 10 minutes. Performance on the 9HPT is scored as the amount of time required to place and remove nine pegs from the testing instrument with each hand scored separately. Performance on the BBT is scored as the number of blocks moved from one of the testing instrument's bins to the other, again with each hand scored separately. Both tests have face validity as tests of upper extremity dexterity. At first glance, both would seem to be measuring the same function, but the 9-Hole Peg Test requires finer dexterity; Goodkin et al. (1988) have shown that better sensitivity is obtained if both are used. Intra- and interrater reliability is extremely high and a 20% change in baseline performance time has been shown to occur by chance less than 5% of the time. Goodkin and colleagues originally suggested than the 9HPT and BBT could be combined with the EDSS to improve sensitivity for detecting change in neurologic impairment in patients participating in controlled clinical trials (Goodkin et al., 1988, 1992). These investigators subsequently demonstrated that a composite outcome of the 9HPT and EDSS was more sensitive than the EDSS for detecting sustained change in neurologic impairment in patients enrolled in a phase II clinical trial of oral methotrexate for chronic progressive MS (Goodkin et al., 1995). Similar findings have been reported in a phase III trial of interferon beta-1a in patients with relapsing MS (Goodkin et al., 1996). If replicated by others, composite outcomes of upper extremity testing and the EDSS are likely to be more widely used in future MS clinical trials. Other quantitative tests of neurologic function (Syndulko et al., 1993), including quantitative isometric strength assessments, may also be useful for constructing composite outcomes that are more sensitive for detecting change in neurologic impairment (Noseworthy et al., 1996).

Instruments to Measure MS-Related Disability

The Incapacity Status Scale (ISS)

The ISS was developed from the PULSES profile (physical condition, upper limb function, lower limb function, sensory function, excretory function, support factors) (Granger, Albracht, & Hamilton, 1979) and the Barthel Index (Mahoney & Barthel, 1965). The ISS is a patient interview and scoring is based on current level of function. The validity of this instrument may be compromised by inaccurate reporting of performance ability and disability may result in part from problems that are not disease-specific. The ISS provides a description of performance on each of the following items: stair climbing, ambulation, transfers, bowel function, bladder function, bathing, dressing, grooming, feeding, vision, speech and hearing, all medical problems, mood and thought disturbance, mentation, fatigue, and sexual function. Scoring of each item is from 0 (normal) to 4 (most dysfunction). Weighting of the scores is arbitrary. This instrument has not been widely used in MS clinical trials.

The Functional Independence Measure (FIM)

The FIM is an updated version of the Barthel Index (Mahoney & Barthel 1965) and the Brief Symptom Inventory (BSI) (Derogatis & Melisaratos, 1983). The FIM has been compared to the ISS as a predictor of general life satisfaction and minutes of help required each day by MS patients. Multiple regression analyses reveal that the predictors most likely associated with need for help are transfers from tub and shower (FIM), vision (ISS), and ambulatory status (FIM). With vision removed from the regression, multiple FIM items are predictive of help required, including transfers from a chair or bed, memory, ambulatory status, dressing lower body, bladder management, and eating. FIM items associated with general life satisfaction included toileting, dressing lower body, and climbing stairs. The ISS and FIM may provide a more informative outcome in assessing the results of rehabilitation than controlled clinical trials of experimental therapeutics; however, the FIM is included as a secondary outcome measure in a phase III trial of interferon beta-1a in relapsing MS (Jacobs et al., 1996). Data from this study are awaited with interest and will help to clarify the role of the FIM in future MS clinical trials (see also Chapter 7).

Instruments to Measure MS-Related Incapacity

The Environmental Status Scale (ESS)

The ESS provides an assessment of social dysfunction in the context of one's cultural setting. It consists of seven items scored from 0 (normal) to 5 (most dysfunction). These items include work status, financial/economic status, personal residence, personal assistance requirement, transportation, community services, and social activities. Some of the items are imprecisely defined (i.e., mild, moderate, severe), which contributes to limitations similar to those presented for the EDSS. Since scoring is based on performance, an individual capable of work but unemployed will receive the worst dysfunction score for work status if the evaluator believed the customary role for that individual in his or her social environment to be full-time employment. The ESS has not been widely used in MS clinical trials. The ESS may provide a more informative outcome in assessing the results of rehabilitation than controlled clinical trials of experimental therapeutics (Stewart, Kidd, & Thompson, 1955; Solari et al., 1993).

References

Alexander L. New concept of critical steps in course of chronic debilitating neurologic disease in evaluation of therapeutic response. *Arch Neurol Psychiatry* 1951;66:253–58.

Arkin H, Sherman IC, Weinberg SL. Tetraethylammonium chloride in the treatment of multiple sclerosis. *Arch Neurol Psychiatry* 1950;64:536–45.

Beatty WW, Goodkin DE. Screening for cognitive impairment in multiple sclerosis: an evaluation of the Mini-Mental State Examination. *Arch Neurol* 1990;47:297–304.

Charcot JM. *Lectures on diseases of the nervous system* (trans. G. Sigerson; first series lectures 6,7,8 delivered 1868). London: The New Sydenham Society, 1877:157.

Cook SD, Troiano R, Zito G, et al. Effect of total lymphoid irradiation in chronic progressive multiple sclerosis. *Lancet* 1986;1:1405–1409.

Derogatis LR, Melisaratos N. The brief symptom inventory: an introductory report. *Psychol Med* 1983:13:595–605.

Engell T. A clinico-pathoanatomical study of multiple sclerosis. *Acta Neurol Scand* 1988;78:39–44.

Goodkin DE. Unique problems in multiple sclerosis clinical trial design: strategies for clinical investigators. In: "Tools for practice and research: understanding neuroepidemiology." American Academy of Neurology 45th annual meeting course #242, 4/26/93.

Goodkin DE, Cookfair D, Wende K, Bourdette D, Pullicino P, Scherokman B, Whitham R, and the Multiple Sclerosis Collaborative Study Group. Inter- and intrarater scoring agreement using grades 1.0–3.5 of the Kurtzke Expanded Disability Status Scale (EDSS). *Neurology* 1992;42:859–63.

Goodkin DE, Herndon RM, Jacobs LD, et al. Intramuscular interferon beta-1a (IFNB-1a) in relapsing multiple sclerosis: analyses of quantitative upper extremity testing. *Neurology* 1996;46:A136.

Goodkin DE, Hertsgaard D, Seminary J. Upper extremity function in multiple sclerosis: improving assessment sensitivity with Box-and-Block and Nine-Hole Peg Tests. *Arch Phys Med Rehabil* 1988;69:850–54.

Goodkin DE, Rudick RA, VanderBrug-Medendorp S, et al. Low-dose (7.5 mg) oral methotrexate (MTX) for chronic progressive multiple sclerosis: design of a randomized placebo-controlled trial with sample size benefits from composite outcome variable. Preliminary data on toxicity. *Online J Curr Clin Trials* [serial online] 1992 Sep 25;1992 (Doc No 19); [7723 words; 89 paragraphs].

Goodkin DE, Rudick RA. Low-dose, oral methotrexate for the treatment of chronic progressive multiple sclerosis. In: Goodkin DE, Rudick RA (eds.). *Treatment of multiple sclerosis: advances in trial design, results and future perspectives.* In press.

Goodkin DE, Rudick RA, VanderBrug-Medendorp S, et al. Low-dose (7.5 mg) oral methotrexate is effective in reducing the rate of progression of neurological impairment in patients with chronic progressive multiple sclerosis. *Ann Neurol* 1995;37:30–40.

Granger CV, Albracht GL, Hamilton BB. Outcome of comprehensive medical rehabilitation: measurement by PULSES profile and the Barthel index. *Arch Phys Med Rehabil* 1979;60:145–54.

Granger CV, Hamilton BB, Sherwin FS. *Guide for the use of the Uniform Data Set for Medical Rehabilitation.* Uniform Data System for Medical Rehabilitation

Project Office, Buffalo General Hospital, Buffalo, New York 14203, U.S.A.

Haber A, LaRocca N (eds.). *Minimal Record of Disability for multiple sclerosis*. New York: National Multiple Sclerosis Society, 1985.

Hauser SL, Dawson DM, Lehrich JR, et al. Intensive immunosuppression in progressive multiple sclerosis: a randomized three-arm study of high dose intravenous cyclophosphamide, plasma exchange and ACTH. *N Engl J Med* 1983;308:173–80.

Herndon RM. The changing pattern of misdiagnosis in multiple sclerosis. In: Herndon RM, Seil FJ (eds.). *Multiple sclerosis: current status of research and treatment*. New York: Demos, 1994:149–56.

Jacobs LD, Cookfair DL, Rudick RA, et al. Intramuscular interferon beta-1a for disease progression in relapsing multiple sclerosis. *Ann Neurol* 1996;39:285–94.

Kurtzke JF. A new scale for evaluating disability in multiple sclerosis. *Neurology* 1955;5:580–83.

Kurtzke JF. Rating neurologic impairment in multiple sclerosis: an expanded disability status scale (EDSS). *Neurology* 1983;33:1444–52.

Mahoney FI, Barthel DW. Functional evaluation: the Barthel Index. *MD State Med J* 1965;14:61–65.

Mathiowetz V, Volland G, Kashman N, Weber K. Adult norms for the Box and Block Test of manual dexterity. *Am J Occup Ther* 1985;39:386–91.

Mathiowetz V, Volland G, Kashman N, Volland G. Adult norms for Nine Hole Peg Test of finger dexterity. *Occup Ther J Res* 1985;5:24–38.

Noseworthy JH, Rodriguez M, Weinshenker BG, et al. Isometric muscle strength measurements in a multiple sclerosis treatment trial: comparison with the clinical exam. *Neurology* 1996;46:A254.

Noseworthy JH, Vandervoort MK, Wong CJ, Ebers GC, and the Canadian Cooperative MS Study Group. Interrater variability with the Expanded Disability Status Scale (EDSS) and Functional Systems (FS) in a multiple sclerosis clinical trial. *Neurology* 1990;40:971–75.

Poser CM, Paty DW, Scheinberg L, et al. New diagnostic criteria for multiple sclerosis: guidelines for research protocols. *Ann Neurol* 1983;13:227.

Rudick RA, Schiffer RB, Schwetz KM, Herndon RM. Multiple sclerosis: the problem of misdiagnosis. *Arch Neurol* 1986;43:578–93.

Schumacher GA, Beebe G, Kibler RF, et al. Problems of experimental trials of therapy in multiple sclerosis: report by the panel on the evaluation of experimental trials of therapy in multiple sclerosis. *Ann NY Acad Sci* 1965;122:552–68.

Sipe JC, Romine JS, Koziol JA, McMillan R, Zyroff J, Beutler E. Cladribine in treatment of chronic progressive multiple sclerosis. *Lancet* 1994;344:9–13.

Solari A, Amato MP, Bergamasch R, et al. Accuracy of self-assessment of the Minimal Record of Disability in patients with multiple sclerosis. *Acta Neurol Scand* 1993;83:43–46.

Stewart G, Kidd D, Thompson AJ. The assessment of handicap: an evaluation of the Environmental Status Scale. *Disability and Rehabilitation* 1995;17:312–16.

Syndulko K, Tourtellotte WW, Baumhefner RW, Ellison GW, Myers LW, Belendiuk G, Kondraske GV. Neuroperformance evaluation of multiple sclerosis disease progression in a clinical trial: implications for neurological outcomes. *J Neuro Rehab* 1993;7:153–76.

The IFNB Multiple Sclerosis Study Group. Interferon beta-1b is effective in relapsing-remitting multiple sclerosis. I. Clinical results of a multicenter, randomized, double-blind, placebo-controlled trial. *Neurology* 1993;43:655–61.

The IFNB Multiple Sclerosis Study Group and the University of British Columbia MS/MRI Analysis Group. Interferon beta-1b in the treatment of multiple sclerosis. *Neurology* 1995;45:1277–85.

Weiss W, Stadlan EM. Design and statistical issues related to testing experimental therapy in multiple sclerosis. In: Rudick RA, Goodkin DE. *Treatment of multiple sclerosis: trial design, results, and future perspectives*. London, Berlin, Heidelberg, New York, Paris, Tokyo, Hong Kong, Barcelona, Budapest: Springer Verlag, 1992:91–122.

CHAPTER 6 Assessment of the Elderly with Dementia

*Richard Camicioli, M.D.,
and Katherine Wild, Ph.D.*

Dementia is a syndrome of persistent cognitive dysfunction caused by impairment in multiple domains (Cummings & Benson, 1992). A number of formal definitions are available, including the Diagnostic and Statistical Manual (most recently DSM-IV) (APA, 1994). Dementia has numerous potential causes, some of which are amenable to treatment (Clarfield, 1988). The most common type of dementia is Alzheimer's disease (AD) (McKhann et al., 1984). While there is currently no cure for AD, optimal management and counseling require an accurate diagnosis. Early diagnosis not only facilitates future planning by families but may allow treatable entities to be uncovered prior to the accumulation of excess disability. Once a diagnosis is made, appropriate follow-up can ensure optimal care. These goals are facilitated by the use of appropriate clinical scales.

Clinical scales cannot be used without due consideration of the clinical history obtained from the patient and their informant. Memory impairment, cognitive change, personality change, functional impairment, or other complaints consistent with the diagnosis of dementia should prompt an assessment directed at establishing a diagnosis. The scales to be discussed provide an important starting point for these diagnostic considerations.

Despite the importance of dementia as a public health problem, standardized approaches to assessment are not widely used in clinical practice (Brodaty et al., 1994). Among the possible reasons for this may be the lack of recognition of the utility of standardized assessment, a lack of familiarity with available instruments, the limitations of commonly used instruments, and time constraints of busy clinical practices.

Objective evaluation allows the clinician to compare performance at different times in a standardized and reliable fashion. Use of these measures has been shown to be superior to clinicians' impressions (Cooper et al., 1992; Knopman & Gracon, 1994; Wind et al., 1994). In mild dementia documented objective change on a standardized instrument may allow early detection of dementia in an appropriate clinical context. Once the diagnosis is established, standardized tools allow better evaluation of changes over time and improved assessment of acute change (Galasko et al., 1991). Another advantage of standardized scales is improved communication among professionals. Use of common tools may actually save time by obviating the need for repeating an exam done by another clinician.

Decisions concerning which measure to use should be based on a clear understanding of its properties. Instruments vary in sensitivity and specificity (Hazzard et al., 1994). Sensitivity is a measure of a test's ability to identify cases. It is defined as the number of subjects with a given diagnosis detected by a test, divided by the total number of subjects with the diagnosis in the population under study. Specificity refers to the number of subjects without a given diagnosis with a negative test result, divided by the total number of subjects without the diagnosis in the population under study. A sensitive test is very good at detecting cases, so that if a subject is not classified as having the diagnosis by the test, they are unlikely to have the diagnosis. In other words, a negative result rules out the disorder. A specific test is good at eliminating a diagnosis, so that a positive result obtained with a specific test would rule in the diagnosis. The population under consideration determines the predictive value of a positive or negative test score (Nardone, 1996).

In this chapter we discuss the utility of selected scales for detecting and following progression in patients with dementia. We consider scales that measure (1) cognitive function, (2) functional status, (3) global function, and (4) aspects of behavior. We discuss the strengths and weaknesses of each and explain how to use selected instruments. Our goal is to make standardized instruments readily available to clinicians in practice outside of research centers.

The scales for this section were chosen from the literature using Medline and PsychInfo searches, a review of recently published textbooks on geriatric medicine (Hazzard et al., 1994), geriatric neurology (Albert & Knoefel, 1994; Barclay, 1993; Katzman & Rowe, 1992), and dementia (Katzman & Kawas, 1994; Whitehouse, 1993; Cummings & Benson, 1992), and recent reviews on assessment of the elderly (Fleming et al., 1995; Siu, 1991; White & Davis, 1990). This compilation is a selective one, and readers should refer to the secondary sources and the primary literature for a comprehensive review. The scales are relatively simple to administer and are in wide use. Validity and reliability data have been published and are discussed.

Cognitive Assessment Instruments

Several brief scales are available for the assessment of cognitive function in patients with dementia. One must keep in mind that dementia is defined by involvement of more than one cognitive domain

(see Table 6-1). The brief scales discussed test limited domains, and therefore they should be supplemented by historical information and/or additional testing to reach a diagnosis of dementia or to exclude such a diagnosis.

The Mini-Mental State Examination (MMSE) is a widely used mental status scale (Folstein et al., 1975). Numerous studies have demonstrated its test characteristics (Tombaugh & McIntyre, 1992). The Short Blessed Orientation-Memory-Concentration (BOMC) test is another instrument that is somewhat briefer than the MMSE (Katzman et al., 1983). Other brief instruments suitable for office use include the Short Test of Mental Status (Kokmen et al., 1991), the Short Portable Mental Status Questionnaire (Pfeiffer, 1975), and the Mental Status Questionnaire (Kahn et al., 1960).

All of these scales lack sensitivity for detecting early dementia. The problem of early detection can be circumvented in several ways. Some authors have modified the MMSE (Mayeux et al., 1981; Teng et al., 1987) by adding tests that have greater sensitivity (Katzman & Rowe, 1992). Others have developed brief batteries of tests that emphasize sensitivity (Fuld, 1978; Knopman & Ryberg, 1989), some of which are based on preexisting neuropsychologic tests (Eslinger et al., 1984).

Expanded cognitive testing instruments offer the potential for early detection of dementia. The Mattis Dementia Rating Scale (DRS) (Mattis, 1976), the Alzheimer's Disease Assessment Scale (ADAS) (Rosen et al., 1984), the Neurobehavioral Cognitive Status Exam (NCSE) (Kiernan et al., 1987), and the Dementia Assessment Battery (Teng et al., 1989) are four such instruments, among others (Lezak, 1995). Although they take longer to perform than the briefer screening instruments, they offer the potential of greater sensitivity for early disease detection and improved assessment of change. In general, they require the purchase or construction of special materials, which may be justified in a clinical practice focusing on the elderly.

Formal neuropsychologic testing, which usually includes tests of multiple cognitive domains, is the best approach to evaluate mildly impaired patients when the diagnosis is in question. Specific test combinations that are particularly useful in detecting or tracking changes in dementia have been published (Lezak, 1995; Locascio et al., 1995; Morris et al., 1989; Parks et al., 1993). Reexamining patients using standardized instruments at regular intervals permits the documentation of progressive decline that strongly supports the diagnosis of

Table 6-1. Elements of the Mental Status Examination Relevant for the Diagnosis of Dementia

Cognitive Domain	Tests (Examples)
Memory	3, 4, 10, or longer word list: registration, recall, and recognition
Orientation	To person, place, time
Attention	Digit span (forward, reverse)
	Serial subtractions
	Reversals (days of the week, months of the year, etc.)
Visuospatial	Clock drawing
	Figure drawing and copying
Language	Fluency, grammar, and content of spontaneous speech
	Naming
	Repetition
	Comprehension
	Reading
	Writing
Praxis	Multiple step commands
Executive function and reasoning	Calculations
	Similarities and differences
	Proverb interpretation
	Problem solving
	Judgment

dementia. Psychometric tests with well-defined properties may offer the best way to do this, although the briefer instruments have been used for the same purpose.

Another disadvantage of all of the brief instruments, shared with most psychometric tests, is that severely impaired subjects may not be able to perform the test. At the extremes of the scoring range, the patient's disease may progressively worsen without detectable change in scores (i.e., a patient cannot score worse than zero). Approaches to dealing with severely impaired patients are not as well worked out, but recently several tools that are sensitive to change in severely impaired patients have been described (Albert & Cohen, 1992; Cole & Dastoor, 1987; Saxton et al., 1990). Functional, global, and behavioral scales, discussed in subsequent sections of this chapter, are essential in tracking meaningful change in severely impaired patients. In this section, we focus our discussion on the MMSE and the

Blessed scales and their modifications as the most commonly used instruments in clinical practice.

The Mini-Mental State Examination (MMSE)

The MMSE (Appendix 1) was developed as a brief tool for grading the level of cognitive impairment in the elderly (Folstein et al., 1975). It is currently used for this purpose, as well as in screening for dementia (Fratiglioni et al., 1992; Ganguli et al., 1993; Paykel et al., 1994). It has been used in clinical trials for Alzheimer's disease as a tool to grade initial dementia severity as well as to measure the effect of medications, although it may not be sensitive enough to change for the latter use (Knopman & Gracon, 1994). Other measures such as the ADAS may be better suited to detect change. Nevertheless, the established properties of this scale, its widespread use, and its brevity make it an excellent choice for office use.

Description

The MMSE is a 30-point scale, consisting of several orientation questions (10 points); a registration and recall task (6 points); an attention task (5 points); a multistep command (3 points); two naming tasks (2 points); a repetition task (1 point); a reading comprehension task (1 point); a written sentence (1 point); and a visual construction task (1 point). The reading comprehension task involves the patient reading the sentence "CLOSE YOUR EYES" and performing this command. The construction task involves copying interlocking pentagons. These items are generally printed on the form used to facilitate administration of the test.

Administration

The patient is asked the questions directly by the examiner. A watch, a plain piece of paper, and a pencil are the only equipment required.

Time to Administer

The MMSE takes 5 to 10 minutes to administer.

Reliability and Validity

The MMSE has been validated in a number of ways. It has face validity in that it tests cognitive domains important to the diagnosis of dementia: orientation, language, memory, attention, and construction abilities. It has convergent validity as indicated by the high correlation with other brief instruments, including the short Blessed Orientation-Memory-Concentration Test (BOMC) (Murden et al., 1991). Scores on the MMSE and the BOMC correlate with the pathologic changes at autopsy in patients with AD (Terry et al., 1991).

Internal consistency of the MMSE is quite good, with Cronbach's alpha ranging from .54 to .96 (Tombaugh & McIntyre, 1992), depending on the patient population. Test-retest and interrater reliability are also excellent. There is a practice effect with repeated administration of the MMSE or the BOMC (Galasko et al., 1993).

Special Considerations

As with all mental status tests, optimal patient cooperation should be obtained. At the outset the patient should be made comfortable with the examiner. A conversation regarding recent events and autobiographical details usually puts the patient at ease and offers the opportunity to informally assess language, as well as memory for recent events.

It is useful to provide the patient with a non-threatening introduction to the formal testing. For example, one could say, "Now I am going to ask you some questions that will test your memory and thinking. Some of the questions are very easy, while others are harder for everyone. Please do the best you can, but don't worry if you can't get an answer."

Demographic factors such as age, socioeconomic group, race (Murden et al., 1991), gender, and education (Uhlmann & Larson, 1991) all affect performance on mental status tests, including the MMSE (Crum et al., 1993). With fewer than nine years of education the cut-off for suspecting dementia on the basis of mental status tests alone should be adjusted downward from 23/24 to 21/22 in order to minimize false-positive classification (Liu et al., 1994). Age and education adjusted norms may also be used (Crum et al., 1993).

The MMSE has been translated and adapted for use with Spanish- and Chinese-speaking people (Liu et al., 1994; Mungas et al., 1996).

Advantages

The MMSE is quite easy to administer and takes minimal training. It has been validated in numerous studies (Tombaugh & McIntyre, 1992). Although up to 20% of patients with dementia in some studies may score above the recommended cut-off of 23/24, it is more sensitive to dementia than routine clinical judgment. Follow-up of patients (Braekhus et al., 1995) and appropriate reliance on clinical history should increase its diagnostic accuracy.

A validated version of the MMSE is available for administration by telephone (Roccaforte et al., 1992). Overall, the MMSE makes an excellent choice for office use. By keeping its limitations in mind, clinicians can use it to advantage in assessing cognitive status in dementia.

Disadvantages

One disadvantage of the MMSE is its insensitivity to the early changes of dementia. This is due in part to its heavy weighting toward orientation and memory, which makes the test especially insensitive in cases that present with difficulties in cognitive domains other than memory. The test relies on verbal responses, which is a problem in patients with language disorders such as aphasia or dysarthria due to motor problems as seen in motor neuron disease. Compared with usual practice, however, it represents a considerable improvement.

The MMSE is insensitive to cognitive impairment in cerebrovascular disease (Grace et al., 1995), multiple sclerosis (Swirsky-Sacchetti et al., 1992), and Parkinson's disease (Rothlind & Brandt, 1993). It fails to assess cognitive functions that are often impaired in these diseases such as executive function (Elias, 1995) and attention, which are best tested using different instruments (Royall, 1994).

Blessed Orientation-Memory-Concentration Test (BOMC)

Blessed and colleagues (1968) were the first to examine the relationship between cognitive measures and neuropathologic changes in dementia. The scale that they developed to measure cognitive and functional status has been subsequently modified for use in numerous clinical studies. Modified versions of the cognitive aspects of their scale are quite useful in clinical practice (Katzman & Rowe, 1992). We discuss the use of a short version of the Blessed Orientation-Memory-Concentration Test because it provides a brief alternative to the MMSE and its psychometric properties have been well documented. It is contrasted with the longer Blessed Information-Memory-Concentration Test (BIMC), which was adapted from the original version for use in the United States (Fuld, 1978) (see Appendix 2).

Description

The short BOMC (Appendix 3) consists of 6 items, compared to 26 in the full-length BIMC. There are three orientation items, one of which is administered along with two additional distractors between a registration and recall task. The distractor tasks also test concentration. Each item is given a weighting that allows the calculation of a total possible score of 28. The long BIMC includes additional orientation, memory, and attention items.

Administration

The scale is administered to the patient directly as part of a mental status evaluation.

Time to Administer

Administration takes about five minutes.

Reliability and Validity

Fuld (Fuld, 1978) has validated the scale in a population admitted to a skilled nursing facility. Results on the short test ($r = .54$, $p < 0.001$) and the long version ($r = .59$, $p < .001$) correlate with the autopsy findings of Alzheimer's disease. The Blessed scales have been shown to correlate with the Clinical Dementia Rating Scale, an integrated rating of overall function (Davis et al., 1990). Unfortunately, sensitivity, specificity, and population-based predictive values have not been reported.

Advantages

The use of a reproducible, valid instrument is advantageous. The BOMC scale is much briefer than the MMSE by virtue of the elimination of a large number of questions that address orientation. As it is presented, subjects do not have to use their limbs. This allows it to be used with patients with motor disabilities sparing speech. It has been adapted for a telephone interview (Kawas et al., 1995).

Disadvantages

This test has both floor and ceiling effects. It cannot be used to make the diagnosis of dementia because it only tests a limited number of cognitive domains. It must be supplemented with tests in other domains in order to establish a diagnosis. Katzman (Katzman & Rowe, 1992) recommends using it in conjunction with tests of specific cognitive domains: (1) a construction task, such as clock drawing (Mendez et al., 1992; Spreen & Strauss, 1991; Tuokko et al., 1992); (2) a verbal fluency task, such as listing as many animals as possible in one minute (Spreen & Strauss, 1991); (3) a multistep command, such as taking a piece of paper, folding it, placing it in an envelope, and preparing the envelope for mailing; and (4) a test of naming, such as naming a pen and its component parts or naming body parts. Together with the clinical history, these provide a reasonable overall assessment of cognitive function.

Short Test of Mental Status

The Short Test of Mental Status (Appendix 4) was developed at the Mayo Clinic by Kokmen (Kokmen et al., 1991). Although not in wide use, it tests cognitive functions other than memory, making it potentially more sensitive to early dementia. Although longitudinal studies have not been published, it is distinctive enough that it merits consideration for routine use.

Description

The test is administered to the patient. Scores range from 0, indicating maximally poor performance, to 38, indicating perfect performance. There are eight domains: orientation (8 points); attention (7 points); immediate recall (4 points); calculation (4 points); abstraction (3 points); construction (4 points); information (4 points); and delayed recall (4 points).

Administration

The Short Test of Mental Status is administered directly to the patient as part of the mental status evaluation.

Time to Administer

This test takes about five minutes to administer.

Reliability and Validity

The scale was administered to a group of patients with dementia and control subjects along with the MMSE, the BIMC, the Mattis DRS, and neuropsychologic testing. It correlates significantly with these, indicating convergent validity. Notably it correlated well with neuropsychologic testing and the Mattis Dementia Rating Scale (Kokmen et al., 1991).

Sensitivity was 0.86 for detecting dementia using a cut-off of less than 29/38 for subjects 80 to 89 years of age and 0.94 using a cut-off of less than 28/38 for subjects older than 90 years of age.

Advantages

The cognitive domains tested using this scale resemble those tested by other scales discussed. By testing calculation and abstraction, this test is unique among the brief instruments. This scale incorporates a four-word memory list and clock drawing, affording the potential for improved sensitivity for detection of dementia.

Disadvantages

Although this test may be an improvement in some domains compared to the MMSE and the BIMC, language function is not tested in detail. The test is biased to testing memory and orientation. Patients who have more focal impairment may do well on these items, yet may be significantly impaired. This test needs to be validated in other populations to test its overall utility. To our knowledge, it has not been validated in pathologically confirmed cases.

Functional Status Instruments

Functional status is a patient-based measure that refers to a person's ability to perform tasks in the real world. Functional assessment is usually divided into activities of daily living (ADLs) and instrumental activities of daily living (IADLs) (see Table 6-2). These tasks are a necessary part of daily living; if a patient cannot perform them, they must be performed by a caregiver. ADLs refer to basic self-care tasks such as dressing or eating. These tasks are

Table 6-2. Examples of Items in a Functional Assessment: Activities of Daily Living (ADLs) and Instrumental Activities of Daily Living (IADLs)

Activities of Daily Living	Instrumental Activities of Daily Living
Rising from bed	Using the telephone
Walking	Transportation (beyond residence)
Dressing	Shopping
Bathing or showering	Cooking meals
Grooming (hair, shaving, teeth, etc.)	Housework and home maintenance
	Handling money
Eating	Hobbies and employment
Toileting	Taking medications

impaired only in more severely affected patients. IADLs are more complex tasks such as using the telephone or cooking. These tasks are more cognitively demanding and consequently are impaired earlier in the course of dementia. Impairment in instrumental activities of daily living has been used as an early indicator of dementia (Barberger-Gateau et al., 1992; Barberger-Gateau et al., 1993).

Cognitive and physical impairments can affect performance in both ADLs and IADLs. It is important for both practical and research purposes to determine which aspect of a person's illness is contributing to impairment in daily life functioning. Some may be amenable to remediation at the individual or environmental level.

Determining a person's functional status can be achieved through direct questioning of a patient or caregiver, testing in a clinic, or observation in the home. Because a patient's self-reported function is unreliable (Kiyak et al., 1994), the most practical approach for the medical practitioner is to question a caregiver. In some cases consultation with an occupational or physical therapist can be invaluable in determining how a patient performs in a simulated or actual home environment. One should distinguish what the patient actually does from what the patient can do; both are important. The former refers to real needs (which the caregiver is providing), whereas the latter is a measure of that which might potentially be achieved (through rehabilitation, for example).

Although many scales are available to assess function, few validated scales have been developed for use in patients with dementia. Some available scales include the Barthel Activities of Daily Living Scale (Wade, 1992); the Blessed Dementia Scale (Appendix 5) (Blessed et al., 1968); the Bristol Activities of Daily Living Scale (Bucks et al., 1996); the Cleveland Scale of Activities of Daily Living (Mace et al., 1993; Paterson et al., 1992); the Direct Assessment of Functional Status (Loewenstein et al., 1989); the Katz Activities of Daily Living scale (Wade, 1992); the Physical Self-Maintenance and Instrumental Activities of Daily Living Scale of Lawton and Brody (Lawton & Brody, 1969; Reed et al., 1989); the Rapid Disability Rating Scale-2 (Linn & Linn, 1987); the Scale of Functional Capacity (Pfeffer et al., 1982); and the Structured Assessment of Independent Living (Mahurin et al., 1991).

We discuss two scales selected on the basis of documented validity, reliability, and ease of administration: the Older Americans Resources and Services Procedures (OARS) functional assessment scale (Fillenbaum, 1988) and the Functional Assessment Staging Test (FAST) (Sclan & Reisberg, 1992). Several comprehensive scales are available for the rehabilitation or research setting, which we do not discuss.

Modified OARS Instrument

This scale is a modification of an extensive multidimensional assessment instrument that was validated for practical use (Fillenbaum, 1985) (Appendix 6). Subscales of this instrument focus on activities of daily living and instrumental activities of daily living (Fillenbaum, 1988). Measures of ADLs are more useful in moderately or severely demented patients (Reed et al., 1989).

Description

In applying the modified OARS instrument, questions should be addressed to caregivers of patients with dementia. As formulated, the scale addresses the capabilities of the patient as assessed by a caregiver. There are 9 items that address ADLs and 7 items that address IADLs, each on a 3-point scale. A score of 0 indicates complete independence on an item, a score of 1 indicates slight impairment or need for help, and a score of 2 indicates full dependence on the assistance of others. The exception to this approach is the question regarding incontinence as an ADL, which is graded with respect to severity. Each part has been validated as described below.

Administration

The caregiver is usually questioned separately from the patient in order to facilitate honest responses without distressing the patient. For example, the caregiver is asked if the patient "Can use the telephone without help?" If the answer is negative, the score on that item is either 1 or 2. The criterion for independence should be applied strictly. For instance, if someone needs assistance or needs reminding to take medications, the score is 1. Next one asks if the task can be performed with slight assistance or full assistance. If the patient cannot perform the task at all, even with full assistance, the score is 2.

Time to Administer

Five to ten minutes are required for asking about ADLs and IADLs.

Reliability and Validity

The OARS scale has been extensively validated with a sample of more than 6,000 people (Fillenbaum, 1988; Fillenbaum, 1985). A physical therapist examined patients in their homes to determine their self-care capacity, which was compared to the instrument with an excellent agreement between approaches (Kendall's τ = .83; r = .89). The OARS scale incorporates items from Lawton and Brody's scale for Instrumental Activities of Daily Living and the Physical Self-Maintenance Scale (Appendix 7) (Lawton & Brody, 1969; Reed et al., 1989), suggesting concurrent validity. Test-retest reliability and interrater reliability data have both been published. Overall, the reliability coefficient for ADLs is .84 (Fillenbaum, 1988), whereas that for IADLs is .87. The scale has obvious content validity in that the items selected are relevant to daily self-care and the ability to live independently.

Special Considerations

It is important not to ask these questions of demented patients directly. While mildly impaired patients may be accurate, one cannot be sure of their accuracy without asking a caregiver.

Advantages

The scale has been very well studied in a wide range of individuals with a broad spectrum of disabilities. It is valid and reliable. The scales from which this tool has been derived are widely used.

Disadvantages

It is critical to have a reliable caregiver or patient for the administration of this scale. It has not been validated on a population with Alzheimer's disease, although it has been used in a broad spectrum of people, including patients with cognitive impairment. By asking caregivers about the patient's capabilities, the scale may be biased toward overestimating function. Other scales may avoid this bias by addressing actual performance (Wade, 1992).

Functional Assessment Staging (FAST)

The Functional Assessment Staging (FAST) (Appendix 8) is a scale that was developed specifically for functional assessment of elderly people with dementia (Sclan & Reisberg, 1992).

Description

The FAST is an ordinal scale ranging from 1, indicating normal function, to 7, indicating severe dementia. Levels 6 and 7 are divided into specific subscales yielding 16 possible ratings (Sclan & Reisberg, 1992). Each level is indicated by a functional description with adequate detail for clinical scoring

Administration

The FAST score is derived from a caregiver interview.

Time to Administer

Administration of the FAST takes from 15 to 20 minutes.

Reliability and Validity

The FAST was developed by clinicians experienced in the care of patients with dementia. It has face validity as well as convergent validity with psychometric measures and other clinical measures (Sclan & Reisberg, 1992). The intraclass correlation coefficient for interrater agreement was 0.86 (p < 0.01), which represents a high rate of agreement. Correlation with psychometric tests is high, with a range from −0.60 to −0.79 (p < 0.001) (Reisberg et al., 1994). The correlation with the MMSE is 0.83 (Reisberg et al., 1992). The coefficient of reproducibility was 0.99, indicating excellent validity (Sclan & Reisberg, 1992). Progression of disease can be assessed with the FAST.

Special Considerations

By emphasizing functional elements in everyday performance, the FAST allows the clinician to identify areas of difficulty that may be related to caregiving. It is possible that individual patients would not progress in an orderly, hierarchical fashion. The application of this scale in such circumstances is not entirely clear.

Advantages

This scale provides reliable ratings for the early stages of dementia but remains sensitive to differences between subjects in the severe range of cognitive performance, an advantage shared with other functional scales that measure activities of daily living. The FAST can be used to stage patients whose behavioral symptoms interfere with cognitive testing.

Disadvantages

Its application to non-AD dementia has been studied to a limited extent. The relationship between the FAST and other functional scales is not clear inasmuch as studies examining convergent validity are not available.

Global Assessment Instruments

Global measures that give an overall idea of a patient's status are useful both as a summary measure integrating cognitive and functional status and to communicate to families. Global measures have long been used to stage the severity of disease. While global scales have been used when patients have already been diagnosed with dementia, they may also be useful in guiding the earliest steps in diagnosis by integrating all the available clinical information. Two such systems are the Clinical Dementia Rating Scale (CDR) and the Global Deterioration Scale (GDS). They both span the range of severity from mildly to severely impaired. Moreover, both of these scales are responsive to disease progression, which is an essential feature for a scale to be used in grading severity of disease.

Clinical Dementia Rating (CDR)

Description

The CDR (Appendix 9)consists of six domains (memory, orientation, judgment and problem solving, home and hobbies, community affairs, and personal care), each of which is graded on a scale of 0 to 3 (Hughes et al., 1982). Possible scores are: 0 = no impairment; 0.5 = questionable dementia; 1 = mild dementia; 2 = moderate dementia; 3 = severe dementia. While the memory domain is weighted above all others, it is not the sole determinant of the final score.

Administration

Ratings are obtained through a combination of caregiver interview and direct patient assessment. It is important to obtain examples of the patient's behavior in each of the domains while obtaining the functional history. Examples can be presented to the caregiver to facilitate grading if they cannot provide them (see Table 6-3 for questions useful as probes for the CDR). The caregiver should be asked about autobiographic details of the patient and examples of recent activities or events attended by the patient in order to probe the patient's memory in a separate interview. The patient interview is used to refine the gradation in the cognitive domains by mental status testing. Although a standard mental status examination such as the MMSE can be incorporated into the patient interview, additional assessment of memory (especially for recent and remote events), insight (into the memory disorder, for example), problem solving, and abstract reasoning should be performed to grade these domains (see Table 6-4 for examples). An overall CDR score is obtained through a system that assigns a priority to the memory subscore.

The score is the same as the memory score unless at least three of the other items are higher or lower than the memory score, in which case the score is the same as the majority of the items. The exception to this scoring occurs when two items are to one side of the memory score and three items are on the other side. In that situation the score is the same as the memory score (Morris, 1993). When the memory score is 0.5, a score of 0 cannot be obtained; the score must be 0.5 or 1, depending on the score on the other items. If the memory score is 0 but 2 other items are scored 1 or more, then the CDR score would be 0.5.

Time to Administer

An accurate assessment, interviewing the caregiver and the patient independently, takes a minimum of 20 to 30 minutes.

Reliability and Validity

Face validity of the scale follows from the fact that the scale was developed directly from established clinical criteria for the diagnosis of dementia. The scale has also been validated against pathologically verified cases of Alzheimer's disease (Morris et al., 1988) and with prospectively assessed subjects with mild cognitive impairment (Morris et al., 1996). High interrater reliability was found in studies of physicians (Burke et al., 1988) and nonphysicians (McCulla et al., 1989) (weighted kappa = 0.87).

Table 6-3.   Probe Questions for Caregiver Portion of the CDR Interview (adapted from unpublished materials provided by John Morris, M.D.).

1. Memory
   √ Does the patient have problems with her/his thinking or memory? Is this consistent? Does it interfere with everyday activities now? Has it worsened in the last year? Give some examples.
   √ Can the patient recall a short shopping list?
   √ Does the patient recall recent events? What about remote events (such as birthdays, anniversaries, major holidays, places of work)?
   √ Does the patient recall details of events?
   √ Can you give an example of an event which the patient attended in the last week/month, or any unusual event from the last week/month? Provide some details so that I can ask the patient about them later.
   √ Where was the patient born? What is her/his birthday?
   √ Where did the patient go to school? What was the name of the school?

2. Orientation
   √ Does the patient get lost in the home? In the neighborhood? Beyond your neighborhood?
   √ Does the patient usually know where s/he is?
   √ Does the patient usually know the day, month, date, and year?

3. Judgment and Problem Solving
   √ How is the patient's problem solving? Can you give an example? Examples include handling money (e.g., leaving a tip, using a checkbook), or household repairs.
   √ How do you think the patient would handle a household emergency?
   √ How does the patient do in social situations? Does s/he ever interact inappropriately?

4. Home and Hobbies
   √ Has the patient given up his/her job or any chores or hobbies? Give examples of activities that s/he has given up. Good examples include cooking, using appliances, yard work, games.
   √ What is the patient able to do?

5. Community Affairs
   √ What was the patient's last employment?
   √ Why did s/he retire?
   √ Does the patient attend activities outside of the home? Examples of such activities include driving, group discussions, and shopping.

6. Self-Care
   √ Is the patient able to take care of him/herself in terms of everyday activities?
   √ Does the patient need prompting?
   √ Does the patient need assistance in dressing, hygiene, and personal care?

Special Considerations

The caregiver who has the most contact with the patient should be interviewed. Others may not be able to give accurate information. Although the global score is not particularly sensitive to change, sensitivity can be improved by using the total score, which is easily generated by adding the domain scores.

Advantages

The CDR is clinically based. It rates domains beyond psychometric testing, thereby integrating cognitive and functional domains. It is valid and reliable. A sum of the scores gives an overall quantitative severity rating, which could potentially be used for following disease progression. The scale is multidimensional and can be used

Table 6-4. Additional Questions for the Patient Portion of the CDR Interview (adapted from unpublished materials provided by John Morris, M.D.)

1. Memory

    √ Can you give an example of an event that you attended in the last week/month, or any unusual event from the last week/month?

    √ Provide some details (may prompt for the occasion, names of people who were there, and so on).

    √ What was your last employment?

    √ Why did you retire?

    √ Where did you go to school? What was the name of the school?

    √ Where did you grow up?

    √ Where were you born? What is your birthday?

    Use MMSE, Blessed, or other standardized instrument.

2. Orientation

    Use MMSE, Blessed, or other standardized instrument.

3. Judgment and Problem Solving

    I am going to ask you how some words are alike. For example, a pen a pencil are alike because they are both used for writing.

    √ How are an apple and an orange alike?

    √ How are a chair and a table alike?

    √ How are painting and music alike?

    √ What would you do if you arrived in a strange city and you wanted to find a friend whom you knew lived in that city?

    √ How many nickels are there in a dollar?

    √ How many quarters are there in $6.75?

    √ Can you subtract 3 from 21 and keep subtracting 3 from the answer you get?

with people in the community and in institutions.

Another advantage is that it formalizes clinically relevant history taking. This has been applied in a recent study that used the CDR to screen for dementia (Juva et al., 1995). These authors found the sensitivity of the CDR to be 0.95 with a specificity of 0.94. These data suggest that the CDR might make an excellent assessment tool for research studies and clinical practice.

Disadvantages

One disadvantage of this scale is its inability to make distinctions as severely impaired patients continue to deteriorate. Future versions of the CDR will include more gradation at the higher level of severity, but validation of the extended scale is not yet published.

Another potential issue is the lack of language, affect, and problem behavior domains. These items are reflected in the functional domains graded on the CDR. Moreover, changes in affect and problem behaviors occur at all stages of the disease and are therefore not features that can be used for staging. Subgroups of patients may have prominent behavioral characteristics, language impairment, or motor dysfunction as a consequence of specific pathological or neurochemical features that may be evident at an early stage. Although these features may have prognostic implications, they are present early and may persist through the course of disease in individual patients, arguing against inclusion of these items in a staging system. One group of investigators has validated a scale that includes language and behavior domains (Tuokko, 1993)—the Functional Rating Scale (FRS), which is adapted from the CDR.

Global Deterioration Scale (GDS)

The Global Deterioration Scale (GDS) (Appendix (10) was developed by Reisberg and colleagues for staging patients with dementia (Reisberg et al., 1982). It is a widely used scale that has been extensively studied (Eisdorfer et al., 1992).

Description

The Global Deterioration Scale is a hierarchically organized 7-level scale, with a score of 1 representing the absence of cognitive decline and a score of 7 indicating very severe cognitive impairment. It has a parallel structure to the FAST and can be related to traditional global ratings based on cognitive status.

Administration

The scale is derived from a caregiver interview.

Time to Administer

An accurate assessment takes approximately 20 minutes.

Reliability and Validity

Concurrent validity was established for the Global Deterioration Scale by Reisberg (Reisberg et al., 1994) by comparing scores on the Global Deterioration Scale with performance on the MMSE. Reisberg and colleagues also showed that the Global Deterioration Scale correlates significantly ($p < 0.05$) with psychometric tests ($r = .30$ to .60), the Inventory of Psychic and Somatic Complaints—Elderly (IPSC-E; $r = .30$ to .70), CT scan measures ($r = .50$ for sulcal enlargement and .60 for ventricular dilatation), and cerebral blood flow ($r = .70$ to .80) (Reisberg et al., 1988). Longitudinal change can also be assessed (Reisberg et al., 1986).

Interrater reliability for the Global Deterioration Scale is quite high, ranging from 0.82 to 0.97 in different studies (Reisberg et al., 1994).

Special Considerations

The caregiver who has the most contact with the patient should be interviewed. Others may not be able to give accurate information. The scale is applicable to patients living in nursing facilities where the caregivers are the nursing staff. In this situation it may be difficult to find an individual who knows the patient well enough to apply the scale. In such circumstances nursing notes may be relied on. It is generally useful to discuss individual items that might be mentioned in the nursing notes with a caregiver who knows the patient.

Advantages

This scale remains one of the few validated, reliable staging systems for patients with dementia. It can easily be related to a simpler three-stage system: mild (GDS = 2–3); moderate (GDS = 4–5); severe (GDS = 6–7). Furthermore, it is relatively easy to apply (Reisberg et al., 1982). The available version of the Global Deterioration Scale has been validated in patients with severe dementia, an advantage over other available scales.

Disadvantages

Unlike the CDR, in which the structure helps with documenting a dementia diagnosis, this scale is structured such that it presumes a diagnosis of dementia. This is not a major problem because in everyday practice this is usually the case.

To our knowledge, the Global Deterioration Scale has not been validated in pathologically verified cases of Alzheimer's disease.

Behavior/Psychopathology Assessment

Personality and behavior changes are well-documented features of the dementias. Both the American Psychiatry Association's criteria for dementia (APA, 1994) and the NINCDS-ADRDA diagnostic criteria for AD (McKhann et al., 1984) state that changes in personality and behavior are supportive of the diagnosis of dementia. Many new instruments are available to assess various aspects of psychopathology in demented elderly. Some have been developed specifically for use with dementia patients, while others have more general applications. Recent articles have reviewed a broad range of behavioral and psychiatric assessment tools (Teri & Logsdon, 1995; Weiner et al., 1996). This section focuses on those most widely used and/or relevant to dementia in its consideration of measures of psychopathology.

BEHAVE-AD

The Behavioral Pathology in Alzheimer's Disease Rating Scale (BEHAVE-AD) was developed to assess potentially remediable behaviors in patients with AD, independent of cognitive symptomatology (Reisberg et al., 1987). It was intended for use in prospective studies of pharmacologic interventions in the treatment of behavioral symptoms in AD. Items were selected based on chart reviews of outpatients with a diagnosis of Alzheimer's disease. It continues to be a widely used instrument for the assessment of behavioral disturbance.

Description

The BEHAVE-AD is a 25-item scale covering the following domains: paranoid and delusional ideation, hallucinations, activity disturbances, aggressiveness, diurnal rhythm disturbances, affective disturbance, and anxieties and phobias. There is an additional item providing a global rating of behavioral disturbance. Items are rated on a 4-point scale based on a clinical interview with a reliable informant. Each item is rated as not present or by descriptive categories of increasing severity, which are specific to each item. Some items have fairly distinct categories, while others are on a continuum of severity. For example, purposeless activities are rated in terms of the degree of restraint or physical harm resulting from the activity as indicators of severity of the behavior.

Administration

The caregiver is interviewed by a clinician either in person or by telephone interview. Some of the items, such as one related to delusions of infidelity, are more easily rated by spousal caregivers than by other family members or paid caregivers.

Time to Administer

The administration time has been estimated to be approximately 45 minutes (Weiner et al., 1996). Typically, the more numerous the difficult behaviors, the longer the interview.

Reliability and Validity

In a comparison of the BEHAVE-AD, the Brief Psychiatric Rating Scale, and the Cornell Scale for Depression in Dementia, the BEHAVE-AD was found to have the most items rated as occurring frequently in AD patients but not in control subjects (Mack & Patterson, 1994). Eighty-seven percent of those patients were reported to have at least one symptom from the BEHAVE-AD rated as present.

Content validity is based on derivation of items from chart review.

Interrater agreement ranged from 81% to 100% across the 25 items, with an overall agreement of 94% (Mack & Patterson, 1994). When corrected for chance agreement, kappa statistics ranged from 0.29 to 1.00, with a median of 0.70.

Special Considerations

Some items of the BEHAVE-AD make it more suitable for use with spouse caregivers. Similarly, some items assume that the patient lives at home, making this instrument inappropriate for use in nursing homes or assisted living situations. While it provides a good overview of most behavioral disturbances, it is less comprehensive in some domains than other instruments.

Advantages

The items of the BEHAVE-AD address most of the behaviors reported to occur frequently in patients with AD. This scale is a sensitive measure of change in behavioral pathology and has good reliability.

Disadvantages

The items of this scale do not assess frequency of behavior. While caregiver distress or burden can be extrapolated from severity ratings, it is not directly evaluated. Of particular concern is the means of rating severity; for some items the behaviors used to describe severity may be indirectly related to the behavior in question. For example, anger or aggression are frequently used as a benchmark of severity for individual items, although aggressiveness is a separate domain within the scale. Other items indicate severity in terms of impact on caregiver (e.g., "disturbing to caregiver" vs. "intolerable to caregiver").

CERAD Behavior Rating Scale for Dementia (BRSD)

The Consortium to Establish a Registry for Alzheimer's Disease (CERAD) developed this scale to assess a wide range of psychopathology in patients with AD. The CERAD BRSD (Appendix 11) is based on clinical experience and a review of existing instruments and literature to elicit information covering symptoms relevant to dementia (Tariot et al., 1995).

Description

The BRSD consists of 51 items, most of which are rated on a frequency scale ranging from 0 (has not occurred since illness began) to 4 (present 16 days or more in the past month). Ratings are also available for behaviors that have occurred since the illness began but not in the past month. Five items (e.g., changes in appetite and weight) are rated only as present, absent, or having occurred but not in the past month. At the completion of the interview, the clinician rates the validity of the informant's responses. Scores are not totaled, but number of items endorsed can be summed for a rough index of behavioral pathology.

Administration

The patient's informant is questioned by a trained examiner or clinician. Positive responses on certain items require further probing.

Time to Administer

A thorough interview can take approximately 30 to 45 minutes.

Reliability and Validity

Validation of the scale has not yet been performed. However, in the original sample of 303 patients the number of items endorsed increased with increasing dementia severity. Global assessments of behavior or personality change were associated with a greater number of behavior problems on the BRSD. A factor analysis yielded 8 clinically relevant domains: depressive features, psychotic features, defective self-regulation, irritability/agitation, vegetative features, apathy, aggression, and affective lability.

Interrater reliability was calculated for a subset of 104 patients for whom the BRSD was scored simultaneously by two raters. Agreement ranged from 91% to 100% across items.

On the basis of these analyses, the instrument has been modified. Some items have been discarded because of very low frequency of occurrence; others have been reworded to be more inclusive.

Advantages

This scale was developed for use with AD patients. It has been administered to a large sample of carefully characterized subjects with probable Alzheimer's disease. It covers a broad range of psy-chopathology in mildly to moderately impaired patients. Response choices are unambiguous and include the opportunity to report behaviors that have occurred since the illness began but not in the recent past.

Disadvantages

The length of the BRSD makes it impractical in some settings. Many patients will not manifest a large number of the behaviors described, yet the scale must be administered in its entirety. It has yet to be validated on the full range of dementia severity, notably those with very mild or very severe dementia. As a research instrument, it lacks an adequate scoring system.

The Neuropsychiatric Inventory (NPI)

The Neuropsychiatric Inventory (NPI) (Cummings et al., 1994) was developed to assess behavioral disturbances in patients with dementia. Ten domains were selected for evaluation based on the frequency of their occurrence and their potential for distinguishing among the dementias. The NPI was reviewed by a panel of experts who rated the ability of the individual items to capture the important features of each behavioral domain.

Description

This instrument consists of 10 behavioral domains: delusions, hallucinations, dysphoria, anxiety, agitation/aggression, euphoria, disinhibition, irritability/lability, apathy, and aberrant motor behavior. Each domain includes a screening item and 7 to 8 subquestions. For example, if an informant responds in the affirmative to an initial question about hallucinations, 7 additional items describing unusual sensory experiences are administered. If the respondent indicates that a behavior does not occur, the subsequent items in that domain are skipped. Each domain is rated in terms of frequency and severity, yielding a score based on the most aberrant or problematic behavior(s) within that domain. A maximum composite score of 120 is possible for the total NPI.

Administration

Information is obtained from an informed caregiver who is familiar with the patient's premorbid behavior. Daily contact with the patient is considered necessary to be able to respond adequately.

Time to Administer

The format of the NPI, whereby screening questions are sufficient for behaviors that are not present, makes it an efficient way to assess these domains. Administration can take 30 minutes or less, depending on the number of behavioral domains probed.

Reliability and Validity

Content validity was based on ratings by a panel of experts on the adequacy of assessment within each domain. Concurrent validity was determined in a comparison of the NPI with comparable subscales of the BEHAVE-AD. Significant correlations demonstrated that the instruments are describing similar psychopathology. A comparison of AD patients with healthy controls yielded significant differences in scores on all 10 behavioral domains. Overall scores on the NPI were associated with dementia severity.

Interrater agreement ranged from 89% for apathy to 100% for several other subscale scores. Overall test-retest correlations were 0.79 for frequency and 0.86 for severity; all subscale test-retest reliabilities yielded significant correlations. Cronbach's coefficient alpha was 0.88, demonstrating good internal consistency among items of the NPI.

Advantages

The screening approach allows time for more detailed questioning of areas relevant to a particular patient while not belaboring areas that are less germane. This is one of the few scales that was developed with the intention of distinguishing among the dementias based on behavior changes, although as yet those studies have not been performed. The NPI is distinct from others in its assessment of behaviors' frequency, severity, and impact on caregiver.

Disadvantages

It may occur that a caregiver denies problems based on the screening item but would respond in the affirmative to probe items within that domain. These would be missed by use of the screening approach.

While the scales described thus far were developed to provide comprehensive assessments of

behavioral disturbances in dementia patients, the remaining instruments have as their goal the quantification of particular domains of psychopathology. One scale provides a detailed assessment of agitated behaviors, while depressive symptomatology is the focus of several instruments, two of which are described below.

Cohen-Mansfield Agitation Inventory (CMAI)

Agitation has been operationally defined by Jiska Cohen-Mansfield as "inappropriate verbal, vocal, or motor activity that is not judged by an outside observer to result directly from the needs or confusion of the agitated individual" (Cohen-Mansfield & Billig, 1986a). The Cohen-Mansfield Agitation Inventory (CMAI) (Cohen-Mansfield, 1986b) was originally developed as a research instrument for use in nursing homes. Items were selected based on the perceptions of nurses and a review of the literature. A community-based version added several items specific to that population.

Description

The current form of the CMAI consists of 29 items rated on a 7-point scale of frequency, from never to several times an hour. Behaviors are rated on the basis of the prior two weeks. A factor analysis revealed three factors: aggressive behavior (hitting, grabbing, pushing), physically nonaggressive behavior (pacing, repetitive mannerisms, trying to get to a different place), and verbally agitated behavior (complaining, screaming, constant requests for attention). A 14-item short form has been developed, in which behaviors are rated on a 5-point scale. Computation of total scores is not recommended; factor scores or analyses of individual items may provide more meaningful information.

Administration

The CMAI may be self-administered by a caregiver or can be completed by interviewing the informant.

Time to Administer

It should take no longer than 15 to 20 minutes to administer the 29 items in an interview, while caregiver self-administration tends to take less time.

Reliability and Validity

Several studies have reported reliability and validity data for the CMAI. Concurrent validity has been demonstrated by significant correlations with scores on the Nursing Home Behavior Problems Scale (0.91) (Ray et al., 1992) and the Behavioral and Emotional Activities Manifested in Dementia (BEAM-D) (0.91, 0.79, and 0.92 for three nursing home shifts) (Miller et al., 1995). The three factors originally described have been confirmed in other nursing home populations (Miller et al., 1995).

The original manual provides reliability data based on nursing home assessments. Average inter-rater agreement across items ranged from 0.88 to 0.92 across three residential units.

Advantages

The items of the CMAI, by referring to specific observable behaviors, do not rely on caregivers' interpretations of emotional states or causality of symptoms. Each behavior is intended to include multiple closely related behaviors, many of which are described in expanded items. For example, an item concerning the inappropriate handling of objects offers exemplars to assist the informant. Research has shown this to be a reliable measure of behavioral disturbance in nursing home patients.

Disadvantages

While the CMAI offers a comprehensive assessment of a particular domain of behavioral disturbances, it does not address several other symptoms, including disturbances of mood, hallucinations, delusions, and problems of impulse control. Although the original form has been adapted for use with people residing in a community, reliability data are not yet available with that population.

Cornell Scale for Depression in Dementia (CSDD)

Unlike other measures of depression that are more widely used, such as the Beck Depression Inventory (Beck et al., 1961) and the Hamilton Depression Rating Scale (Hamilton, 1960), the Cornell Scale for Depression in Dementia (CSDD) (Appendix 12) was developed specifically for use with dementia patients (Alexopoulos et al., 1988b). As the items of this scale are based primarily on observations, it excludes symptoms that cannot be reliably observed. This measure was designed not as a diagnostic tool but for assessment of mood disturbance in pharmacologic studies.

Description

This 19-item scale assesses 5 domains of mood disturbance: mood-related signs, behavioral disturbance, physical signs, cyclic functions, and ideational disturbance. Ratings are based on interviews with both patient and informant, although primary emphasis is given to caregiver input. Items are rated on a 3-point scale based on observations in the prior week: absent, mild or intermittent, or severe. There is also an "unable to evaluate" response choice. The clinician is instructed to disregard responses based on physical disability or illness, such as in rating weight loss or multiple physical complaints. Recommended cut-off scores are 8 for mild depression and 12 for moderate depression.

Administration

Following interviews with patient and caregiver, the clinicians provide ratings of each behavior. In instances of discrepancy between the two sources of information, greater weight is given to the caregiver's responses.

Time to Administer

Interview of both patient and caregiver should take no longer than 30 minutes.

Reliability and Validity

In a comparison of 5 depression measures, Logsdon and Teri (1995) found the CSDD to be the most sensitive measure in the detection of depression. Scores on the CSDD were able to distinguish between patients with diagnoses of major and minor depression, regardless of the severity of their dementia. Alexopoulos and colleagues (1988a) validated the CSDD in a nondemented patient sample and found that scores discriminated among the diagnostic categories of major depression vs. minor depression vs. other psychiatric diagnoses.

Interrater reliability across items has been reported to range from .82 to 1.00, with overall reliability of .74 (Alexopoulos et al., 1988a). A Kuder-

Richardson coefficient for internal consistency was .98. Mack and Patterson (1994) report interrater agreement across items to range from 0.78 to 1.00. They caution, however, that the restricted range of choices inflates interrater agreement.

Advantages

As one of the few measures of depression in dementia, this scale is particularly suited for AD patients. It contains few items that focus on somatic signs and symptoms that occur commonly in elderly nondepressed patients. Unlike another widely used instrument, the Hamilton Dementia Rating Scale, it does not rely exclusively on patient self-reports, which are notably unreliable in patients with moderate to severe dementia.

Disadvantages

Ratings are based on behaviors in the week prior to the assessment, which may fail to capture behaviors that occur sporadically but are troublesome. The 3-point frequency/severity scale is unlikely to detect subtle changes in behavior. In some instances, it may be difficult to rate symptoms independent of other medical conditions, which may make this scale less appropriate with dementia patients who have comorbidities. Like other measures of specific domains, the CSDD does not provide a comprehensive assessment of the range of behavioral disturbances frequently described in dementia patients.

The Geriatric Depression Scale (GDS)

The Geriatric Depression Scale (GDS) was developed for use with nondemented elderly (Yesavage et al., 1983). It has been widely used in a variety of geriatric populations.

Description

This is a 30-item questionnaire with a yes/no response format. Items are worded to minimize a response bias so that both positive and negative responses can be indicative of depressive symptomatology. Suggested cut-off scores are 11 for mild depression and 14 for moderate depression.

Administration

The GDS is a self-report inventory.

Time to Administer

It should take no longer than 10 minutes to read and respond to the 30 questions. Respondents with more severe dementia might need to have the test items read aloud. (See the following discussion of use of this instrument with severely impaired dementia patients.)

Reliability and Validity

When compared with other measures of depression, Geriatric Depression Scale scores correlated significantly with the Beck Depression Inventory (0.80), the Hamilton Depression Rating Scale (0.32), the Cornell Scale for Depression in Dementia (0.36), and the Center for Epidemiological Studies Depression Scale (0.69) (Logsdon & Teri, 1995). In that study, caregiver surrogate ratings on the Geriatric Depression Scale were found to perform as well as the original self-report measure in describing depressive symptoms in demented elderly. A study of nursing home residents found the Geriatric Depression Scale to have lower sensitivity and specificity in patients with severe levels of dementia (McGivney et al., 1994). They report sensitivity and specificity values as follows: for residents with MMSE scores > 14, sensitivity (84%) and specificity (91%); for MMSE scores < 14, sensitivity (27%) and specificity (69%). They conclude that first determining the level of dementia will greatly improve the utility of the Geriatric Depression Scale in detecting depression.

Advantages

The Geriatric Depression Scale has been shown to be a valid and reliable measure of depression in older adults. It is sensitive to both major and minor depression. As a self-report inventory, it is able to assess mood and internal states that are not amenable to observation. A version that has been modified to be used as a caregiver report has been reported to be equally sensitive and reliable.

Disadvantages

This instrument was not developed for use with demented patients. As a self-report, it is of questionable utility with more severely demented patients whose insight is impaired. Use of the Geriatric Depression Scale in an institutionalized population needs further validation, given the high rate of dementia in nursing home residents.

Summary

We have discussed scales for the assessment of four aspects of dementia: cognition, functional abilities, global function, and behavior. For office use the MMSE and a brief assessment of functional abilities are most useful for initial assessment and follow-up. This could be supplemented by the Clinical Dementia Rating Scale or the Global Deterioration Scale for longitudinal assessment. On the other hand, clinical trials should use a cognitive scale, such as the Alzheimer's Disease Assessment Scale (ADAS), which is more sensitive to clinical change. Early detection of dementia should include tests, such as expanded word lists, that are more sensitive to the earliest manifestations of degenerative dementias. Behavioral assessment is an essential part of the assessment of dementia. All patients should have an assessment of mood using one of the proposed instruments during the diagnostic evaluation. This should be repeated periodically or when the caregiver or patient expresses a complaint that could be explained on the basis of depression. The proposed scales can be used to track the response of a depressed patient to antidepressant medications. It is essential that instruments that grade mood are included in clinical trials. Abnormal behaviors should also be assessed. The Neuropsychiatric Inventory may find use in both the clinic and clinical trials because it is relatively simple to use and may be sensitive enough to change to be useful in longitudinal follow-up. In the clinical practice setting it may necessary to break up the complete evaluation over several visits. The physician need not perform all of the evaluations if adequately trained personnel are available to perform assessments. Clinical trials are usually designed to maximize the use of nonphysician personnel in the assessment of dementia.

In conclusion, clinical scales are an important complement to the routine history and physical examination in the assessment of patients with dementia. These can readily be incorporated into clinical practice and they are an essential part of clinical trials.

Acknowledgment. Supported by grants from the Department of Veterans' Affairs and the Oregon Alzheimer's Disease Center of Oregon Health Sciences University (NIA grant #AG08017). Dana Jones and Joan Pennock assisted in preparing the manuscript.

References

Albert M, Cohen C. The test for severe impairment: an instrument for the assessment of patients with severe cognitive dysfunction. *J Am Ger Soc* 1992;40:449–53.

Albert M, Knoefel J (eds.). *Clinical neurology of aging,* 2nd ed. New York: Oxford University Press, 1994.

Alexopoulos G, Abrams R, Young R, Shamoian C. Cornell scale for depression in dementia. *Biological Psychiatry* 1988b;23:271–84.

Alexopoulos G, Abrams R, Young R, Shamoian C. Use of the Cornell scale in nondemented patients. *J Am Ger Soc* 1988a;36:230–36.

American Psychiatric Association. *Diagnostic and statistical manual of mental disorders: DSM-IV,* 4th ed. Washington, DC: American Psychiatric Association, 1994.

Barberger-Gateau P, Commenges D, Gagnon M, Letenneur L, Sauvel C, Dartigues J. Instrumental activities of daily living as a screening tool for cognitive impairment and dementia in elderly community dwellers. *J Am Ger Soc* 1992;40:1129–34.

Barberger-Gateau P, Dartigues J, Letenneur L. Four instrumental activities of daily living score as a predictor of one-year incident dementia. *Age and Ageing* 1993;22:457–63.

Barclay L (ed.). *Differential diagnosis of gait disorders and falls.* Philadelphia: Lea & Febiger, 1993.

Beck A, Ward C, Mendelson M. An inventory for measuring depression. *Arch Gen Psychiatry* 1961;4:561–71.

Blessed G, Tomlinson B, Roth M. The association between quantitative measures of dementia and of senile change in the cerebral gray matter of elderly subjects. *Brit J Psychiatry* 1968;114:797–811.

Braekhus A, Laake K, Engedal K. A low, "normal" score on the mini-mental state examination predicts development of dementia after three years. *J Am Ger Soc* 1995;43:656–61.

Brodaty H, Howarth G, Mant A, Kurrle S. General practice and dementia—a national survey of Australian GPs. *Med J Australia* 1994;160:10–14.

Bucks R, Ashworth D, Wilcock G, Siegfried K. Assessment of activities of daily living in dementia: development of the Bristol activities of daily living scale. *Age and Ageing* 1996;25:113–20.

Burke W, Miller J, Rubin E, et al. Reliability of the Washington University clinical dementia rating. *Arch Neurol* 1988;45:31–32.

Clarfield A. The reversible dementias: do they reverse? *Ann Int Med* 1988;109:476–86.

Cohen-Mansfield J. Agitated behaviors in the elderly—II. Preliminary results in the cognitively deteriorated. *J Am Ger Soc* 1986b;34:722–27.

Cohen-Mansfield J, Billig N. Agitated behaviors in the elderly—I. A conceptual review. *J Am Ger Soc* 1986a;34:711–21.

Cole M, Dastoor D. A new hierarchic approach to the measurement of dementia. *Psychosomatics* 1987;28:298–304.

Cooper B, Bickel H, Schaufele M. The ability of general practitioners to detect dementia and cognitive impairment in their elderly patients: a study in Mannheim. *Int J Ger Psychiatry* 1992;7:591–98.

Crum R, Anthony J, Bassett S, Folstein M. Population-based norms for the mini-mental state examination by age and education level. *JAMA* 1993;269:2386–91.

Cummings J, Benson D. *Dementia—a clinical approach,* 2nd ed. Boston: Butterworth-Heinemann, 1992.

Cummings J, Mega M, Gray K, Rosenberg-Thompson S, Carusi D, Gornbein J. The neuropsychiatric inventory: comprehensive assessment of psychopathology in dementia. *Neurology* 1994;44:2308–14.

Davis P, Morris J, Grant E. Brief screening tests versus clinical staging in senile dementia of the Alzheimer type. *J Am Ger Soc* 1990;38:129–35.

Eisdorfer C, Cohen D, Paveza G, et al. An empirical evaluation of the global deterioration scale for staging Alzheimer's disease. *Am J Psychiatry* 1992;149:190–94.

Elias J. Normal versus pathological aging: are we screening adequately for dementia? *Exp Aging Res* 1995;21:97–100.

Eslinger P, Damasio A, Benton A. *The Iowa screening battery for mental decline.* Iowa City: University of Iowa Press, 1984.

Fillenbaum G. *Multidimensional functional assessment of older adults: the Duke older Americans resources and services procedures.* Hillsdale, NJ: Lawrence Erlbaum Associates, 1988.

Fillenbaum G. Screening the elderly: a brief instrumental activities of daily living measure. *J Am Ger Soc* 1985;33:698–705.

Fleming K, Adams A, Petersen R. Dementia: diagnosis and evaluation. *Mayo Clin Proc* 1995;70:1093–1107.

Folstein M, Folstein S, McHugh P. "Mini-mental state"—a practical method for grading the cognitive state of patients for the clinician. *J Psychiatric Res* 1975;12:189–98.

Fratiglioni L, Grut M, Forsell Y, Viitanen M, Winblad B. Clinical diagnosis of Alzheimer's disease and other dementias in a population survey. *Arch Neurol* 1992;49:927–32.

Fuld P. Psychological testing in the differential diagnosis of the dementias. In: Katzman R, Terry R, Bick K (eds.). *Aging: Alzheimer's disease.* New York: Raven Press, 1978:185–93.

Galasko D, Abramson I, Corey-Bloom J, Thal L. Repeated exposure to the mini-mental state examination and the information-memory-concentration test results in a practice effect in Alzheimer's disease. *Neurology* 1993;43:1559–63.

Galasko G, Corey-Bloom J, Thal L. Monitoring progression in Alzheimer's disease. *J Am Ger Soc* 1991;39:932–41.

Ganguli M, Belle S, Ratcliff G, Seaberg E, Huff F, von der Porten K, Kuller L. Sensitivity and specificity for dementia of population-based criteria for cognitive impairment: the moVIES project. *J Gerontol* 1993;48:M152–M161.

Grace J, Nadler J, White D, Guilmette T, Giuliano A, Monsch A, Snow M. Folstein vs modified mini-mental state examination in geriatric stroke. *Arch Neurol* 1995;52:477–84.

Hamilton M. A rating scale for depression. *J Neurol Neurosurg Psychiatry* 1960;23:56–62.

Hazzard W, Eierman E, Blass J, Ettinger W Jr, Halter J. *Principles of geriatric medicine and gerontology,* 3rd ed. San Francisco: McGraw-Hill, 1994.

Hughes C, Berg L, Danizger W, Coben L, Martin R. A new clinical scale for the staging of dementia. *Brit J Psychiatry* 1982;140:566–72.

Juva K, Sulkava R, Erkinjuntti T, Ylikoski R, Valvanne J, Tilvis R. Usefulness of the clinical dementia rating scale in screening for dementia. *International Psychogeriatrics* 1995;7:17–24.

Kahn R, Goldfarb A, Pollack M, Peck A. Brief objective measures for the determination of mental status in the aged. *Am J Psychiatry* 1960 (October):326–28.

Katzman R, Brown T, Fuld P, Peck A, Schechter R, Schimmel H. Validation of the short orientation-memory-concentration test of cognitive impairment. *Am J Psychiatry* 1983;140:734–39.

Katzman R, Kawas C (eds.). *The epidemiology of dementia and Alzheimer's disease.* New York: Raven Press, 1994.

Katzman R, Rowe J. *Principles of geriatric neurology.* Philadelphia: F.A. Davis, 1992.

Kawas C, Karagiozis H, Resau L, Gorrada M, Brookmeyer R. Reliability of the Blessed telephone information-memory-concentration test. *J Ger Psychiatry Neurol* 1995;8:238–42.

Kiernan R, Meuller J, Langston J, Van Dyke C. The neurobehavioral cognitive status examination: a brief but differentiated approach to cognitive assessment. *Ann Int Med* 1987;107:734–39.

Kiyak H, Teri L, Borson S. Physical and functional health assessment in normal aging and in Alzheimer's disease: self-reports vs family reports. *The Gerontologist* 1994;34:324–30.

Knopman D, Gracon S. Obervations on the short-term "natural history" of probable Alzheimer's disease in a controlled clinical trial. *Neurology* 1994;44:260–65.

Knopman D, Ryberg S. A verbal memory test with high predictive accuracy for dementia of the Alzheimer's type. *Arch Neurol* 1989;46:141–45.

Kokmen E, Smith G, Peterson R, Tangalos E, Ivnik R. The short test of mental status: correlations with standardized psychometric testing. *Arch Neurol* 1991;48:725–28.

Lawton M, Brody E. Assessment of older people: self-maintaining and instrumental activities of daily living. *J Am Ger Soc* 1969:179–86.

Lezak M. *Neuropsychological assessment,* 3rd ed. New York: Oxford University Press, 1995.

Linn M, Linn B. The rapid disability rating scale-2. *J Am Ger Soc* 1987;30:378–82.

Liu H, Teng E, Hsu T, et al. Performance on a dementia screening test in relation to demographic variables. *Arch Neurol* 1994;51:910–15.

Locascio J, Growdon J, Corkin S. Cognitive test performance in detecting, staging, and tracking Alzheimer's disease. *Arch Neurol* 1995;52:1087–99.

Loewenstein D, Amigo E, Duara R, et al. A new scale for the assessment of functional status in Alzheimer's disease and related disorders. *J Gerontology* 1989;44:P114–P121.

Logsdon R, Teri L. Depression in Alzheimer's disease patients: caregivers as surrogate reporters. *J Am Ger Soc* 1995;43:150–55.

Mace N, Whitehouse P, Smyth K. Management of patients with dementia. In: Whitehouse P (ed.). *Dementia.* Philadelphia: F.A. Davis, 1993:400–11.

Mack J, Patterson M. The evaluation of behavioral disturbances in Alzheimer's disease: the utility of three rating scales. *J Ger Psychiatry Neurol* 1994;7:101–17.

Mahurin R, DeBettignies B, Pirozzolo F. Structured assessment of independent living skills: preliminary report of a performance measure of functional abilities in dementia. *J Gerontology* 1991;42:P58–P66.

Mattis S (ed.). *Status examination for organic mental syndrome in the elderly patient.* New York: Grune & Stratton, 1976.

Mayeux R, Stern Y, Rosen J, Leventhal J. Depression, intellectual impairment, and Parkinson disease. *Neurology* 1981;31:645–50.

McCulla M, Coats M, Van Fleet N, Duchek J, Grant E, Morris J. Reliability of clinical nurse specialists in the staging of dementia. *Arch Neurol* 1989;46:1210–11.

McGivney S, Mulvihill M, Taylor B. Validating the GDS depression screen in the nursing home. *J Am Ger Soc* 1994;42:490–92.

McKhann G, Drachman D, Folstein M, Katzman R, Price D, Stadlan E. Clinical diagnosis of Alzheimer's disease: report of the NINCDS-ADRDA work group under the auspices of Department of Health and Human Services task force on Alzheimer's disease. *Neurology* 1984;34:939–43.

Mendez M, Ala T, Underwood K. Development of scoring criteria for the clock drawing task in Alzheimer's disease. *J Am Ger Soc* 1992;40:1095–99.

Miller R, Snowdon J, Vaughn R. The use of the Cohen-Mansfield agitation inventory in the assessment of behavioral disorders in nursing homes. *J Am Ger Soc* 1995;43:546–49.

Morris J. The clinical dementia rating (CDR): current version and scoring rules. *Neurology* 1993;43(11):2412–14.

Morris J, Heyman A, Mohs R, Hughes M. The consortium to establish a registry for Alzheimer's disease (CERAD) Part 1. Clinical and neuropsychological assessment of Alzheimer's disease. *Neurology* 1989;39:1159–65.

Morris J, McKeel D, Fulling K, Torack R, Berg L. Validation of clinical diagnostic criteria for Alzheimer's disease. *Ann Neurol* 1988;24:17–22.

Morris J, Storandt M, McKeel D Jr, Rubin E, Price J, Grant E, Berg L. Cerebral amyloid deposition and diffuse plaques in "normal" aging: evidence for presymptomatic and very mild Alzheimer's disease. *Neurology* 1996;46:707–19.

Mungas D, Marshall S, Weldon M, Haan M. Age and education correction of mini-mental state examination for English and Spanish-speaking elderly. *Neurology* 1996;46:700–706.

Murden R, McRae T, Kaner S, Bucknam M. Mini-mental state exam scores vary with education in blacks and whites. *J Am Ger Soc* 1991;39:149–55.

Nardone D. Cognitive impairment in primary care. *Ann Int Med* 1996;124:273.

Parks R, Zec R, Wilson R. *Neuropsychology of Alzheimer's disease and other dementias.* New York: Oxford University Press, 1993.

Paterson M, Mack J, Neundorfer M, Smith R, Smyth D, Whitehouse P. Assessment of functional ability in Alzheimer's disease: a review and preliminary report on the Cleveland scale for activities of daily living. *Alzheimer Disease and Associated Disorders* 1992;6:145–63.

Paykel E, Brayne C, Huppert F, et al. Incidence of dementia in a population older than 75 years in the United Kingdom. *Arch Gen Psychiatry* 1994;51:325–32.

Pfeffer R, Kurosaki T, Harrah C, Chance J, Filos S. Measurement of functional activities in older adults in the community. *J Gerontology* 1982;37:323–29.

Pfeiffer E. A short portable mental status questionnaire for the assessment of organic brain deficit in elderly patients. *J Am Ger Soc* 1975;23:433–41.

Ray W, Taylor J, Lichtenstein M, Meador K. The nursing home behavior problem scale. *Journal of Gerontology: Medical Sciences* 1992;47:M9–M16.

Reed B, Jagust W, Seab J. Mental status as a predictor of daily function in progressive dementia. *The Gerontologist* 1989;29(6):804–807.

Reisberg B, Borenstein J, Salob S, Ferris S, Franssen E, Georgotas A. Behavioral symptoms in Alzheimer's disease: phenomenology and treatment. *J Clin Psychiatry* 1987;48:9–15.

Reisberg B, Ferris S, de Leon M, Crook T. Global deterioration scale (GDS). *Psychopharmacol Bull* 1988;24:661–63.

Reisberg B, Ferris S, de Leon M, Crook T. The global deterioration scale for the assessment of primary progressive dementia. *Am J Psychiatry* 1982;139:1136–39.

Reisberg B, Ferris S, Shulman E. Longitudinal course of normal aging and progressive dementia of the Alzheimer's type: a prospective study of 106 subjects over a 3.6 year mean interval. *Prog Neuropsychopharmacol Biol Psychiatry* 1986;10:571–78.

Reisberg B, Ferris S, Torossian C, Kluger A, Monteiro I. Pharmacologic treatment of Alzheimer's disease: a methodologic critique based upon current knowledge of symptomatology and relevance for drug trials. *International Psychogeriatrics* 1992;4:9–42.

Reisberg B, Sclan S, Franssen E, Kluger A, Ferris S. Dementia staging in chronic care populations. *Alzheimer Disease and Associated Disorders* 1994;8:S188–S205.

Roccaforte WH, Burke W, Bayer B, Wengel S. Validation of a telephone version of the mini-mental state examination. *J Am Ger Soc* 1992;40:697–702.

Rosen W, Mohs R, Davis K. A new rating scale for Alzheimer's disease. *Am J Psychiatry* 1984;141:1356–64.

Rothlind J, Brandt J. A brief assessment of frontal and subcortical function in dementia. *J of Neuropsychiatry and Clin Neurosciences* 1993;5:73–77.

Royall D. Precis of executive dyscontrol as a cause of problem behavior in dementia. *Exp Aging Res* 1994;20:73–103.

Saxton J, McGonigle-Gibson K, Swihart A, Miller V, Boller F. Assessment of the severely-impaired patient: description and validation of a new neuropsychological test battery. *Psychological Assessment: A Journal of Consulting and Clinical Psychology* 1990;2:298–303.

Sclan S, Reisberg B. Functional assessment staging (FAST) in Alzheimer's disease: reliability, validity, and ordinality. *International Psychogeriatrics* 1992;4:55–69.

Siu A. Screening for dementia and investigating its causes. *Ann Int Med* 1991;115:122–32.

Spreen O, Strauss E. *A compendium of neuropsychological tests.* New York: Oxford University Press, 1991.

Swirsky-Sacchetti T, Field H, Mitchell D, Seward J, Lublin F, Knobler R, Gonzales C. The sensitivity of the mini-mental state exam in the white matter dementia of multiple sclerosis. *J Clin Psychol* 1992;48:779–86.

Tariot P, Mack J, Patterson M, et al. The behavior rating scale for dementia of the consortium to establish a registry for Alzheimer's disease. *Am J Psychiatry* 1995;152:1349–57.

Teng E, Chui H, Schneider L, Metzger L. Alzheimer's dementia: performance of the mini-mental state examination. *J Consult Clin Psychol* 1987;55:96–100.

Teng E, Wimer C, Damasio R, Eslinger P, Folstein M, Tune L, Whitehouse P, Bardolph E, Chui H. Alzheimer's dementia: performance on parallel forms of the dementia assessment battery. *J Clin Neuropsychol* 1989;11:899–912.

Teri L, Logsdon R. Methodologic issues regarding outcome measures for clinical drug trials of psychiatric complications in dementia. *J of Ger Psy and Neuro* 1995;8:S8–S17.

Terry R, Masliah E, Salmon D, et al. Physical basis of cognitive alterations in Alzheimer's disease: synapse loss is the major correlate of cognitive impairment. *Ann Neurol* 1991;30:575–80.

Tombaugh T, McIntyre N. The mini-mental state examination: a comprehensive review. *J Am Ger Soc* 1992;40:922–35.

Tuokko H. Psychosocial evaluation and management of the Alzheimer's patient. In: Parks R, Zec R, Wilson R (eds.). *Neuropsychology of Alzheimer's disease and other dementias.* New York: Oxford University Press, 1993:565–88.

Tuokko H, Hadjistavropoulos T, Miller J, Beattie B. The clock test: a sensitive measure to differentiate normal elderly from those with Alzheimer's disease. *J Am Ger Soc* 1992;40:579–84.

Uhlmann R, Larson E. Effect of education on the mini-mental state examination as a screening test for dementia. *J Am Ger Soc* 1991;39:876–80.

Wade D. *Measurement in neurologic rehabilitation.* New York: Oxford University Press, 1992.

Weiner M, Koss E, Wild K, Folks D, Tariot P, Luszczynska H, Whitehouse P. Measures of psychiatric symptoms in Alzheimer patients: a review. *Alzheimer Disease and Associated Disorders* 1996;10:20–30.

White H, Davis P. Cognitive screening tests: an aid in the care of elderly outpatients. *J Gen Int Med* 1990;5:438–45.

Whitehouse P. *Dementia.* Philadelphia: F.A. Davis, 1993.

Wind A, Van Staveren G, Schellevis F, Jonker F, Jonker C, Van Eijk J. The validity of the judgement of general practitioners on dementia. *International J Ger Psychiatry* 1994;9:543–49.

Yesavage J, Brink T, Rose T. Development and validation of a geriatric depression screening scale: a preliminary report. *J Psychiatric Res* 1983;17:37-49.

Appendix 1

MINI-MENTAL STATE EXamination

ORIENTATION

Maximum Score	Score	
5	( )	What is the (year)(season)(date)(day)(month)?
5	( )	Where are we: (state)(county)(town)(hospital)(floor)?

REGISTRATION

3	( )	Name 3 objects: 1 second to say each. Then ask the patient all 3 after you have said them. Give 1 point for each correct answer. Then repeat them until he learns all 3. Count trials and record.

Trials _____

ATTENTION AND CALCULATION

5	( )	Serial 7's, 1 point for each correct. Stop after 5 answers. Alternatively, spell "world" backwards.

RECALL

3	( )	Ask for the 3 objects repeated above. One point for each correct answer

LANGUAGE

9	( )	Identify and name a pencil and a watch (2 points) Repeat the following "No ifs, ands, or buts" (1 point) Follow a 3-stage command. "Take a paper in your right hand, fold it in half, and put it on the floor " (3 points) Read and obey the following:

Close your eyes (1 point)

Write a sentence (1 point)
Copy design (angles must intersect properly as shown)(1 point)

Total Score _____

ASSESS level of consciousness along a continuum _____

alert   drowsy   stupor   coma

INSTRUCTIONS FOR ADMINISTRATION

ORIENTATION

(1) Ask for the date. Then ask specifically for parts omitted, e.g., "can you tell me what season it is?" One point for each correct.

(2) Ask in turn "Can you tell me the name of this hospital?" (town, county, etc.) One point for each correct.

REGISTRATION

Ask the patient if you may test his memory. Then say the names of 3 unrelated objects, clearly and slowly, about 1 second for each. After you have said all 3, ask him to repeat them. This first repetition determines his score (0–3) but keep saying them until he can repeat all 3, up to 6 trials. If he does not eventually learn all 3, recall cannot be meaningfully tested.

ATTENTION AND CALCULATION

Ask the patient to begin with 100 and count backwards by 7. Stop after 5 subtractions (93, 86, 79, 72, 65). Score the total number of correct answers.

If the patient cannot or will not perform this task, ask him to spell the word "world" backwards. The score is the number of letters in correct order. E.g., dlrow = 5, dlorw = 3

RECALL

Ask the patient if he can recall the 3 words you previously asked him to remember. Score 0–3.

LANGUAGE

Naming: Show the patient a wrist watch and ask him what it is. Repeat for pencil. Score 0–2.

Repetition: Ask the patient to repeat the sentence after you. Allow only one trial. Score 0 or 1.

Three-stage command: Give the patient a piece of plain blank paper and repeat the command. Score 1 point for each part correctly executed.

Reading: On a blank piece of paper, print the sentence "close your eyes," in letters large enough for the patient to see clearly. Ask him to read it and do what it says. Score 1 point only if he actually closes his eyes.

Writing: Give the patient a blank piece of paper and ask him to write a sentence for you. Do not dictate a sentence; it is to be written spontaneously. It must contain a subject and verb and be sensible. Correct grammar and punctuation are not necessary.

Copying: On a clean piece of paper, draw intersecting pentagons, each side about 1 inch and ask him to copy it exactly as it is. All 10 angles must be present and 2 must intersect to score 1 point. Tremor and rotation are ignored.

Estimate the patient's level of sensorium along a continuum, from alert on the left to coma on the right.

Ref. Folstein MF, Folstein SE and McHugh, 1975

Appendix 2

BLESSED INFORMATION-MEMORY-CONCENTRATION TEST (BIMC)

INFORMATION	POINTS
Name	1
Age	1
Time (hour)	1
Time of day	1
Day of week	1
Date	1
Month	1
Year	1
Place—Name	1
Street	1
Town	1
Type of place (home, hospital, etc.)	1
Recognition of persons (doctor, nurse, receptionist patient, relative—any two available	2 (1 each)

MEMORY

(1) Personal

Date of birth	1
Place of birth	1
School attended	1
Occupation	1
Name of siblings or name of wife	1
Name of any town where patient worked	1
Name of employers	1

(2) Non-personal

*Date of World War I	1
*Date of World War II	1
Name of Monarch	1
Name of Prime Minister	1

Name and Address (5 minute recall)
Mr. John Brown
42 West St.
Gateshead

CONCENTRATION

Months of year backward	2	1	0
Counting 1–20	2	1	0
Counting 20–1	2	1	0
Test 5 minute recall item	5		

*1/2 for approximation within 3 years
Note—for Europeans and Canadians WWII is 1939–45, for U.S. 1941–45
In U.S. use President and Governor

Appendix 3

SHORT (SIX-ITEM) ORIENTATION-MEMORY-CONCENTRATION TEST

Items	Maximum Error	Score		Weight		
1. What year is it now?	1	_____	X	4	=	_____
2. What month is it now?	1	_____	X	3	=	_____
Repeat this phrase: John Brown 42 Market Street Chicago						
3. About what time is it (within 1 hour)?	1	_____	X	3	=	_____
4. Count backwards 20–1.	2	_____	X	2	=	_____
5. Say the months in reverse order.	2	_____	X	2	=	_____
6. Repeat the phrase just given.	5	_____	X	2	=	_____
				Total =		_____

Score of 1 for each incorrect response; maximum weighted error score = 24.

Ref. Katzman et al., 1983

Appendix 4

SHORT TEST OF MENTAL STATUS

Name_____ Date_____

Number:_____ Education_____yrs.

Handedness R__ L__   Sex M__ F__

1. Orientation	Name, address, current location (bldg), city, state, date (day) month, year	_____ (8)
2. Attention	Digit span (present 1/s: record longest correct span) 2-9-6-8-3, 5-7-1-9-4-6, 2-1-5-9-3-6-2	_____(7)
3. Immediate recall	Four unrelated words Learn: "apple, Mr. Johnson, charity, tunnel" (No. of trail needed to learn all four:____)	_____(4)
4. Calculation	5×13, $65 - 7$, $58 \div 2$, $29 + 11$	_____(4)
5. Abstraction	Similarities: orange/banana, dog/horse, table/bookcase	_____(3)
6. Construction	Draw a clock face showing 11:20	_____(2)
	Copy	_____(2)
7. Information	President; first president; define an island; No of weeks/year	_____(4)
8. Recall	The four words "apple, Mr. Johnson, charity, tunnel"	_____(4)
Total score		_____(38)

Subtract 1, 2, or 3 if there were more than 1 trial required to learn the four words.   _____

Adjusted Total Score   _____(38)

Appendix 5

BLESSED DEMENTIA SCALE

Information obtained as much as possible from relative or close and continual contact with patient. Inquiries were directed toward defining changes in capacity, habits and personality. Allowance was made in scoring for physical disabilities that would restrict activities.

Scoring—0 = competent, $1/2$ = partial competence, 1= total incompetence in the particular activity

CHANGES IN PERFORMANCE OF EVERYDAY ACTIVITIES		*POINTS*	
1.	Inability to perform household tasks	1	$1/2$	0
2.	Inability to cope with small sums of money	1	$1/2$	0
3.	Inability to remember short list of items, e.g. shopping list	1	$1/2$	0
4.	Inability to find way about indoors	1	$1/2$	0
5.	Inability to find way about familiar streets	1	$1/2$	0
6.	Inability to interpret surroundings (e.g., to recognize	1	$1/2$	0
	whether in hospital, or at home, to discriminate between patients,	1	$1/2$	0
	doctors and nurses, relatives and hospital staff, etc.)	1	$1/2$	0
7.	Inability to recall recent events (e.g. recent outings, visits of			
	relatives or friends etc.)	1	$1/2$	0
8.	Tendency to dwell in the past	1	$1/2$	0

9.	Eating	
	Cleanly with proper utensils	0
	Messily with spoon only	2
	Simple solids, e.g., biscuits	2
	Has to be fed	3

10.	Dressing	
	Unaided	0
	Occasionally misplaced buttons, etc.	1
	Wrong sequence, commonly forgetting items	2
	Unable to dress	3

11.	Continence	
	Complete sphincter control	0
	Occasionally wets bed	1
	Frequently wets bed	2
	Doubly incontinent	3

Change in Personality, Interests, Drive

	No change	0
12.	Increased rigidity	1
13.	Increased egocentricity	1
14.	Impairment in feelings for others	1
15.	Coarsening of affect	1

16.	Impairment of emotional control, e.g., increased petulance and irritability	1
17.	Hilarity in inappropriate situations	1
18.	Diminished emotional responsiveness	1
19.	Sexual misdemeanor (appearing *de novo* in old age)	1
	Interest retained	0
20.	Hobbies relinquished	1
21.	Diminished initiative or growing apathy	1
22.	Purposeless hyperactivity	1

Appendix 6

ADCO
MODIFIED ACTIVITIES OF DAILY LIVING/ INSTRUMENTAL ACTIVITIES OF DAILY LIVING (ADL/ IADL)
OARS Methodology Adaptation

Office Use Only

Clinic Site Patient ID#   Patient Designation Evaluation #

Patient Name _____ Medical Record # _____

Evaluation Date [M][D][Y] Evaluating Clinician _____

Name of Person Completing Form _____ Date Completed _____

Activities of Daily Living - ADL

Assistance Needed

Unless otherwise specified, Score:
0 None
1 Slight
2 Full

1. Eating ⌴
2. Dressing and undressing ⌴
3. Combing hair and shaving ⌴
4. Walking ⌴
5. Getting in and out of bed ⌴
6. Bathing or showering ⌴
7. Toileting ⌴
8. Incontinence ⌴

Score:
0 Never
1 Once or twice/ week
2 Three or more times/ week

9. Needs help with shopping, bathing, housework, and/ or getting around? ⌴

Total ADL Score ⌴

Instrumental Activities of Daily Living - IADL

Assistance Needed

Score:
0 None
1 Slight
2 Full

1. Using telephone ⌴
2. Traveling by car, bus, or taxi ⌴
3. Shopping for food and clothing ⌴
4. Preparing meals ⌴
5. Doing housework ⌴
6. Taking own medicine ⌴
7. Handling own money ⌴

Total IADL Score ⌴

Appendix 7

Physical Self-Maintenance Scale (PSMS)

The Physical Self-Maintenance Scale (PSMS) is a valuable tool to assess and monitor the Alzheimer's patient. The PSMS rates the patient's competence in six activities of daily living. Total scores range from 6 to 30, with lower scores indicating less impairment.

Patient's Name: _____   Date: _____

Check *one* response to each of the following items which best describes this patient. Add the number of points and fill in total score at bottom.

1. Toilet
1 ☐ Cares for self at toilet completely, no incontinence.
2 ☐ Needs to be reminded, or needs help in cleaning self, or has rare (weekly at most) accidents.
3 ☐ Soiling or wetting while asleep more than once a week.
4 ☐ Soiling or wetting while awake more than once a week.
5 ☐ No control of bowels or bladder.

2. Feeding
1 ☐ Eats without assistance.
2 ☐ Eats with minor assistance at mealtimes, and/or with special preparation of food, or help in cleaning up after meals.
3 ☐ Feeds self with moderate assistance and is untidy.
4 ☐ Requires extensive assistance for all meals.
5 ☐ Does not feed self at all and resists efforts of others to feed him/her.

3. Dressing
1 ☐ Dresses, undresses, and selects clothes from own wardrobe.
2 ☐ Dresses and undresses self if clothes are preselected.
3 ☐ Needs some assistance in dressing even when clothes are preselected.
4 ☐ Needs major assistance in dressing but cooperates with efforts of others to help.
5 ☐ Completely unable to dress self and/or resists efforts of others to help.

4. Grooming (neatness, hair, nails, hands, clothing)
1 ☐ Always neatly dressed, well-groomed without assistance.
2 ☐ Grooms self adequately with occasional minor assistance, eg, shaving.
3 ☐ Needs moderate and regular assistance or supervision in grooming.
4 ☐ Needs total grooming care but can remain well-groomed after help from others.
5 ☐ Actively negates all efforts of others to maintain grooming.

5. Physical Ambulation
1 ☐ Goes about grounds or city.
2 ☐ Ambulates within residence or within about a one block radius.
3 ☐ Ambulates with assistance of another person or using railing, cane, walker, or wheelchair.
4 ☐ Sits unsupported in chair or wheelchair but cannot propel self without help.
5 ☐ Bedridden more than half the time.

6. Bathing
1 ☐ Bathes self (tub, shower, sponge bath) without help.
2 ☐ Bathes self with help in getting in and out of tub.
3 ☐ Washes face and hands easily but cannot bathe rest of body.
4 ☐ Does not wash self but is cooperative with those who bathe him/her.
5 ☐ Does not try to wash self and/or resists efforts to keep him/her clean.

☐ **Total Score**

Appendix 8

FUNCTIONAL ASSESSMENT STAGING (FAST)[1]

(Check highest **consecutive** level of disability.)

1. ☐   No difficulty, either subjectively or objectively.

2. ☐   Complains of forgetting location of objects. **Subjective work difficulties.**

3. ☐   Decreased job functioning evident to co-workers. Difficulty in traveling to new locations. **Decreased organizational capacity.***

4. ☐   **Decreased ability to perform complex tasks,** e.g., planning dinner for guests, handling personal finances (such as forgetting to pay bills), difficulty marketing, etc.*

5. ☐   **Requires assistance in choosing proper clothing** to wear for the day, season, or occasion, e.g., patient may wear the same clothing repeatedly, unless supervised.*

6. ☐   (a)   **Improperly putting on clothes without assistance or cuing** (e.g., may put street clothes on over night clothes, or put shoes on wrong feet, or have difficulty buttoning clothing) occasionally or more frequently over the past weeks.*

   ☐   (b)   Unable to bathe properly (e.g., **difficulty adjusting bath-water temperature)** occasionally or more frequently over the past weeks.*

   ☐   (c)   **Inability to handle mechanics of toileting** (e.g., forgets to flush the toilet, does not wipe properly or properly dispose of toilet tissue) occasionally or more frequently over the past weeks.*

   ☐   (d)   **Urinary incontinence** (occasionally or more frequently over the past weeks).*

   ☐   (e)   **Fecal incontinence** (occasionally or more frequently over the past weeks).*

7. ☐   (a)   Ability to speak limited to approximately **a half a dozen intelligible different words or fewer,** in the course of an average day or **in the course of an intensive interview.**

   ☐   (b)   Speech ability limited to the use of **a single intelligible word** in an average day or **in the course of an intensive interview** (the person may repeat the word over and over).

   ☐   (c)   Ambulatory ability lost (**cannot walk without personal assistance).**

   ☐   (d)   **Cannot sit up without assistance** (e.g., the individual will fall over if there are no lateral rests [arms] on the chair).

   ☐   (e)   **Loss of ability to smile.**

   ☐   (f)   **Loss of ability to hold up head independently.**

* Scored primarily on the basis of information obtained from a knowledgeable informant and/or caregiver.

[1] Reisberg, B. Functional assessment staging (FAST). Psychopharmacology Bulletin, 1988; 24:653–659.

Appendix 9

Clinical Dementia Rating (CDR)

	None **0**	Questionable **0.5**	Impairment Mild **1**	Moderate **2**	Severe **3**
Memory	No memory loss or slight inconstant forgetfulness	Consistent slight forgetfulness; partial recollection of events; "benign" forgetfulness	Moderate memory loss; more marked for recent events; defect interferes with everyday activities	Severe memory loss; only highly learned material retained; new material rapidly lost	Severe memory loss; only fragments remain
Orientation	Fully oriented	Fully oriented except for slight difficulty with time relationships	Moderate difficulty with time relationships; oriented for place at examination; may have geographic disorientation elsewhere	Severe difficulty with time relationships; usually disoriented to time, often to place	Oriented to person only
Judgment and Problem Solving	Solves everyday problems and handles business and financial affairs well; judgment good in relation to past performance	Slight impairment in solving problems, similarities, and differences	Moderate difficulty in handling problems, similarities, and differences; social judgment usually maintained	Severely impaired in handling problems, similarities, and differences; social judgment usually impaired	Unable to make judgments or solve problems
Community Affairs	Independent function at usual level in job, shopping, and volunteer and social groups	Slight impairment in these activities	Unable to function independently at these activities although may still be engaged in some; appears normal to casual inspection	No pretense of independent function outside home Appears well enough to be taken to functions outside a family home	Appears too ill to be taken to functions outside a family home
Home and Hobbies	Life at home, hobbies, and intellectual interests well maintained	Life at home, hobbies, and intellectual interests slightly impaired	Mild but definite impairment of function at home; more difficult chores abandoned; more complicated hobbies and interests abandoned	Only simple chores preserved; very restricted interests, poorly maintained	No significant function in home
Personal Care	Fully capable of self-care		Needs prompting	Requires assistance in dressing, hygiene, keeping of personal effects	Requires much help with personal care; frequent incontinence

Score only as decline from previous usual level due to cognitive loss, not impairment due to other factors.

Appendix 10

GLOBAL DETERIORATION SCALE (GDS)[1]

(Choose the most appropriate global stage based upon cognition and function.)

☐ 1.   No subjective complaints of memory deficit. No memory deficit evident on clinical interview.

☐ 2.   **Subjective complaints of memory deficit**, most frequently in following areas:
   (a)   forgetting where one has placed familiar objects;
   (b)   forgetting names one formerly knew well.

No objective evidence of memory deficit on clinical interview.
No objective deficit in employment or social situations.
Appropriate concern with respect to symptomatology.

☐ 3.   **Earliest clear-cut deficits.**

Manifestations in more than one of the following areas:
   (a)   patient may have gotten lost when travelling to an unfamiliar location.
   (b)   co-workers become aware of patient's relatively poor performance.
   (c)   word and/or name finding deficit become evident to intimates.
   (d)   patient may read a passage or book and retain relatively little material.
   (e)   patient may demonstrate decreased facility remembering names upon introduction to new people.
   (f)   patient may have lost or misplaced an object of value.
   (g)   concentration deficit may be evident on clinical testing.

Objective evidence of memory deficit obtained **only with an intensive interview.**
Decreased performance in demanding employment and social settings.
Denial begins to become manifest in patient.
Mild to moderate anxiety frequently accompanies symptoms.

☐ 4.   Clear-cut deficit on careful clinical interview.

Deficit manifest in following areas:
   (a)   decreased knowledge of current and recent events.
   (b)   may exhibit some deficit in memory of one's personal history.
   (c)   concentration deficit elicited on serial subtractions.
   (d)   decreased ability to travel, **handle finances**, etc.

Frequently no deficit in following areas:
   (a)   orientation to time and place.
   (b)   recognition of familiar persons and faces.
   (c)   ability to travel to familiar locations.

Inability to perform complex tasks.
Denial is dominant defense mechanism.
Flattening of affect and withdrawal from challenging situations.

Appendix 11

ADCO
Blessed Dementia Rating Scale
(BDRS - CERAD Version)

Office Use Only

| Clinic Site | Patient ID# | Patient Designation | Evaluation # |

Patient Name _____   Medical Record # _____

Evaluation Date |__|__||__|__||__|__| Evaluating Clinician _____
  M   D   Y

Name of Person Completing Form _____   Date Completed _____

Memory and Performance of Everyday Activities

Loss of Ability

| Unless otherwise specified, score: |
| 0 None |
| 0.5 Some |
| 1 Severe |

1. Ability to perform household tasks |__|.|__|

2. Ability to cope with small sums of money |__|.|__|

3. Ability to remember short list of items (e.g. , shopping list) |__|.|__|

4. Ability to find way around indoors (patient's home or other familiar locations) |__|.|__|

5. Ability to find way around familiar streets |__|.|__|

6. Ability to grasp situations or explanations |__|.|__|

7. Ability to recall recent events |__|.|__|

8. Tendency to dwell in the past |__|.|__|

> **Score:**
> 0 None
> 0.5 Some
> 1 Frequent

Subscore |__|.|__|

Habits

Assistance Needed

9. Eating

   Score:
   0 Feeds self without assistance |__|
   1 Feeds self with minor assistance
   2 Feeds self with much assistance
   3 Has to be fed

10. Dressing

    Score:
    0 Unaided |__|
    1 Occasionally misplaces buttons, etc., requires minor help
    2 Wrong sequence, forgets items, requires much assistance
    3 Unable to dress

11. Toileting

    Score:
    0 Clean, cares for self at toilet |__|
    1 Occasional incontinence, or needs to be reminded
    2 Frequent incontinence, or needs much assistance
    3 No control

Subscore |__|

Total BDRS Score |__|__|.|__|
  (0-17)

Appendix 12

CORNELL SCALE FOR DEPRESSION IN DEMENTIA

Name _____ Age___ Sex___ Date _____

Address _____Telephone _____

Inpatient ___   Nursing home resident ___   Outpatient ___

Scoring System

a = unable to evaluate   1 = mild or intermittent
0 = absent   2 = severe

Ratings should be based on symptoms and signs occurring during the week prior to interview. No score should be given if symptoms result from physical disability or illness.

A. Mood-Related Signs

1. Anxiety   a. 0 1 2
    anxious expression, ruminations, worrying
2. Sadness   a. 0 1 2
    sad expression, sad voice, tearfulness
3. Lack of reactivity to pleasant events.   a. 0 1 2
4. Irritability   a. 0 1 2
    easily annoyed, short tempered

B. Behavioral Disturbance

5. Agitation   a. 0 1 2
    restlessness, hand wringing, hair pulling
6. Retardation   a. 0 1 2
    slow movements, slow speech, slow reactions
7. Multiple physical complaints.   a. 0 1 2
    (score 0 if GI symptoms only)
8. Loss of interest   a. 0 1 2
    less involved in usual activities (score only if change occurred
    acutely, i.e., in less than 1 month)

C. Physical Signs

9. Appetite loss   a. 0 1 2
    eating less than usual
10. Weight loss   a. 0 1 2
    (score 2 if greater than 5 lbs. in 1 month)
11. Lack of energy   a. 0 1 2
    fatigues easily, unable to sustain activities
    (score only if change occurred acutely, i.e., in
    less than 1 month)

D. Cyclic Functions

12. Diurnal variation of mood symptoms worse in the morning   a. 0 1 2
13. Difficulty falling asleep   a. 0 1 2
    later than usual for this individual

14. Multiple awakenings during sleep   a. 0 1 2
15. Early morning awakening   a. 0 1 2
    earlier than usual for this individual

E. Ideational Disturbance

16. Suicide   a. 0 1 2
    feels life is not worth living, has suicidal wishes, or
    makes suicide attempt
17. Poor self-esteem   a. 0 1 2
    self-blame, self-depreciation, feelings of failure
18. Pessimism   a. 0 1 2
    anticipation of the worst
19. Mood-congruent delusions   a. 0 1 2
    delusions of poverty, illness, or loss

Ref. Alexoupoulos et al., 1988

CHAPTER 7 Clinical Stroke Scales

Wayne M. Clark, M.D.,
and J. Maurice Hourihane, M.B., M.R.C.P.I.

The ideal method of assessing a patient's deficit following a stroke has not yet been determined. Early clinical stroke therapy trials relied heavily on detailed neurologic scales such as the NIH Stroke Scale (NIHSS) to quantify a patient's deficits. Arbitrary levels of improvement, e.g., 4 points in the total scale score, were set as primary efficacy endpoints and were used to test whether a drug was therapeutically beneficial. It soon became clear that such arbitrary endpoints may not be clinically meaningful in terms of the patient's recovery. For example, a severe stroke patient could have a 4-point improvement on the NIHSS and yet remain confined to bed. Further, the various numeric ratings for each subset of the scales are arbitrary and may not accurately reflect the impact such deficits have on the patient. For instance, a moderate aphasia is given 2 points on the NIHSS, the same as a hemisensory numbness. For these reasons, beginning in the early 1990s, there has been a general trend toward assessing patients' level of function using a variety of functional outcome assessments as opposed to relying solely on detailed neurologic examination scores. This change is illustrated by the recently published NIH tPA stroke treatment study results (NINDS rt-PA Stroke Study Group, 1995). In part 1 of the study primary efficacy was assessed using a 4-point improvement on the NIHSS, whereas in part 2 various functional outcome measures were used to determine the final efficacy for the tPA treated patients.

Functional outcome testing measures are generally much easier to administer and have far fewer gradations than scales based on neurologic examination. Taking this simplified outcome assessment to an extreme, the most reliable efficacy endpoint would be to determine if the patient is normal or abnormal. This 2-point functional outcome assessment has been advocated by some investigators (Zivin & Waud, 1992). A problem with the simplified outcome assessments is that patients can achieve a fairly normal score and still have significant cognitive deficits. A patient may be able to perform all activities of daily living (ADLs) and still have problems with cortical functioning and be unable to return to his or her prior level of employment. A combination of these two techniques, with weighting given to functional outcome as well as more detailed neurologic evaluations, would be the ideal method of determining outcome. To date, such a method has not been validated.

This chapter reviews both the detailed neurologic deficit stroke scales and the commonly used functional outcome scales that are currently employed in stroke therapeutic efficacy trials.

Neurologic Deficit Stroke Scales

National Institutes of Health Stroke Scale (NIHSS)

The NIHSS (Table 7-1) was developed by investigators at the University of Cincinnati Stroke Center to quantify neurologic status in stroke patients. This scale is in widespread use in a variety of stroke therapy efficacy trials.

Description

The NIHSS was developed to quantify neurologic deficit status in stroke patients and is based on a scale originally devised at the University of Cincinnati Stroke Center (Brott et al., 1989a; Goldstein et al., 1989). It was revised in 1994 to measure both affected and nonaffected sides (Lyden et al., 1994). Its primary use is to determine drug efficacy comparing initial evaluations at baseline in acute stroke patients to three-month follow-up assessment performed by the same examiner. The NIHSS is a 24-point scale (11 items), with zero being a normal score. Patients receive points depending on different areas of deficit. They are scored on their initial actual performance, not on what the evaluator thinks they should be able to do. In general, patients are also given the worst possible score if they are unable to perform a task. A patient who is completely mute from severe aphasia also receives 2 points for severe dysarthria even though he or she cannot actually speak at all. In general, patients who score higher than 15 points are assumed to have had a major stroke; a score of 4–15 points is indicative of a moderate stroke, and less than 4 points is considered a mild stroke. This less than 4-point criterion is frequently used by stroke studies to exclude patients with minimal deficit. In several studies an additional assessment of distal motor function has been added.

Validation

The NIHSS has high interrater reliability among neurologists, emergency room physicians, house officers, and stroke research nurses (Goldstein et al., 1989). It has also been shown to have high criterion validity by predicting stroke lesion size on brain computed tomography (Brott et al., 1989a,b). This scale has been clinically validated in several drug therapy stroke trials (Brott et al., 1992; Haley et al., 1993; Haley et al., 1993).

Administration

The NIHSS is performed during the bedside neurologic evaluation. Although the exam could be performed by anyone with neurologic examination experience, it is now recommended that it be administered only by individuals who have passed a certification tape examination. Although many stroke studies require a board certified neurologist to perform the test, it can actually be performed by neurologists, ER physicians, or neurologic nurses, provided that they have passed the certification examination. This certification process improves intrarater reliability.

The test takes approximately 5 minutes to administer and another 5 minutes to record the proper scores.

Special Considerations

One of the main advantages of the NIHSS is that there is an associated training tape and certification examination. The tape consists of 6 patient examples for which a neurologist points out the proper scoring of the case (Lyden et al., 1994). Following the viewing of this training tape, the individual sees 6 new cases and scores them appropriately. The scoring sheets are sent to a certification center and the individual is notified whether he or she passed the examination. The use of this certification examination greatly increases the reliability of the scale. Individuals interested in obtaining the training and certification tape are directed to contact the National Institute of Neurological Disorders and Stroke or the National Stroke Association.

Advantages/Disadvantages

The advantage of the NIHSS is that it can be rapidly performed in the acute stroke setting. It has been well validated in a large number of studies. The training tape, along with the certification exam, is an added feature that insures high reliability between raters. The scale is easy to learn; with the aid of the training tape, people can become highly

Table 7-1.   The Modified National Institutes of Health Stroke Scale.

Item	Name	Response
1A	Level of consciousness	0 = Alert 1 = Not alert, but arousable easily 2 = Not alert, obtunded 3 = Unresponsive
1B	Questions	0 = Answers both correctly 1 = Answers one correctly 2 = Answers neither correctly
1C	Commands	0 = Performs both tasks correctly 1 = Performs one task correctly 2 = Performs neither task correctly
2	Gaze	0 = Normal 1 = Partial gaze palsy 2 = Total gaze palsy
3	Visual fields	0 = No visual loss 1 = Partial hemianopsia 2 = Complete hemianopsia 3 = Bilateral hemianopsia
4	Facial palsy	0 = Normal 1 = Minor paralysis 2 = Partial paralysis 3 = Complete paralysis
5	Motor arm a. Left b. Right	0 = No drift 1 = Drift before 10 seconds 2 = Falls before 10 seconds 3 = No effort against gravity 4 = No movement
6	Motor leg a. Left b. Right	0 = No drift 1 = Drift before 5 seconds 2 = Falls before 5 seconds 3 = No effort against gravity 4 = No movement
7	Ataxia	0 = Absent 1 = One limb 2 = Two limbs
8	Sensory	0 = Normal 1 = Mild loss 2 = Severe loss
9	Language	0 = Normal 1 = Mild aphasia 2 = Severe aphasia 3 = Mute or global aphasia

Table 7-1.   *(continued)*

Item	Name	Response
10	Dysarthria	0 = Normal
		1 = Mild
		2 = Severe
11	Extinction/inattention	0 = Normal
		1 = Mild
		2 = Severe

There are 15 items in this version of the NIHSS. Complete scale with instructions can be obtained from the National Institute of Neurological Disorders and Stroke (Lyden et al., 1994).

competent in its use following a single afternoon training session.

A disadvantage of the NIHSS scale is that it is not good for posterior circulation strokes. The scale is weighted toward language-related functions and, as such, individuals who have mainly brainstem features may receive scores that are less severe despite significant deficits.

Summary

The NIHSS is the most commonly used clinical rating score for acute stroke patients. This scale has been well validated in stroke patients and provides an additional advantage of having a training tape available. Its ease of use and associated training tape make it the most widely recommended scale for evaluating acute stroke patients in the United States. It shows the weakness of all neurologic scores in that changes in the exam may not accurately reflect meaningful changes in the patient's status.

Scandinavian Stroke Scale (SSS)

The SSS was developed to test therapeutic efficacy of hemodilution treatment in acute middle cerebral artery stroke (Scandinavian Stroke Study Group, 1985; Scandinavian Stroke Study Group, 1987; Lindenstrøm et al., 1991). The scale is currently in widespread use to determine therapeutic efficacy of a variety of potential stroke treatments in Europe.

Description

The SSS is a 9-item scale consisting of both a prognostic score and a long-term score. The prognostic score includes measures of consciousness, gaze palsy, and limb weakness. It is designed to stratify patients into several groups, depending on their prognosis for survival. The long-term score is meant for repeated evaluations of the patient during follow-up. The long-term score does not include consciousness or gaze palsy but does include limb strength, aphasia, facial palsy, orientation, and gait (see Table 7-2). Limb strength is rated only on the symptomatic side. Unlike the NIH score, visual fields, ocular motor function, and sensation are not included. A score of 48 indicates normal performance on the long-term exam. The SSS is most suitable for assessing deficits in the carotid artery.

Validation

The SSS has been shown to have high interrater and intrarater reliability (Lindenstrøm et al., 1991). It has been clinically validated in several stroke studies (Scandinavian Stroke Study Group, 1985; Scandinavian Stroke Study Group, 1987; Lindenstrøm et al., 1991).

Administration

The score is calculated during the bedside neurologic exam. Anyone with neurologic examination experience could administer it, although it has only been validated for neurologists. It takes approximately 5 minutes to administer.

Special Considerations

Acute stroke patients with scores of 40 or greater on the SSS long-term have a high likelihood of spontaneous recovery. Scores of less than 40 resulted in incomplete recovery. Therefore, the 40 point cut-off is frequently used as an inclusion criterion for acute stroke trials.

Advantages/Disadvantages

The SSS is easy to administer and can be performed with minimal prior training as part of the neurologic evaluation. It is one of the few scales that includes gait as one of the items to be tested. Gait evaluation is an important component of the patient's outcome. One of the main disadvantages is that the scale is weighted heavily toward middle cerebral artery stroke, so a patient with a substantial brainstem infarction may not be adequately assessed.

Summary

The SSS is an easily administered neurologic scoring scale for acute middle cerebral artery stroke patients. It has been well validated and is in widespread use in several European stroke studies.

Orgogozo Scale

The Orgogozo scale, also called the Neurological Scale for Middle Cerebral Artery Infarction, is a neurologic deficit scale designed to test the degree of deficit in middle cerebral artery infarction patients.

Table 7-2. The Unified Neurological Stroke Scale (Combination of the Scandinavian Stroke Scale and the Orgogozo Scale)

Item		SSS	Orgogozo
Consciousness	Normal/fully conscious	6	15
	Somnolent/drowsiness	4	10
	Reacts to verbal command	2	10
	Stupor (reacts to pain only)	0	5
	Coma	0	0
Orientation	Correct for time, place, person	6	—
	Two of these	4	—
	One of these	2	—
	Completely disoriented	0	—
Speech/verbal	Normal/no aphasia	10	10
Communication	Limited vocabulary or incoherent speech/difficult	6	5
	More than yes-no but not longer sentences/difficult	3	5
	Only yes-no or less/extremely difficult or impossible	0	0
Eye movements/ eyes and head shift	No gaze palsy/none	4	10
	Gaze palsy/gaze failure	2	5
	Conjugate eye deviation/forced	0	0
Facial palsy	None/dubious/slight paresis	2	5
	Present/paralysis or marked paresis	0	0
Gait	Walks at least 5 m without aids	12	—
	Walks with aids	9	—
	Walks with help of another person	6	—
	Sits without support	3	—
	Bedridden/wheelchair	0	—
Arm: motor power/ raising	Raises with normal strength/normal	6	10
	Raises with reduced strength/possible	5	10
	Raises with flexion in elbow/incomplete	4	5
	Can move but not against gravity/impossible	2	0
	Paralysis	0	0
Hand: motor power/ movements	Normal strength/normal	6	15
	Reduced strength/skilled	4	10
	Fingertips do not reach palm/useful	2	5
	Paralysis/useless	0	0
Leg: motor power/ raising	Normal strength	6	15
	Raises with reduced strength/against resistance	5	10
	Raises with flexion of knee/against gravity	4	5
	Can move, but not against gravity/impossible	2	0
	Paralysis	0	0

Table 7-2.   *(continued*

Item		SSS	Orgogozo
Foot dorsiflexion	Against resistance/normal	—	15
	Against gravity	—	5
	Foot drop	—	0
Upper limb tone	Normal (even if brisk reflexes)	—	5
	Overtly spastic or flaccid	—	0
Lower limb tone	Normal (even if brisk reflexes)	—	5
	Overtly spastic or flaccid	—	0

Description

The scale is rated from 0 to 100, with 100 being normal (Orgogozo et al., 1983; Orgogozo & Dartigues, 1986) (see Table 7-2). The scale is weighted heavily to measure hemiplegia due to middle cerebral artery infarction. As such, patients receive scores for both upper and lower extremity weakness and abnormalities of tone. Facial abnormalities are given minimal weighting, and there are no assessments of confusion, visual fields, or sensory deficits. Consciousness is rated on a 3-point scale.

Validation

Interrater reliability is very high even when the scale is used by less trained personnel (Orgogozo & Dartigues, 1991). The items have good construct validity and have been shown to be a powerful predictor of neurologic outcome (Orgogozo & Dartigues, 1986). The scale has been changed from its original form to improve interrater reliability (Orgogozo & Dartigues, 1986).

Administration

Due to the additional tone and detailed motor assessments for this scale, some expertise with a general neurologic evaluation is required of the examiner. This scale can be performed in approximately 10 minutes.

Advantages/Disadvantages

The main advantage of the Orgogozo scale is the detailed assessment of the patient's motor weakness. A disadvantage is the minimal assessment of neurologic items outside of motor weakness. An additional disadvantage is that it has not been used in any large clinical drug trials.

Summary

Although it is a potentially important method of determining motor outcome of a patient, the Orgogozo scale is not in widespread use. Several of the other stroke scales are easier to learn and have greater clinical validation.

Canadian Neurologic Scale

The Canadian neurologic scale (Table 7-3) was designed as a simple clinical instrument to be used by neurologists and nonphysicians alike to evaluate and monitor the neurologic status of acute stroke patients (Côté et al., 1989; Côté et al., 1986).

Description

The 8-item scale measures level of consciousness, orientation, speech, motor function, and facial weakness for a maximum score of 10 points in the normal patient. A separate section measuring motor response is used for patients who have comprehension deficits.

Validation

Validation and reliability have been measured extensively by Côté (Côté et al., 1988). Criterion validity was shown in that the test was able to accurately predict morbidity and mortality; patients with low total scores had higher mortality at six months, along with a greater incidence of recurrent strokes (Côté et al., 1989). Interobserver agreement levels of 0.92 have been reported with this scale (Côté et al., 1989). The scale has been used in several clinical trials evaluating neuroprotective efficacy.

Advantages/Disadvantages

The advantages of the Canadian neurologic scale include its ease of administration, which enables even nonphysicians to administer the test with high reproducibility. A disadvantage is that the scale is weighted toward anterior circulation strokes.

Summary

The Canadian neurologic scale is simple to administer and is a highly reliable method of assessing neurologic deficit. It appears to have interobserver reliability and has good construct validity.

Toronto Stroke Scale

The Toronto stroke scale (Table 7-4) was developed to assess neurologic deficit in acute stroke patients as part of a steroid therapy efficacy trial (Norris, 1976).

Description

The Toronto stroke scale is a 317-point (11 categories) assessment measuring consciousness, motor weakness, sensory impairment, visual field

Table 7-3.   Canadian Neurologic Scale

Mentation	Level Consciousness	Alert	3.0
	Drowsy		1.5
	Orientation	Oriented	1.0
	Disoriented/Non Applicable		0.0
	Speech	Normal	1.0
	Expressive Deficit		0.5
	Receptive Deficit		0.0
Section A1	**Motor Functions**	**Weakness**	
No	Face	None	0.5
Comprehension	Present		0.5
Deficit	Arm: Proximal	None	1.5
	Mild		1.0
	Significant		0.5
	Total		0.0
	Arm: Distal	None	1.5
	Mild		1.0
	Significant		0.5
	Total		0.0
	Leg: Proximal	None	1.5
	Mild		1.0
	Significant		0.5
	Total		0.0
	Leg: Distal	None	1.5
	Mild		1.0
	Significant		0.5
	Total		0.0
Section A2	**Motor Response**		
Comprehension	Face	Symmetrical	0.5
Deficit	Asymmetrical		0.0
	Arms	Equal	1.5
	Unequal		0.0
	Legs	Equal	1.5
	Unequal		0.0

Table 7-4. Toronto Stroke Scale

1. Consciousness	Alert	0			
	Drowsy	1			
	Stupor	2	x	25	0–100
	Light coma	3			
	Deep coma	4			
2. Paresis	Face	0–3	x	1	0–3
	Arm	0–4	x	3.5	0–14
	Leg	0–4	x	2.5	0–10
3. Sensory loss	Face	0–2	x	1.5	0–3
	Arm	0–2	x	6	0–12
	Leg	0–2	x	4.5	0–9
4. Hemianopia		0–2	x	3	0–6
5. Aphasia	Mild, moderate, severe, total	0–4	x	10	0–40
6. Higher cortical function	Frontal	0–2	x	12	0–48
	Parietal	0–2	x		
7. Dementia		0–3	x	3	0–9
8. Forced gaze		0–2	x	2	0–4
9. Incoordination		0–3	x	3	0–9
10. Dysarthria		0–3	x	2	0–6
11. Dysphagia		0–2	x	4	0–8

deficit, aphasia, higher cortical functions, confusion, gaze function, incoordination, dysarthria, and dysphagia. Each item is measured from 0 to 4, reflecting the amount of deficit.

Validation

The Toronto stroke scale has not been extensively validated. It did appear to accurately reflect neurologic impairments as part of the original therapy trial. It also has been compared to several other stroke studies and has high correlation (Brown et al., 1990).

Administration

Due to the complexity of the Toronto stroke scale, it probably needs to be administered by a neurologist trained in cerebrovascular disease. The time of administration ranges from 10 to 20 minutes, depending on the severity of the case.

Special Considerations

The Toronto stroke scale is one of the more comprehensive neurologic scales. As such, strokes of any vascular territory appear to be assessed as part of this scale.

Advantages/Disadvantages

The main advantage of the Toronto stroke scale is that it can be used outside of the middle cerebral artery territory. Disadvantages include the fact that it is relatively difficult to learn to administer and has had little validation in terms of testing in clinical trials.

Summary

The Toronto stroke scale is a comprehensive neurologic deficit assessment scale. It is relatively difficult to learn and there is little reported experience with its use.

Hemispheric Stroke Scale

The Hemispheric stroke scale was designed to test neurologic deficit as part of an acute stroke therapy trial using hemodilution (Adams et al., 1987).

Description

The Hemispheric stroke scale is a 100-point (19 items) neurologic assessment scale. This comprehensive scale measures level of consciousness, language, cortical function, motor function, and sensory capacity, with higher scores reflecting more deficits. Due to the length and complexity of the scale, it is not included here. Readers are referred to the original paper by Adams and colleagues (Adams et al., 1987). The Hemispheric stroke scale actually includes the Glasgow coma scale.

Validation

The Hemispheric stroke scale has been shown to have good construct validity in comparison to the Glasgow coma scale ($r = 0.89$), as well as both the Toronto stroke scale and the Mathew scale (Brown et al., 1990; Adams et al., 1987). Intraobserver reliability has not been reported.

Administration

The Hemispheric stroke scale should take 15-30 minutes to administer. Due to the complexity of the neurologic evaluation, a neurologist with cerebrovascular training is probably required.

Special Considerations

Due to testing at least some higher cortical functions, the Hemispheric stroke scale may be more sensitive for nondominant cortical infarctions.

Advantages/Disadvantages

Due to the relative large amount of neurologic information obtained, the Hemispheric stroke scale can be used to measure strokes in a variety of vascular territories. Its disadvantages are similar to those of the Toronto scale in that it is relatively difficult to administer and time-consuming, and several of the scores appear to test redundant information.

Summary

The Hemispheric stroke scale is a comprehensive neurologic deficit assessment scale. Although it appears to have fairly high construct validity, it has not been validated in recorded therapeutic stroke trials.

Mathew Stroke Scale

The Mathew stroke scale (Table 7-5) was originally designed to test neurologic deficit as part of an

Table 7-5. The Mathew Stroke Scale

Factor	Score	Factor	Score
Mentation		Motor Power*	
Level of consciousness			
fully conscious	8	normal strength	5
lethargic but mentally intact	6	contracts against resistance	4
obtunded	4	elevates against gravity	3
stuporous	2	flicker	2
comatose	0	no movements	0
Orientation		**Performance or disability status scale**	
oriented x 3	6	normal	28
oriented x 2	4	mild impairment	21
oriented x 1	2	moderate impairment	14
disoriented	0	severe impairment	7
		death	0
Speech		**Reflexes**	
normal	23	normal	3
incoherent words	15	asymmetrical or pathological reflexes	2
expressive or impressive words	10	clonus	1
speechless	0	no reflexes elicited	0
Cranial Nerves			
Homonymous hemianopsia		**Sensation**	
intact	3	normal	3
mild	2	mild sensory abnormality	2
moderate	1	severe sensory abnormality	1
severe	0	no response to pain	0
Conjugate/deviation of eyes			
intact	3		
mild	2		
moderate	1		
severe	0		
Facial weakness			
intact	3		
mild	2		
moderate	1		
severe	0		

* Each limb separately.

acute stroke study testing the therapeutic efficacy of glycerol.

Description

The Mathew stroke scale is a comprehensive neurologic scale measuring cognition, cranial nerve function, motor power, global disability status, reflexes, and sensation. It is a 100-point scale (10 items), with lower scores reflecting more severe deficit (Mathew et al., 1972). A modified Mathew scale has been used in recent studies of nimodipine or hemodilution for acute stroke (Gelmers et al., 1988a; Killer et al., 1990).

Validation

The Mathew stroke scale has high construct validity in that it has been shown to be highly correlated with several other stroke scales. It has also been shown to be predictive of long-term outcome (Frithz et al., 1976). It appears to have fairly poor interobserver reliability, with several of the items in the scale having only "slight" interobserver agreement (Gelmers et al., 1988b). The scale has also been shown to have low internal consistency compared to other measures (Brown et al., 1990). It has had fairly extensive validation in several clinical studies (Gelmers et al., 1988a; Koller et al., 1990).

Administration

Due to the neurologic complexity of the Mathew stroke scale, a neurologist with cerebrovascular training is required. The test takes approximately 15 minutes to administer.

Advantages/Disadvantages

An advantage of the Mathew stroke scale is that it should be able to detect strokes in many vascular territories due to its relative comprehensive nature. Disadvantages include the relatively poor interobserver agreement on several of the items, the time required to administer the test, and the need for specialized neurologic training to properly perform the test.

Summary

The Mathew stroke scale is a comprehensive neurologic deficit assessment scale. It has good construct validation in several clinical therapeutic trials, but it appears to have poor intraobserver relia-

bility and requires specialized neurologic training to administer.

European Stroke Scale

The European stroke scale (Table 7-6) is a recently developed test designed to detect therapeutic effects in acute stroke treatment trials. The scale is intended to test only middle cerebral artery stroke and is heavily weighted toward motor items (Hantson et al., 1994).

Description

The European stroke scale was designed for clinical stroke trials in patients with middle cerebral artery stroke. The scale can be used both for matching patients into severity groups and for long-term efficacy evaluations similar to the SSS. It consists of 14 items selected on the basis of prognostic value: level of consciousness, comprehension, speech, visual field, gaze, facial movement, maintenance of arm position, arm raising, wrist extension, finger strength, maintenance of leg position, leg flexing, foot dorsal flexion, and gait. A normal individual will score 106 on this scale. The scale is similar to the NIHSS except that there are more levels for consciousness evaluation and there is an inclusion of a gait assessment (Hantson et al., 1994).

Validation

The European stroke scale has high construct validity, showing correlations with the other neurologic stroke scales ranging between 0.93 and 0.95. The scale also correlated well with long-term functional recovery measured by the Barthel Index. There was high interrater and intrarater reliability in a development study (Hantson et al., 1994). This scale has not been validated in published clinical therapeutic trials to date.

Administration

Given its similarity to the NIHSS, it appears that both physicians and nurses could learn to administer the European stroke scale. The average time of administration is 8 minutes.

Advantages/Disadvantages

Advantages include ease of administration and the ability of nonneurologists to learn the scale.

Table 7-6. The European Stroke Scale

LEVEL OF CONSCIOUSNESS		
-alert, keenly responsive		10
-drowsy, but can be aroused by minor stimiulation to obey, answer, or respond		8
-requires repeated stimulation to atten, or is lethargic or obtunded, requiring stroke or painful stimulation to make movements		6
-cannot be roused by any stimulation, does react purposefully to painful stimuli		4
-cannot be roused by any stimulation, does react with decerebration to painful stimuli		2
-cannot be roused by any stimulation, does not react to painful stimuli		0
COMPREHENSION		
Verbally give the patient the following commands:		
1. Stick out your tongue	-patient performs 3 commands	8
2. Put your finger (of the unaffected side) on your nose	-patient performs 2 or 1 commands	4
3. Close your eyes	-patient does not perform any commands	0
IMPORTANT: DO NOT DEMONSTRATE!		
SPEECH		
The examiner makes a conversation with the patient (how is the patient feeling, did he/she sleep well, for how long has the patient been in the hospital...)	-normal speech	8
	-slight word-finding diffiiculties, conversation is possible	6
	-severe word-finding difficulties, conversation is difficult	4
	-only yes or no	2
	-mute	0
VISUAL FIELD		
The examiner stands at arm's length and compares the patient's field of vision by advancing a moving finger from the periphery inwards. The patient must fixate on the examiner's pupil. (First with one and then with the other eye closed)	-normal	8
	-deficit	0
GAZE		
The examiner steadies the patient's head and asks him/her to follow his finger	-normal	8
The examiner observes the resting eye position and subsequently the full range of movements by moving the index finger from the left to the right and vice versa.	-median eye position, deviation to one side impossible	4
	-lateral eye position, return to midline possible	2
	-lateral eye position, return to midline impossible	0
FACIAL MOVEMENT		
The examiner observes the patient as he/she talks and smiles, noting any asymmetrical elevation of one corner of mouth, flattening of nasolabial fold. Only the muscles in the lower half of the face are assessed.	-normal	8
	-paresis	4
	-paralysis	0
ARM (maintain outstretched position)		
The examiner asks the patient to close the eyes and actively lifts the patient's arms into position so that they are outstretched at 45° in relation to the horizontal plane with both hands in mid-position so that the palms face each other. The patient is asked to maintain this position for 5s after the examiner withdraws the arms. Only the affected side is evaluated.	-arm maintains position for 5s	4
	-arm maintains position for 5s, but affected arm pronates	3
	-arm drifts before 5s pass and maintains a lower position	2
	-arm can't maintain position, but attempts to oppose gravity	1
	-arm falls	0
ARM (raising)		
The patient's arm is rested next to the leg with the hand in the mid-position	-normal	4
The examiner asks the patient to raise the arm outstretched to 90°	-straight arm, movement not full	3
	-flexed arm	2
	-trace movements	1
	-no movement	0
EXTENSION OF THE WRIST		
The patient is tested with the forearm supported and the ha nd unsupported, relaxed in pronation. The patient is asked to extend the hand.	-normal (full isolated movement, no decrease in strength)	8
	-full isolated movement, reduced strength	6
	-movement not isolated and /or full	4
	-trace movements	2
	-no movement	0
FINGERS		
The examiner asks the patient to form with both hands and as strongly as possiblea pinch grip with the thumb and forefinger and to try to resist a weak pull. The examiner checks the strength of this grip by pulling the pinch with one finger.	-equal strength	8
	-reduced strength on affected side	4
	-pinch grip impossible on affected side	0
LEG (maintain position)		
The examiner actively lifts the patient's affected leg into position so that th e thigh forms an angle of 90° with the bed, with the shin parallel with the bed. The examiner asks the patient to close the eyes and to maintain this position for 5s without support	-leg maintains position for 5s	4
	-leg drifts to intermediate position by the end of 5s	2
	-leg drifts to bed within 5 s, but not immediately	1
	-leg falls to bed immediately	0
LEG (flexing)		
The patient is in the supine position with the legs outstretched. The examiner asks the patient to flex the hip and knee.	-normal	4
	-movement against resistance, reduced strength	3
	-movement against gravity	2
	-trace movements	1
	-no movement	0
DORSIFLEXION OF THE FOOT		
The patient is tested with the leg outstretched. The examiner asks the patient to dorsiflex the foot.	-normal (leg outstretched, full movement, full strength)	8
	-leg outstretched,full movement, reduced strength	6
	-leg outstretched,movement not full or knee flexed or foot in supination	4
	-trace movements	2
	-no movements	0
GAIT	-normal	10
	-gait has abnormal aspect and/or distance/speed limited	8
	-patient can walk with aid	6
	-patient can walk with the physical assistance of person(s)	4
	-patient cannot walk, but can stand supported	2
	-patient cannot walk or stand	0

Disadvantages include the fact that it is not in widespread use, so results obtained with the scale may not be directly comparable to those from other scales.

Summary

The European stroke scale is a recently developed scale designed to test therapeutic effects in acute stroke therapy trials. It appears to have good validity and good prognostic ability, but further experience in clinical trials is needed before widespread use can be recommended.

Unified Neurological Stroke Scale

The Unified Neurological stroke scale is a newly developed "composite" scale for the assessment of acute stroke patients.

Description

The Unified Neurological stroke scale is a combination of the Orgogozo scale and the Scandinavian stroke scale (see Table 7-2). An alternate way of looking at it is that it is the Scandinavian stroke scale with the addition of assessments of foot dorsal flexion and extremity tone.

Validation

Both construct and predictive validity were determined in a study by Edwards and colleagues (Edwards et al., 1995; Orgogozo et al., 1992; Brown et al., 1990). Not surprisingly, there was high construct validity as assessed by correlations with the Scandinavian scale and the Orgogozo scale. The Unified Neurological stroke scale was also shown to be a good predictor of functional outcome for both ischemic stroke and hemorrhagic stroke. In this study, the investigators also looked at the use of this scale for subarachnoid hemorrhage and traumatic brain injury and found it to be a less reliable predictor of outcome than it is in stroke. The scale has also been shown to have high interrater agreement (Treves et al., 1994).

Administration

The Unified Neurological stroke scale probably needs to be administered by a neurologist because of the inclusion of the tone assessments. The time of administration would only require 1 minute additional to that required by the SSS, i.e., it should be done in less than 15 minutes.

Advantages/Disadvantages

The Unified Neurological stroke scale appears to have good reliability and good construct validity. It appears to be an improvement over the Scandinavian scale alone, with only minimal additional time being required to administer it compared to the Scandinavian scale. An additional advantage of the Unified Neurological stroke scale is that it is the only scale that has been validated in terms of assessing patients with intracerebral hemorrhage. Disadvantages include the fact that it is not in widespread use and therefore has not been validated in published therapeutic efficacy trials.

Summary

The Unified Neurological stroke scale is a newly developed composite scale that appears to be valid in both ischemic stroke and intracerebral hemorrhage. Further work is needed to determine if it will prove useful in therapeutic efficacy trials.

Conclusion

A large number of stroke scales have been developed to assess neurologic deficits following acute stroke. These scales range from relatively simple and rapid measurements, i.e., the Canadian stroke scale, to much more detailed time-consuming assessments, such as the Toronto stroke scale and the Hemispheric stroke scale. Many of these scales are designed primarily to assess middle cerebral artery strokes and almost all are heavily weighted toward motor function. All of the scales appear to have fairly high construct validity and many of them have shown good predictive validity. The NIHSS and the Canadian stroke scale have had the largest amount of work done assessing inter- and intraobserver reliability, both of which have been found to be very good. The NIHSS and the SSS appear to be the most frequently used for current stroke clinical trials.

Although each neurologic deficit stroke scale has its proponents and merit, overall we think that the NIHSS is currently the preferred scale given its widespread use, high reliability, and the availability of a training tape. If a simpler scale is desired, the Canadian stroke scale would be the choice, whereas if a more comprehensive scale is desired, the Unified Neurological stroke scale appears to offer a good balance between detailed assessment and ease of use.

Functional Outcome Scales

As opposed to the previously discussed stroke scales, which attempt to define a patient's neurologic examination, the various functional outcome scales attempt to quantify the patient's functional status as measured by ability to perform tasks of daily living. There are two general categories of outcome scales. The first is global assessment. Such scales give broad-based gestalt assessments of the overall functional status of a patient. The second type of outcome scale involves more detailed testing of either routine activities of daily living (ADLs) or more detailed instrumental activities of daily living (IADLs). ADL scales measure performance of functions that are used for independent living. One of the advantages of such scales is that they can be administered by any health care professional and can actually be done through conversation with family or patient over the telephone. A general disadvantage is that they are impractical in the acute stroke setting, where it is inappropriate to test several of the activities.

Overall, functional outcome scales have been receiving more attention in several ongoing clinical trials. As is evidenced in the tPA NIH study (NINDS rt-PA Stroke Study Group, 1995), several companies have abandoned neurologic stroke scales as their primary endpoint and have gone on to functional outcome assessments. The driving force behind this trend is the belief that while a drug may improve a finding on a neurologic exam, e.g., improve a patient by 4 points on the NIHSS, the patient may have no meaningful improvement in terms of ability to function. It is the patient's ability to resume his or her prior activities of daily life that patients, providers, and insurance companies measure as the "gold standard" for measuring the effectiveness of a drug.

Global Outcome Scales

Glasgow Outcome Scale

This 5-point global outcome scale (Table 7-7) was originally designed as a companion to the Glasgow coma scale (Jennett et al., 1979; Jennett et al., 1975). The scale has been extensively used in studies of head injury and nontraumatic coma (Jennett et al.,

1979; Levy et al., 1991). It is in widespread use in many clinical therapeutic stroke trials.

Description

The Glasgow outcome scale is a 5-point scale with 1 = dead and 5 = good recovery. Although the scale is simple to administer, having only 5 scores, there is sometimes confusion in that there is no clear demarcation between some of the levels. This is particularly true in some cases between the severe disability and moderate disability scores.

Administration

The Glasgow outcome scale can be administered by any trained health care worker; it takes only seconds to complete.

Validation

The Glasgow outcome scale has high reliability in several studies of head injury, but reliability assessments in stroke population have not been extensively published. Interestingly, it has actually been used as a "gold standard" to measure whether several of the clinical stroke scales previously discussed had good construct validity (Côté et al., 1989).

Advantages/Disadvantages

Advantages include ease of use and the ability of nonstroke neurologists to fill out the form. Disadvantages include the relative lack of proven construct validity in stroke, along with the problem of poor demarcation between several of the categories.

Summary

The Glasgow outcome scale is in widespread use in clinical stroke trials. It is easy to administer and appears to provide a good overview of a patient's functional outcome.

Modified Rankin Scale

The Modified Rankin scale (Table 7-8) is a 5-point global assessment categorization of patients' function based on the ability to perform activities of daily life.

Table 7-7. Glasgow Outcome Scale

SCORE	Circle the appropriate score
1	DEAD
2	PERSISTENT VEGETATIVE STATE. Patient exhibits no obvious cortical function.
3	SEVERE DISABILITY. (Conscious but disabled). Patient depends upon others for daily support due to mental or physical disability or both.
4	MODERATE DISABILITY. (Disabled but independent). Patient is independent as far as daily life is concerned. The disabilities found include varying degrees of dysphasia, hemiparesis, or ataxia, as well as intellectual and memory deficits and personality changes.
5	GOOD RECOVERY. Resumption of normal activities even though there may be minor neurological or psychological deficits.

Table 7-8. The Modified Rankin Scale

Grade	Description
0	No symptoms at all.
1	No significant disability despite symptoms: able to carry out all usual duties and activities.
2	Slight disability: unable to carry out all previous activities but able to look after own affairs without assistance.
3	Moderate disability: requiring some help, but able to walk without assistance.
4	Moderately severe disability: unable to walk without assistance, and unable to attend to own bodily needs without assistance.
5	Severe disability: bedridden, incontinent, and requiring constant nursing care and attention.

Description

Groups are ranked from 0 = no symptoms to 5 = severe disability (Rankin et al., 1957; van Swieten et al., 1988). Ratings are given as to how much assistance the patient requires to achieve various levels of function. Some clinical stroke trials also add a grade 6 for patients who have expired. Similar to the Glasgow outcome scale, the Modified Rankin sometimes suffers from poor demarcation between its various levels. As an example, a patient with a middle cerebral artery stroke could have severe disability in many categories yet still be scored as only "moderate" in that he or she frequently is able to ambulate without assistance.

Administration

The Modified Rankin scale can be administered by a neurologist or other health care professional.

Validation

The Modified Rankin scale has been reported to have moderate interobserver reliability. It has had significant use in several stroke therapeutic outcome trials (Tomasello et al., 1982; Bonita & Beaglehole, 1988).

Activities of Daily Living Scales

Barthel Index

The Barthel Index (Table 7-9) is a widely used measure of functional outcome that has been utilized not only in stroke but also in a multitude of neurologic disorders (Mahoney & Barthel, 1965; Gresham et al., 1980; Brown et al., 1990; Wade & Hewer, 1987).

Description

The Barthel Index comprises 10 weighted items measuring feeding, bathing, grooming, dressing, bowel control, bladder control, toileting, chair transfer, ambulation, and stair climbing. A maximum score of 100 is normal.

Administration

The Barthel Index can be administered by any health care professional. It takes approximately 5 minutes to administer. The score can be obtained from discussing the questions with the patient, family, or rehabilitation facility nurses.

Validation

The Barthel Index has been extensively studied and has had high construct validation (Brown et al., 1990; Wade & Hewer, 1987). The scale has also been shown to predict length of hospital stay as well as the odds of independent living (Granger et al., 1989; Granger et al., 1989). Barthel Index scores obtained from telephone interview have been shown to correlate highly with those obtained from direct examinations (Shinar et al., 1987). It has also been shown to have high interrater reliability (Shinar et al., 1987).

Advantages/Disadvantages

Advantages include ease of use and the ability to conduct interviews by telephone follow-up. Disadvantages include the fact that the scale only measures very basic functions. Patients can have significant cognitive impairment and still score 100 on the Barthel Index.

Summary

The Barthel Index is a widely used ADL scale with high reliability and construct validation. It is in widespread use as the primary endpoint in many ongoing clinical therapeutic trials.

Activity Index

The Activity Index (Table 7-10) was originally developed using components of other ADL scales to measure the functional outcome of acute stroke patients.

Description

The Activity Index includes 4 mental capacity items, 6 measures of motor function, and 5 measures of ADL. There is a strong correlation between the Activity Index and the Barthel Index (Lindmark, 1988).

Administration

The Activity Index can be administered by any health care professional. No evaluation of whether

Table 7-9. The Barthel Index

<table>
<tbody>
<tr><td>1. Feeding</td><td>10 = Independent. Able to apply any necessary device. Feeds in reasonable time.
5 = Needs help, i.e., for cutting.
0 = Inferior performance.</td></tr>
<tr><td>2. Bathing</td><td>5 = Performs without assistance.
0 = Inferior performance.</td></tr>
<tr><td>3. Personal Toilet (grooming)</td><td>5 = Washes face, combs hair, brushes teeth, shaves (manages plug if electric razor)
0 = Inferior performance.</td></tr>
<tr><td>4. Dressing</td><td>10 = Independent. Ties shoes, fastens fasteners, applies braces.
5 = Needs help but does at least half of task within reasonable time.
0 = Inferior performance.</td></tr>
<tr><td>5. Bowel Control</td><td>10 = No accidents. Able to use enema or suppository if needed.
5 = Occasional accidents or needs help with enema or suppository.
0 = Inferior performance.</td></tr>
<tr><td>6. Bladder Control</td><td>10 = No accidents. Able to care for collecting device if used.
5 = Occasional accidents or needs help with device.
0 = Inferior performance.</td></tr>
<tr><td>7. Toilet Transfers</td><td>10 = Independent with toilet or bedpan. Handles clothes, wipes, flushes, or cleans pan.
5 = Needs help for balance, handling clothes or toilet paper.
0 = Inferior performance.</td></tr>
<tr><td>8. Chair/Bed Transfers</td><td>15 = Independent, including locks of wheelchair and lifting footrests.
10 = Minimum assistance or supervision.
5 = Able to sit, but needs maximum assistance to transfer.
0 = Inferior performance.</td></tr>
<tr><td>9. Ambulation</td><td>15 = Independent for 50 yards. May use assistive devices, except for rolling walker.
10 = With help for 50 yards.
5 = Independent with wheelchair for 50 yards, only if unable to walk.
0 = Inferior performance.</td></tr>
<tr><td>10. Stair Climbing</td><td>10 = Independent. May use assistive devices.
5 = Needs help or supervision.
0 = Inferior performance.</td></tr>
</tbody>
</table>

Table 7-10. Activity Index.

Variable	Score	Variable	Score
MENTAL CAPACITY			
Degree of consciousness		*Left hand*	
Completely awake	8	Normal or nearly normal activity,	
Somnolent	6	isolated gripping and finger	4
Pre-comatose	4	movements	3
Comatose	1	Simple functional grips	2
		Activity without functional value	1
		No activity	
Orientation in time, space and person (identity)		*Left leg*	
Orientation in all three dimensions	6	Normal or nearly normal activity	4
Orientation in two dimensions	4	Activity of some functional value	3
Orientation in one dimension	3	Activity without functional value	2
Disoriented	1	No activity	1
Ability to communicate verbally			
Normal verbal communication	12	**ADL FUNCTION**	
Slight difficulties in communication			
Severe difficulties in communication	8		
No verbal communication			
	4		
	1		
Psychological Activities		*Ambulation*	
Takes initiative him/herself, wants information, etc.	6	Able to walk	6
Takes some initiative, talks to people around	4	Walks if supported by somebody, able to move her/himself about in a wheel-chair	4
Takes no initiative, apathetic	3	Confined to a wheel-chair, able to stand with support of somebody	3
No noticeable psychological activity	1	Confined to bed or wheel-chair, cannot stand even with the support of somebody	1
MOTOR ACTIVITY		*Personal hygiene*	
		Manages personal hygiene by	6
		him/herself	4
		Help needed only for her/his lower toilet	3
		Assists when washing her/himself but needs help both for upper and lower toilet	1
		Does not assist in her/his personal hygiene at all	
Right arm		*Dressing*	
Normal or nearly normal acitivity	4	Dresses her/himself	6
Activity of some functional value	3	Dresses her/himself on the whole, needs help only with stockings/socks, e.g.	4
Activity without functional value	2	Can assist in certain minor elements of the dressing procedure	3
No activity	1	Must be dressed completely by somebody else	1
Right hand		*Feeding*	
Normal or nearly normal activity, isolated gripping and finger movements		Eats completely by her/himself	6
Simple functional grips	4	Eats with some assistance	4
Activity without functional value	3	Is fed	3
No activity	2	Fed by tube or intravenous infusion	1
	1		
Right leg		*Emptying/function of bladder*	
Normal or nearly normal activity	4	Continent	6
Activity of some functional value	3	Occasional failures	4
Activity without functional value	2	Uridome and/or assistance with toilet and bed/pan	3
No activity	1	Incontinent	1
Left arm		*Maximum score*	92
Normal or nearly normal activity	4		
Activity of some functional value	3		
Activity without functional value	2		
No activity	1		

it can be administered by telephone has been reported.

Validation

The Activity Index has shown excellent construct validity in that it correlates highly with the Barthel Index ($r = 0.94$) (Hamrin & Wohlin, 1989). This scale has also been shown to have a good predictive validity in that initial scores on the scale are highly predictive of three-week functional outcome (Hamrin & Wohlin, 1989). The scale has been shown to have high internal consistency (Lindmark, 1988).

Advantages/Disadvantages

Advantages include ease of use and the ability of any health care professional to administer it. Disadvantages include the fact that the scale is not in widespread use in clinical stroke trials.

Summary

Although it is a potential improvement over the Barthel Index, the Activity Index has not received widespread acceptance.

Functional Independence Measure (FIM)

The FIM is a measure of disability. Widely used in the United States, it was originally developed by Uniform Data Systems in Buffalo, New York, based on a large database of patients discharged from rehabilitation facilities (Dodds et al., 1993; Heinemann et al., 1993).

Description

The 18 items of the FIM are organized into 6 subscales and assess 2 dimensions:

1. Physical: eating, grooming, bathing, dressing, toiletry, bowel and bladder control, transferring, and ambulation.
2. Cognitive: communication, social interaction, problem-solving, and memory.

Each of the 18 items is assessed on a 7-point scale ranging from 1 (requiring complete dependence) to 7 (being completely independent). The scale is under copyright protection. Copies can be obtained from the Research Foundation—State University of New York.

Validation

The FIM has been extensively validated in patients who have had either neurologic or orthopedic disabilities (Kidd et al., 1995). It has been shown to have high interrater agreement even when administered by telephone (Ottenbacher et al., 1994). The FIM was recently validated in several stroke outcome studies and was found to be a predictor of long-term stroke outcome (Owen et al., 1995; Segal & Schall, 1994).

Administration

The FIM is usually administered by a rehabilitation physician or nurse. This scale comes with a 24-page instruction manual and is time-consuming to learn. The ratings can be determined through either patient interview or family/provider interview.

Advantages/Disadvantages

Advantages include the fact that it provides a more detailed assessment of the various functional abilities of the patient compared to the Barthel Index. However, it is difficult to learn, and the gradations between the 7-point assistance scale for each item are relatively poorly defined. The FIM is available from the Uniform System for Rehabilitation Project Office, Buffalo General Hospital, 100 High Street, Buffalo, NY 14203.

Summary

The FIM is a comprehensive disability evaluation scale. Although it is in widespread use in the rehabilitation literature, it is not currently frequently utilized in clinical stroke research.

Several other ADL scales are in use in other neurologic diseases. These include the Kennedy self-care evaluation scale (Schoening et al., 1965; Gresham et al., 1980) and the Katz index of ADL (Katz et al., 1963; Katz & Akpom, 1976). These scales have been shown to be highly correlative with the Barthel Index (Wade & Hewer, 1987; Gresham et al., 1980). Both scales utilize performance in ambulation, dressing, personal hygiene, feeding activities, and continence. Since they are not in widespread use in current clinical stroke studies, the reader is referred to the original description of the scales for more details.

The previous scales measure routine activities of daily life. As such, they measure whether a patient can perform basic activities that are required for them to be independent. One of the weaknesses of the ADL scales is that they neglect all aspects of higher cortical function, including such activities as the ability to read, manage money, perform hobbies, drive, and perform general house maintenance functions. In an effort to measure these more complex functions of daily life, measurements of instrumental activities of daily living (IADLs) have been developed. Four such scales have been applied to acute stroke patients. These include the Rivermead ADL Assessment Scale (Whiting & Lincoln, 1980), the Hamrin Activity Index (Holbrook & Skilbeck, 1983), the Frenchay Activities Index (Lincoln & Edmans, 1990), and the Nottingham Extended ADL scale (Nouri & Lincoln, 1987) (Table 7-11). Although they offer a theoretical advantage over the ADL scales previously discussed, they have not received widespread acceptance in the stroke community. To our knowledge, they are not currently employed in any acute stroke therapeutic trial. For this reason, we do not undertake a detailed discussion of each scale in this chapter. Interested readers are referred to a paper by Chong (1995) for an in-depth discussion of these scales as well as a discussion of their validity and reliability.

Functional outcome scales are receiving more attention as primary outcome for various therapeutic trials. Of the scales currently in use, the Modified Rankin, the Glasgow outcome scale, and the Barthel Index all appear to have good construct validity and reliability. These three scales are in widespread use in many acute stroke trials. They are easily administered by any health care professional. A potential weakness is the fact that they do not measure activities that require significant cognitive abilities, so patients who still have major impairments may attain good scores on these scales.

Conclusion

In this chapter we have reviewed both the neurologic deficit scales and the functional outcome scales that are in widespread use in clinical stroke studies. Brief discussions of the validity and reliability of the various scales have been included. For readers interested in a more detailed review of these areas, we recommend the excellent article by Lyden and Lau (1991), in which they critically review many of the stroke scales that are discussed in this chapter. Many ongoing therapeutic trials use a combination of several of the neurologic and outcome scales. Both types of scales have their apparent advantages, with the neurologic scales being able to detect smaller changes in the patient's neurologic exam, whereas the functional outcome scales appear to have more relevance to the patient's ability to function independently. Clearly, both types of scales have their weaknesses, and to date there is no agreement on a single method of determining either an individual patient's outcome or a "gold standard" for measuring a drug's therapeutic efficacy.

The results from the recently completed NIH tPA trial found that all of the endpoints, including the Modified Rankin, Glasgow outcome, Barthel Index, and NIHSS, showed therapeutic benefit (NINDS rt-PA Stroke Study Group, 1995). This suggests that if the effect of a drug is real, any of these scales appear capable of detecting this. Currently, the most widely accepted tests are the Modified Rankin scale and the NIHSS. It is hoped that additional outcome assessments will be employed in the future. These may include measurements of infarct size reduction based on MRI diffusion weighted imaging technology. Finally, several clinical therapeutic trials are now also using pharmacoeconomic assessments as secondary endpoints to assess therapeutic efficacy. In the managed health care environment, such pharmacoeconomic endpoints may actually prove to be the most powerful indicator of a drug's benefit.

Acknowledgment. The authors thank Sandi Hungerford for her excellent assistance in the preparation of this manuscript.

Table 7-11. IADL Scales.

Rivermead Scale	Hamrin Scale	Frenchay Scale	Nottingham Scale
Household 1	Household work	Preparing meals	Mobility
Preparation of hot drink	Make coffee/tea	Washing dishes	Walk outside
Preparation of snack	Simple cooking	Washing clothes	Climb stairs
Cope with money	Dishwashing	Dusting/vacuum cleaning	Get in/out of car
Get in/out of car	Make bed	Cleaning	Walk over uneven ground
Prepare meal	Vacuum cleaning, wash floors	Local shopping	Cross roads
Carry shopping	Easy laundry (by hand or machine)	Social activities	Public transport
Crossing roads	Locomotion	Walks	Kitchen
Transport self to shop	Move from bed to chair	Hobby/sport	Feed self
Public transport	Move about in home	Car/bus travel	Make hot drink
Household 2	Manage stairs	Gardening	Take hot drinks from one room to another
Washing	Walk outdoors	Books	
Ironing	Unlock and close entrance door	Outings	Washing up
Light cleaning		House/car maintenance	Make hot snack
Hang out washing	Psychosocial functions	Employment	Domestic tasks
Bedmaking	Write letters	Manage own money	
Heavy cleaning	Telephone		Wash small items of clothing
	Visit someone		
	Use municipal means of transport	Housework	
		Shopping	
	Go to public premises		Wash full load of clothes
	Shopping		Leisure activities
	Intellectual activities		Read newspapers or books
	Read daily newspapers		
	Listen to news on radio or TV		
	Read books		Telephone
	Keep own accounts		Write letters
			Go out socially
			Manage own garden
			Drive a car

References

Adams RJ, Meador KJ, Sethi KD, Grotta JC, Thomson DS. Graded neurologic scale for use in acute hemispheric stroke treatment protocols. *Stroke* 1987;18:655–69.

Bonita R, Beaglehole R. Recovery of motor function after stroke. *Stroke* 1988;19:1497–1500.

Brott TG, Adams HP, Olinger CP, et al. Measurements of acute cerebral infarction: a clinical examination scale. *Stroke* 1989;20:864–70.

Brott T, Haley EC Jr, Levy DE, et al. Urgent therapy for stroke. Part 1: pilot study of tissue plasminogen activator administered within 90 minutes. *Stroke* 1992;23:632–40.

Brott T, Marler JR, Olinger CO, et al. Measurements of acute cerebral infarction: lesion size by computerized tomography. *Stroke* 1989;20:871–75.

Brown EB, Tietjen GE, Deveshwar RK, et al. Clinical stroke scales: an intra- and interscale evaluation. *Neurology* 1990;40S1:352–55.

Chong DKH. Measurement of instrumental activities of daily living in stroke. *Stroke* 1995;26:1119–22.

Côté R, Battista RN, Wolfson CM. Stroke assessment scales: guidelines for development, validation, and reliability assessment. *Can J Neurol Sci* 1988;115:261–65.

Côté R, Battista RN, Wolfson CM, et al. The Canadian neurological scale: validation and reliability assessment. *Neurology* 1989;39:638–43.

Côté R, Hachinski V, Shurvell BL, Norris JW, Wolfson C. The Canadian neurological scale: a preliminary study in acute stroke. *Stroke* 1986;17:731–37.

Dodds TA, Martin DP, Stolov WC, Deyo RA. A validation of the functional independence measure and its performance among rehabilitation inpatients. *Arch Phys Med Rehabil* 1993;74:531–36.

Edwards DF, Chen YW, Diringer MN. Unified neurological stroke scale is valid in ischemic and hemorrhagic stroke. *Stroke* 1995;26:1852–58.

Frithz G, Werner I. Clinical findings and short-term prognosis in a stroke material. *Acta Med Scand* 1976;199:133–40.

Gelmers HJ, Gorter K, de Weerdt CJ, Wiezer HJA. A controlled trial of nimodipine in acute ischemic stroke. *New Engl J Med* 1988;318:203–207.

Gelmers HJ, Gorter K, de Weerdt CJ, Wiezer HJA. Assessment of interobserver variability in a Dutch multicenter study on acute ischemic stroke. *Stroke* 1988;19:709–11.

Goldstein LB, Bartels C, Davis JN. Interrater reliability of the NIH stroke scale. *Arch Neurol* 1989;46:660–62.

Granger CV, Dewis LS, Peters NC, Sherwood CC, Barrett J. Stroke rehabilitation: analysis of repeated Barthel Index measures. *Arch Phys Med Rehabil* 1979;60:14–17.

Granger CV, Hamilton BB, Gresham GE, Kramer AA. The stroke rehabilitation outcome study: part II. Relative merit of the total Barthel Index score and a four-item subscore in predicting patient outcomes. *Arch Phys Med Rehabil* 1989;70:100–103.

Gresham GE, Phillips TF, Labi MLC. ADL status in stroke: relative merits of three standard indexes. *Arch Phys Med Rehabil* 1980;61:355–58.

Haley EC Jr, Brott TG, Sheppard GL, et al. Pilot randomized trial of tissue plasminogen activator in acute ischemic stroke. *Stroke* 1993;24:1000–1004.

Haley EC Jr, Levy DE, Brott TG, et al. Urgent therapy for stroke. Part 2: pilot study of tissue plasminogen activator administered 91–180 minutes from onset. *Stroke* 1992;23:641–45.

Hamrin E, Wohlin A. Evaluation of the functional capacity of stroke patients through an activity index. *J Clin Physiol* 1989;14:93-100.

Hantson L, de Weerdt W, de Keyser, et al. The European stroke scale. *Stroke* 1994;25:2215–19.

Heinemann AW, Linacre JM, Wright BD, Hamilton BB, Granger CV. Prediction of rehabilitation outcomes with disability measures. *Arch Phys Med Rehabil* 1993;74:566–73.

Holbrook M, Skilbeck C. An activities index for use with stroke patients. *Age Ageing* 1983;12:166–70.

Jennett B, Bond M. Assessment of outcome after severe brain damage: a practical scale. *Lancet* 1975;5:480–84.

Jennett B, Teasdale G, Braakman R, et al. Prognosis of patients with severe head injury. *Neurosurgery* 1979;4:283–89.

Katz S, Akpom CA. A measure of primary sociobiological functions. *Intl J Health Serv* 1976;6:493–507.

Katz S, Ford AB, Moskowitz RW, Jackson BA, Jaffe MW. The index of ADL: a standardized measure of biological and psychosocial function. *JAMA* 1963;185:913–19.

Kidd D, Steward G, Baldry J, et al. The functional independence measure: a comparative validity and reliability study. *Disabil Rehabil* 1995;17:10–14.

Koller M, Haenny P, Hess K. Weniger D, Zangger P. Adjusted hypervolemic hemodilution in acute ischemic stroke. *Stroke* 1990;21:1429–34.

Levy DE, Bates D, Garonna JJ, et al. Prognosis in nontraumatic coma. *Ann Int Med* 1991;94:293–301.

Lincoln NB, Edmans JA. A re-validation of the Rivermead ADL scale for elderly patients with stroke. *Age Ageing* 1990;19:19–24.

Lindenstrøm E. Boysen G, Christiansen LW. a Rogvi-Hansen B, Nielson PW. Reliability of Scandinavian neurological stroke scale. *Cerebrovasc Dis* 1991;1:103–107.

Lindmark B. Evaluation of functional capacity after stroke with special emphasis on motor function and ADL. *Scand J Rehab Med* 1988;21S:1–40.

Lyden P, Brott T, Tilley B, Welch KMA, Maascha EJ, NINDS TPA Stroke Study Group. Improved reliability of the NIH stroke scale using video training. *Stroke* 1994;25:2220–26.

Lyden PD, Lau GT. A critical appraisal of stroke evaluation and rating scales. *Stroke* 1991;22:1345–52.

Mahoney FT, Barthel DW. Functional evaluation: Barthel Index. *Md State Med J* 1965;14:61–65.

Mathew NT, Rivera VM, Meyer JS, Charney JZ, Hartmann A. Double-blind evaluation of glycerol therapy in acute cerebral infarction. *Lancet* 1972;2:1327–29.

National Institute of Neurological Disorders and Stroke rt-PA Stroke Study Group. Tissue plasminogen activator for acute ischemic stroke. *New Engl J Med* 1995;333:1581–87.

Norris JW. Steroid therapy in acute cerebral infarction. *Arch Neurol* 1976;33:69–71.

Nouri FM, Lincoln NB. An extended activities of daily living scale for stroke patients. *Clin Rehab* 1987;1:301–305.

Orgogozo JM, Asplund K, Boysen J. A unified form for neurologic scoring of hemispheric stroke with motor impairment. *Stroke* 1992;23:1678–79.

Orgogozo JM, Calpideo R, Anagnostou CN. Mise au point d'un score neurologique pour l'evaluation clinique des infarctus sylviens. *Presse Med* 1983;12:3039–44.

Orgogozo JM, Dartigues JF. Clinical trials in brain infarction. The question of assessment criteria. In: Battistini N (ed.). *Acute brain ischemia. Medical and surgical therapy.* New York: Raven, 1986:201–208.

Orgogozo JM, Dartigues JF. Methodology of clinical trials in acute cerebral ischemia: survival, functional and neurological outcome measures. *Cerebrovasc Dis* 1991;1(Suppl 1):100–11.

Ottenbacher KJ, Mann WC, Granger CV, et al. Inter-rater agreement and stability of functional assessment in the community-based elderly. *Arch Phys Med Rehabil* 1994;75:1297–1301.

Owen DC, Getz PA, Bulla S. A comparison of characteristics of patients with completed stroke: those who achieve continence and those who do not. *Rehabil Nurs* 1995;20:197–203.

Rankin J. Cerebral vascular accidents in patients over the age of 60: prognosis. *Scott Med J* 1957;2:200–15.

Scandinavian Stroke Study Group. Multicenter trial of hemodilution in ischemic stroke. Backgound and study protocol. *Stroke* 1985;16:885–90.

Scandinavian Stroke Study Group. Multicenter trial of hemodilution in ischemic stroke. *Stroke* 1987;18:691–99.

Schoening HA, Anderegg L, Bergstrom D, et al. Numerical scoring of self-care status of patients. *Arch Phys Med Rehabil* 1965;46:689–97.

Segal ME, Schall RR. Determining function/health status and its relation to disability in stroke survivors. *Stroke* 1994;25:2391–97.

Shinar D, Gross CR, Bronstein KS, et al. Reliability of the activities of daily living scale and its use in the telephone interview. *Arch Phys Med Rehabil* 1987;68:723–28.

Tomasello F, Mariani F, Fieschi C, et al. Assessment of interobserver differences in the Italian multicenter study on reversible cerebral ischemia. *Stroke* 1982;13:32–34.

Treves TA, Karepov VG, Aronovich BD, et al. Interrater agreement in evaluation of stroke patients with the unified neurological stroke scale. *Stroke* 1994;25:1263–64.

van Swieten JC, Koudstall PJ, Visser MC, Schouten HJA, van Gijn J. Interobserver agreement for the assessment of handicap in stroke patients. *Stroke* 1988;19:604–607.

Wade DT, Hewer RL. Functional abilities after stroke: measurement, natural history, and prognosis. *J Neurol Neurosurg Psychiatry* 1987;50:177–82.

Whiting S, Lincoln N. An ADL assessment for stroke patients. *Br J Occup Ther* 1980;43:44–46.

Zivin JA, Waud DR. Quantal bioassay and stroke. *Stroke* 1992;23:767–773.

CHAPTER 8 Assessment of Outcome Following Traumatic Brain Injury in Adults

Zeev Groswasser, M.D.,
Karen Schwab, Ph.D.,
and Andres M. Salazar, M.D.

Assessment of outcome has become one of the major issues in medicine in recent years. The outcome movement has its origins in the need for cost containment and growth of managed care, a renewed sense of competition among health care providers, and studies showing substantial differences in geographic utilization of various medical procedures after controlling for severity of illness (Epstein, 1990). No less important in the field of traumatic brain injury (TBI) is the need for reliable outcome measures with which to compare alternative treatments in clinical research studies.

Outcome measures have changed in recent years from simple physiologic parameters to more complex functional parameters, thus moving from the more standardized medical evaluations to the psychosocial sphere, which is far less well-defined and may be more diversified and varies across cultural and behavioral backgrounds. Rehabilitation medicine has always focused on functional outcome as one of its main goals, utilizing medical processes to achieve the overall well-being of patients, which is better defined in psychosocial terms. Parameters such as mobility, independence in activities of daily living, vocational rehabilitation, and questions concerned with the overall well-being of patients and their families have been the critical issues addressed during the rehabilitation process.

Traumatic brain injury is no exception, especially if we consider its impact on health care systems and individuals. Millions of people are affected each year by this "silent epidemic" (Goldstein, 1990; Teasdale, 1995), which has a profound impact on their lives because of its peak occurrence in young adult men, mostly in their early twenties, the years during which people acquire a profession, start a family, and lay a foundation for the rest of their lives. However, children and senior citizens are important subpopulations of TBI patients; children were considered to have a better chance for recovery due to their alleged greater potential for plasticity and senior citizens were considered as having a worse chance for recovery following TBI.

Treatment of TBI patients is a complex and multi-stage process that starts at the injury site, preferably continues at a hospital provided with a neurosurgical unit and a trauma center (Teasdale, 1995), and then through various other interim institutions, rehabilitation programs, special TBI inpatient and outpatient programs, and follow-up clinics, until the patient is settled back in his environment and family. This long chain requires the definition of outcome at each stage and has high inherent opportunities for miscommunication among the care providers who participate in the process. This is more true today as the whole system is under pressure for cost containment. Assessment at various points in the recovery process uses different measures of outcome and has different goals for the provider of the service or the consumer, i.e., the patient and his family.

Outcome may be defined in entirely different terms by those participating in the process. Definitions used during the acute and the immediate post-acute phase by neurosurgeons may differ substantially from those used by professionals and families engaged in the long course of neurologic rehabilitation. Once the patient returns home, families often discover that a profound change in capacity and personality has taken place and that life has taken a profoundly different course. Many TBI patients are aware of even subtle changes in their functional capacity and may become agitated and depressed because of them. The situation may be even more complex if patients have metacognitive disturbances, i.e., pathologic denial that renders them unaware of the difference and change in their performance and behavior and about the need for further appropriate therapy or supervision.

Cognition and behavior have a greater impact than physical disability on the social function of individuals. This is highlighted in TBI patients, as cognitive and behavioral sequelae are the basic residue of TBI and have a profound impact on rehabilitation and outcome. The growth of neuropsychology made detailed qualitative and quantitative analysis of these deficits more available over the past 20 years and has had a major impact on our understanding and definition of "outcome." Recent advances in neuroimaging and electrophysiology, as well as recent research in brain plasticity and regeneration, also promise to add new dimensions to our understanding of outcome in TBI patients.

The question of assessment of outcome after TBI is closely linked to the question of prognosis. In the very early phase of recovery, questions regarding life and death are the crucial ones. Recovery of consciousness comes next, while recovery of function is the main issue during the later phase. Families and aware TBI patients are very much concerned about the future, thus putting additional pressure on caregivers to provide answers regarding prognosis. Diller (1994)

stated that the ideal situation in medicine is having a patient with a known condition, treated with a known intervention, toward a known outcome. However, in TBI rehabilitation we treat patients with only partial knowledge of their condition, with partial knowledge of the effects of intervention, and with imperfect knowledge of outcomes.

This chapter outlines measures used by different participants in the process, ranging from physicians involved in acute medical assessment and acute care to physical, occupational, and speech therapists, and to patients and their families. It is our belief that there is a significant correlation between objective parameters set by therapists and subjective assessment of quality of life by TBI patients, and that discerning these parameters can be of help in the rehabilitation process and in defining efficacy criteria for rehabilitation research studies.

Measuring Severity and Outcome in the Acute Phase of TBI

Most of the treatment and research on TBI patients during the acute phase is carried out by neurosurgeons and to a lesser extent by neurologists. It is therefore not surprising that most of the data regarding acute phase management and outcome has been generated by neurosurgeons and relates mainly to assessment of severity of injury (Table 8-1). Surviving war veterans sustaining penetrating injuries attracted the greater interest in earlier years, as blunt injuries, mostly due to road accidents and falls, were relatively less common than at present. Mortality of combat injuries with dural tear was about 40% during the First World War (Cushing, 1917, cited by Robotham 1949; Jefferson,

Table 8-1. Acute Phase TBI Severity Measures

Duration of Loss of Consciousness (LOC)
Duration of Posttraumatic Amnesia (PTA)
Glasgow Coma Scale (GCS)
GCS Motor Subscale, Extended GCS
Reaction Level Scale (RLS85)
Injury Severity Scale (ISS), Polytrauma

1919, cited by Robotham 1949), a figure that came down to much lower levels of (7–12.5%) during the Second World War (Robotham, 1949). That war became a turning point in our interest in TBI patients, especially those who survived low velocity penetrating combat injuries. The introduction of antibiotics and better neurosurgical management increased the number of surviving TBI veterans who had to reintegrate into family and community life.

The earliest measures of severity of injury may still be among the best. Duration of loss of consciousness (LOC) and posttraumatic amnesia (PTA) as valid criteria for severity of brain injury, and their relationship to outcome, were recognized early on, as were the differences between blunt and penetrating brain injuries. Terms such as *concussion, contusion,* and *laceration* describing severity of injury were considered of little practical value in closed head injury, "for by far the most important indication of severity was the effect of the injury on consciousness" (Russell & Smith, 1961). Although PTA became a popular measure in assessing severity of injury, determination of exact duration of PTA is usually more difficult than the duration of unconsciousness in most clinical settings.

Roberts conducted a 10–25 year follow-up of a group of severe nonpenetrating TBI patients (PTA >1 week, unconsciousness < 1 month), tracing 62% of the original group. It was the rate of recovery during the first months that most clearly predicted outcome. Disability profiles on a 10-point scale were scored for initial level of neurologic responsiveness, neural lesions, progress, final disability, and for personality changes and memory defects; ultimate outcome was scored in terms of domestic, social, and occupational disability (Roberts, 1976). It is worth noting that even in this early study the exact quantification of changes was considered important and that no single scale could actually represent the full picture of a patient. Furthermore, final outcome was evaluated according to social functioning, i.e., domestic, social, and occupational, and not in strict neurologic terms. It is also of interest to note that Roberts already made clear that the initial apparent severity of injury (the presence of decerebrate rigidity) in the acute stage did not always imply a bad prognosis. Roberts also commented on the term *persistent vegetative state,* introduced by Jennett and Plum (1972), suggesting that in TBI

patients it should be replaced by *decerebrated dementia* (Roberts, 1976).

Glasgow Coma Scale (GCS)

The introduction of the Glasgow Coma Scale (GCS) by Teasdale and Jennett marked a change in the acute assessment of severity of injury. (Teasdale & Jennett, 1974). Ill-defined terms such as *delirium* and *stupor,* much in use for describing changes in consciousness and subject to great interobserver variability, have given place to better defined and more reliable simple bedside subscales that separately assess eyes, verbal, and motor performance. Teasdale stresses that these are different components that may each run an independent course. However, the authors of the GCS were "tempted" to summate the scores of the different components into an overall coma score ranging from 3 to 15 (Teasdale, 1995). Severe TBI patients classified according to GCS score of 8 or less had markedly worse outcome than those scoring 9 and more. The GCS score was considered as an imperfect predictor of eventual productivity status and degree of independence (Vogenthaler et al., 1989). Other associated lesions, such as presence of subdural hematomas, had a profound negative effect on survival and outcome (Gennarelli et al., 1982). Combining the GCS with a variety of complications enhanced outcome predictability (Stein & Spettel, 1995). The fact that the GCS provides an index of severity and has a high reliability and easy bedside applicability gained it universal use, creating a common language that enhanced comparisons of various therapeutic interventions in regard to both survival and outcome.

Shortcomings of the GCS include the difficulties of determining verbal and eye opening score in patients who have extensive facial injuries or are intubated. Partly for this reason, some investigators have used the GCS motor score (score 1 to 6) as a more universally applicable indicator of consciousness. Other scales were subsequently developed to address this issue. Choi and colleagues devised a method to approximate the GCS in patients in whom the verbal response score was unobtainable, such as in intubated patients (Choi, Ward, & Becker, 1983). Most notable among these is the Swedish Reaction Level Scale (Starmark, Stålhammar, & Holmgren, 1988). It has the advantage over the GCS that it is more universally applicable and can be more accurately estimated from medical records in cases in which the initial GCS was never recorded. Although the RLS was properly validated against the GCS, it has not yet gained universal acceptance, perhaps for reasons of historical timing. Another scale in use, especially by trauma center units, is the Injury Severity Score (ISS), which is particularly valuable in cases of polytrauma (Baker, O'Neill, Haddon, & Long, 1974). It should be remembered that severe TBI is associated with other injuries in about 58% of patients, which should be properly treated during the acute phase (Groswasser, Lotem, & Mendelson, 1982; Groswasser, Cohen, & Blankstein, 1990).

Glasgow Outcome Scale (GOS)

It is evident that the assessment of outcome became part and parcel of the management of the acute phase very early. The renewed interest in TBI during the early 1970s prompted the search for a universal outcome measure that would encompass the various aspects of outcome following TBI, which are mostly related to the social domain. The timely introduction of the GOS by Jennett and Bond (Jennett & Bond, 1975), its relative simplicity, its strong association with the GCS, and its relative usefulness for follow-up studies led to its widespread acceptance. It was especially useful in studies conducted by non-rehabilitation professionals addressing questions of survival and, more recently, quality of outcome and life (Young et al., 1981). Disagreement on the GOS among trained observers was considerable, indicating that accurate prediction of the quality of life will be difficult to attain (Maas, Braakman, Schouten, Minderhoud, & van Zommern, 1983). A close look at the GOS categories shows that it is more related to independence in activities of daily living than to return to work, perhaps because work was regarded an unrealistic goal following severe TBI. The GOS was therefore not precise enough for rehabilitation settings (Rao et al., 1990) and of limited value regarding predictability of employment (Uzzell, Langfitt, & Dolinkas, 1987).

However, GCS scores providing confident predictions were available for only the 52–61% of patients in whom data were available up to three days. The higher confidence rate (61%) occurred when prediction was limited to death or survival (Jennett, Teasdale, Braakman, Minderhoud, & Knill-Jones, 1976). There was marginal improve-

ment in predictive power when the motor response subscale of the GCS was combined with assessment of brain stem reflexes in the Glasgow-Liege scale. The 5 selected reflexes—fronto-orbicular, vertical oculocephalic or oculovestibular, pupillary light, horizontal oculocephalic or oculovestibular, and the oculocardiac reflexes—disappear in the order here presented during rostrocaudal deterioration. When GOS was used for evaluating outcome (Born, Albert, Hans, & Bonnal, 1985), the combination of GCS, oculocephalic responses, and age improved predictability of outcome, which was measured as "poor" (combining severely disabled, vegetative, and dead patients) or "good" (combining good and moderate recovery) on the GOS. Although the predictability rose to 87% by the fourth day post-injury, the authors caution against using the prediction charts for clinical decision making, in particular on the sensitive issue of withholding treatment from very severely injured patients.

In recent years both neurosurgeons and the general public have become aware of the probable unfavorable outcomes of the vegetative state (VS), that the application of medical technology may not always be beneficial, and that prediction can influence therapy during the acute phase and before prognosis can be made with higher certainty, at about a week post-injury (Choi et al., 1983). This implies that every TBI patient should receive the best available therapy on admission and thereafter for at least a few days. Using prognostic factors based on probability carries inherent risks of a prophecy that might fulfill itself. Murray and colleagues showed that treatment of TBI patients during the acute phase was markedly influenced by introduction of predictive information and that TBI patients predicted to have the worst outcome received 39% less specific therapy at intensive care units in comparison to those with good prognosis. Although the authors claim that there were no adverse effects on outcome, they clearly state that introduction of a routine prediction instrument can alter patient management and that prognosis was a factor in decisions concerning application of certain kinds of therapy. The response to predictive information should allay concern that an adverse prediction might result in unreasonable early pessimism (Murray et al., 1993). It should also be borne in mind that the current social and political atmosphere for cost containment might have explicit and implicit influences on decision making and use of specific costly therapeutic measures, which might thus affect outcome of individual patients. Given the relatively high in-hospital mortality of severe TBI (30 to 40%), the major concern of acute phase treatment has been improvement of survival and early outcome as assessed within the first months post-injury, mostly in studies using the GOS. This has led to intensive research into the nature of the primary impact damage and the manageable components of secondary injury (Gentleman, Dearden, Midgley, & Maclean, 1993). Early referral to neuro-surgical/trauma units has had a major impact on mortality (Klauber, Marshall, Toole, Knowlton, & Bowers, 1985) and outcome (Groswasser & Cohen, 1985). Better in-hospital care, proper transport, and care of low-risk patients should be considered (Andrews, Piper, Dearden, & Miller, 1993; Colohan et al., 1989; Klauber et al., 1989). The question posed by Langfitt and Gennarelli, "can outcome from head injury be improved?" (Langfitt & Gennarelli, 1982), may have a somewhat more positive answer today in light of the extensive research regarding management of the acute phase and the growing body of evidence that early and timely interventions can reduce the overall damage as well as promote recovery of function.

Levati and colleagues concluded, "as regarding prognosis it is important to stress that no sign, even coma with flaccidity and areflexia, has an absolute value and that no sign can be an absolute criterion if considered independently from time course" (Levati, Farina, Vecchi, Rossanda, & Marrubini, 1982). It is therefore evident that although a great effort was placed on delineating possible relationships between early treatable and nontreatable factors and early as well as late outcome following severe TBI, no such straightforward parameters are at hand for the immediate posttraumatic period. Therefore, patients should be treated vigorously during the immediate posttraumatic period as if they are going to completely recover. The picture may differ at later points in time, and involves complex moral and ethical issues, and medical attitudes regarding quality of life.

Measuring Outcome in the Post-Acute Phase: Providers (Staff) and Consumers (Families and Patients)

During the acute phase treatment of severe TBI patients, physicians, and, to a lesser extent, other allied health professionals play the principal part in treatment and decision making. As time passes and the center stage problems shift from the medical to the psychosocial domain, the voices of family members, and ultimately patients, become more and more important to the process of recovery. It is therefore not surprising that the various participants in this complex process may develop different viewpoints regarding factors and scales that influence and monitor success of the recovery process (Table 8-2).

The post-acute care period of severe TBI patients begins when the patient is in no further need of either a trauma unit or continuous neuro-surgical care. However, this post-acute period might be prolonged, as many patients need care, guidance, and follow-up well beyond discharge from in-hospital rehabilitation or community re-entry programs. This may be so even for patients considered to have good outcome and who are relatively well integrated into "normal life." The need for a continuum of care was already recognized five decades ago. Robotham stated that ideally, following skilled acute treatment, the patient should be

Table 8-2. Post-Acute Care Measures in TBI Rehabilitation

1. Nontreatable Factors
   Age, Premorbid education

2. Admission Criteria and Measurements
   Rancho Los Amigos Cognitive Scale
   Disability Rating Scale (DRS)

3. Measures of Progress During Rehabilitation
   Disability Rating Scale (DRS)
   Functional Independence Measure (FIM)
   Functional Assessment Measure (FAM)
   Functional Assessment Scale (FAS)
   FIM + FAM + FAS

4. Outcome Measures—Society, Families, Patients
   Disability Rating Scale (DRS)
   Katz Adjustment Scale (KAS)
   Sickness Impact Profile (SIP)

5. Outcome Measures—Patients
   Independent Living (home, community)
   Work Status
   Quality of Life
   Rehabilitation Needs and Status Scale

sent to a rehabilitation center to be treated for his physical and mental problems by "doctors who fully understand the underlying problem" and that the closest cooperation must exist between participants in the acute and the post-acute phases (Robotham, 1949).

Severe TBI patients transferred for further in-hospital rehabilitation treatment may still have impaired consciousness or disorientation, or may be suffering from a wide range of CNS-related physical and mental problems. The benefits of early rehabilitation, including a better outcome at lower ultimate cost, have been shown by Cope and Hall (1982). Early rehabilitation with structured, inclusive, well-defined, and simple behavioral norms ("do's and don'ts") may largely decrease late maladaptive phenomena of aggression or the need for psychotherapy and pharmacotherapy to control behavior, and may increase trust and cooperation during the process. On the other hand, the advantages of concentrating rehabilitation in a later time period, when the patient recognizes his or her disabilities and is motivated to work toward recovery, have also been claimed.

During recovery, patients' families, and at later stages the patients themselves, become deeply involved in the rehabilitation process and may evaluate their outcome in different terms from those used by therapists. The evaluation of outcome may be even more diverse at this point since, depending on the complexity of CNS damage, an interdisciplinary team composed of physicians and other allied health professionals from various disciplines is usually involved. It may therefore be expected that each of the participants in the process—the various therapists, family members and patients—will have different temporal objectives. Indeed, many neuropsychologic and behavioral scales and assessments were devised in order to measure the progress of various therapies in TBI patients. It is evident that one of the prerequisites of a successful rehabilitation process will be the setting of goals and intermediate aims that will be common to the parties involved. Objective, understandable, and easy to perform common measures are therefore an integral part of rehabilitation. A comprehensive understanding of the various aspects of TBI is required to properly use these scales. The major sequelae of brain injury include motor deficits (including motor control and behavior), communication disorders (language and speech), cognitive deficits, and behavioral disturbances, all being of prognostic importance regard-

ing outcome, which is currently assessed by independence and employability (Table 8-3) (Groswasser, Mendelson, Stern, Schechter, & Najenson, 1977; Najenson et al., 1975; Schwab, Grafman, Salazar, & Kraft, 1993).

In the early post-acute period, once survival is no longer an issue, a new set of questions arises, debated by staff and families alike and, eventually, by the aware and conscious TBI patient. Questions such as "What will be the final outcome?" "Is he/she going to be the same as prior to injury?" and later "Am I the same person?" are the most common. Unfortunately, there are no straightforward answers to any of these questions in that early phase. This inherent uncertainty may cause concern and may even be a source of tension between staff and families.

In order to monitor change, to decrease uncertainty, and to increase trust during the process, a proper assessment of the surviving patient is needed at the time the patient is transferred to post-acute care. The GOS, while useful as a gross measure of outcome, particularly for assessing acute therapies aimed at improving survival, is nevertheless not detailed enough to be of use in the rehabilitation process (Rao et al., 1990), as it is related to cognitive scores within the first three months of injury but less so thereafter (Brooks, Campsie, Symington, Beattie, & McKinlay, 1986). Other scales have thus evolved for this purpose.

Ideally, a single tool capable of quantitatively and validly measuring temporal related changes through all phases—from intensive care unit to social functioning—would be the perfect one.

The Disability Rating Scale (DRS) was developed by Rappaport and colleagues in order to quantitatively assess severe TBI patients, "particularly through the midzone of recovery spectrum, between early arousal from coma and early sentient

Table 8-3. Long-Term Goals in TBI Rehabilitation

Return to Independent Living
  Home
  Community
Return to Work/School
  Gainful employment
  Homemaker
  Volunteer employment
  Sheltered employment
Assessment by providers of therapy—admission criteria and initial follow-up.

functioning" (Rappaport, Hall, Hopkins, Belleza, & Cope, 1982). The use of the same scale through the recovery process provides consistency over time. The scale is composed of eight items that fall into four categories (Table 8-4).

The first category, which describes arousability, awareness, and responsivity, utilizes the GCS, while the second and third categories, related to cognitive ability for self-care and dependence on others, are actually measures of independence in activities of daily living (ADLs), already in wide use in other scales in rehabilitation medicine. The fourth category is an employability rating and was correctly designed to reflect psychosocial adaptability and was considered to reflect, in a global way, the severity of the residual mental and cognitive disabilities that have an impact on "the individual's ability to compete and to undertake useful work in the marketplace, or to carry out home responsibilities or responsibilities as student" (Rappaport et al., 1982). Employability was described in the following four subcategories: (1) nonrestricted; (2) selected jobs, competitive; (3) sheltered workshop; and (4) unemployable. These four subcategories of employability are very close to those of Najenson and colleagues, who used professional and nonprofessional categories to describe competitive gainful employment (Najenson, Groswasser, Mendelson, & Hackett, 1980; Najenson et al., 1974). The DRS has face validity as well as independent validity and high interobserver agreement. The initial rating was closely related to final outcome, thus showing that patients surviving more severe trauma were left with more disabilities. The pooling of the DRS variables with indices of severity of injury and head injury deficits explained 62% of the total variance of rehabilitation outcome in patients entering a rehabilitation program, which was considered a reasonably high level of prediction considering the variability of functional outcomes (Fleming & Maas, 1994).

The DRS was considered by its authors as possibly helpful in identifying patients who should not be admitted to an intensive hospital rehabilitation program (Rappaport et al., 1982). This conclusion is questionable in view of the benefits of early intervention (Cope & Hall, 1982; Mackay, Bernstein, Chapman, Morgan, & Milazzo, 1992; Rappaport, Herreo-Backe, Rappaport, & Winterfield, 1989) and the above-mentioned explained variance of only 62%. Other authors have found an association between the initial DRS score and discharge score and length of stay. Despite the association found,

the authors state that accurate prediction of length of hospitalization remains difficult (Elliason & Topp, 1984).

Hall and colleagues found that the usefulness of the DRS to monitor changes during rehabilitation was better than that of the GOS (Hall, Cope, & Rappaport, 1985). DRS admission scores were found to be of predictive value, including predicting patients' return to work or school (Fryer & Haffey, 1987; Gouvier, Blanton, LePorte, & Nepomuceno, 1987).

The Functional Independence Measure (FIM) was constructed in order to have a uniform measure in rehabilitation settings and to reflect the cost of disability. The FIM, as earlier the DRS, incorporated items from previous functional scales and had high content and construct validity, especially in stroke patients. Progress of severe TBI patients during in-program rehabilitation as well as during follow-up was assessed with ease (Hall, Hamilton, Gordon, & Zasler, 1993). The FIM is constructed of 18 items, each with a 7-level ordinal scale; 13 are considered to evaluate motor disability and the remaining 5 cognitive deficits (Table 8-5). However, the FIM is not diagnostically specific and underemphasizes the cognitive and psychosocial components, which are by far the dominant sequelae in TBI patients (Hall et al., 1993; Hall & Johnston, 1994).

The Functional Assessment Measure (FAM) was developed as an adjunct to the FIM. It consists of 12 items related to motor, cognitive, and psychosocial aspects more specific to TBI (Table 8-5). Interobserver reliability on the FAM pilot study was considerably lower when compared to the FIM (55% and 81%, respectively). The FIM requires about 40 minutes to complete and needs special training; adding the FAM has not been shown to contribute to prediction of length of stay and costs, and its reliability had yet to be validated (Hall et al., 1993; Hall & Johnston, 1994). Critical problems in TBI rehabilitation such as awareness and behavioral control were not covered by the FIM+FAM combination and had to be added to the evaluation.

The Functional Assessment Scale (FAS), developed at the Rehabilitation Institute of Chicago (Chichowski & Simantel, 1992), addresses the issues of awareness of disability, behavioral control, pragmatics, written expression, reading comprehension, money management, and community recreation reintegration, and was introduced for the evaluation of TBI rehabilitation. The usefulness of the combined FIM+FAM+FAS mea-

Table 8-4.   Disability Rating Scale Categories and Items (1982)

Category	Item
1. Arousability, awareness and responsivity	Eye opening Verbalization Motor responses
2. Cognitive ability for self-care activities	Feeding Toileting Grooming
3. Dependence on others	Level of functioning
4. Psychosocial adaptability	"Employability"

Table 8-5.   FIM and FAM Items

Motor Items

Self-care

Bathing, grooming
Dressing: upper and lower body
Eating, swallowing
Sphincter control, bowel and bladder management

Mobility

Locomotion: walking, stairs, wheelchair
Transfers: bed, chair, wheelchair, auto,
Community mobility

Cognition/Behavior

Communication

Expression, comprehension, reading, writing
Speech intelligibility

Psychosocial adjustment

Emotional status and adjustment to limitations
Social interaction
Employability

Cognitive function

Problem solving, judgment
Orientation and memory
Attention

sure is one of the current issues in TBI research. Another comprehensive scale is the Patient Evaluation and Conference System (PECS), which includes the rehabilitation team goals for patients, but has gained only limited use (Harvey & Jellinek, 1981).

The Rancho Los Amigos Level of Cognitive Functioning Scale (Rancho Scale) described by Hagen (1982) is much in use in referral of patients to different post-acute care facilities and level of care. In combination with length of coma and duration of PTA, it accounted for 79% of the variance of outcome, while other indices of severity (GCS and trauma score) failed to meet the level of 75%. The disability scales (DRS, FIM and FAM motor and cognition) were all well intercorrelated with each other at a level of 78% and any added other single factor increased the explained variance to a level of 92% (Hall et al., 1993).

It is our impression that, given the limited prognostic capacity of currently available predictive measures of late psychosocial outcome from severe TBI, there is at the moment insufficient data to justify exclusion of conscious severe TBI patients from the benefits of an intensive rehabilitation program. The DRS seems to be, at least at the present state of knowledge, the most suitable tool for longitudinal assessment of severe TBI patients.

Assessment by Providers of Therapy— Outcome and Its Predictors

Return to work (RTW) is traditionally considered by those involved in TBI rehabilitation to be the best integrative criterion for a successful recovery process and the "core and raison d'etre" of rehabilitation medicine (Livneh, 1988). This is not surprising since it is individuals who, despite significant disability, are active and productive members of society and are well integrated into their communities, who most often consider themselves to have a high quality of life (Melamed, Stern, Rahmani, Groswasser, & Najenson, 1982). Measures that quantify the client's achievement in work, school, home, and community should be routinely employed to measure what actually matters (Whiteneck, 1994). TBI rehabilitation outcome studies intuitively used career categories as outcome measures following TBI (Najenson et al., 1980; Najenson et al., 1974; Rusk, Block, & Lowman, 1969). The ability to work has been used by numerous authors as a cardinal yardstick for psychosocial recovery (McLean, Dikman, & Temkin, 1993; Rappaport et al., 1989). Leisure time activities were also used, but less frequently (McLean et al., 1993; Oddy, Humphrey, & Uttley, 1978b; Tate, Lulham, Broe, Strettles, & Pfaff, 1989). The growing literature on TBI rehabilitation often uses employment as almost a synonym for successful outcome and has prompted a large body of research aiming at predicting the power of various factors on outcome. The various factors studied include nontreatable ones such as age and premorbid education, premorbid intelligence (Grafman et al., 1988), severity of injury, as well as the influence of various treatment approaches aiming at reducing damage during the acute phase and promoting recovery during later phases. As employment is rather in the social domain, factors such as premorbid education and employment and the chance to return to a previous workplace, although sometimes in a different capacity, appeared to be important predictors in determining outcome (Robertson, 1987).

Age is a well-known independent factor affecting mortality of severe TBI patients and may reflect the higher incidence of mass lesions such as subdural hematomas (Luersen, Klauber, & Marshall, 1988). Earlier studies have set the age of 30 years as the border for good recovery (Overgaard et al., 1973) but more recent studies are more optimistic, claiming that it exerts its effect on vocational outcome in TBI patients only in patients over their mid-forties (Dornan & Schentag, 1995; McMordie, Barker, & Paolo, 1990; Najenson et al., 1974). In other studies age had a significant but marginal impact on outcome (Lokkenberg & Grimes, 1984). Factors such as preexisting systemic diseases, CT findings, and the predisposition of older patients to intracranial mass lesions could not completely account for the age effect. It was concluded that "age effects are intrinsic to the aged brain and that aging impairs the ability of the brain to recover, regardless of etiology" (Vollmer et al., 1991).

Other nontreatable factors were the opportunity to return to a previous job and premorbid education (Robertson, 1987).

Severity of injury assessed by either duration of LOC or PTA has been found to be related to outcome in numerous studies. The relationship of the initial GCS score to outcome was less clear and could not serve as a predictor even in patients unconscious for long periods (Lyle et al., 1986; Sazbon & Groswasser, 1990). The initial GCS score bore little relationship to later cognitive outcome, while PTA was found to be of greater value (Bishara, Partridge, Godfrey, & Knight, 1992; Brooks, Aughton, Bond, & Rivzi, 1980).

Studies of military low velocity penetrating brain injury have shown that most patients with such focal brain wounds have only brief or no loss of consciousness. Such PHI patients with left hemisphere injury also had significantly greater and longer loss of consciousness than those with right-sided injuries, but there was no relationship of loss of consciousness to RTW in those patients, suggesting that LOC is a less valuable measure of injury severity in these unique low velocity focal penetrating brain wounds. The brain areas most associated with unconsciousness are the posterior limb of the left internal capsule, left basal forebrain, midbrain, and hypothalamus (Salazar et al., 1986).

Eight clinical factors outlined by Sazbon and Groswasser to negatively influence recovery of consciousness in severe CHI patients are also closely related to these regions. Six of these, i.e., diffuse body sweating, fever of central origin, abnormal antidiuretic hormone secretion, abnormal motor reactivity, respiratory disturbances, and associated injuries, were already present during the first week after trauma; the other two were late post-traumatic epilepsy and development of hydrocephalus (Sazbon & Groswasser, 1990). However, about 11% of patients who were unconscious for over one month and were subject to an intensive rehabilitation intervention recovered and were gainfully employed (Groswasser & Sazbon, 1990).

Of the four domains of brain function, the motor/physical domain shows the most impressive recovery and is the quickest (McLean et al., 1993). It is thus the communicative, cognitive, and behavioral sequelae that are the most important in determining a "good outcome."

In a recent follow-up study of penetrating head injured Vietnam War veterans, 56% were working at re-evaluation some 14 years after injury and 80% had worked at some point in the five years prior to the evaluation (Schwab et al., 1993). Their occupational distribution also differed little from that of uninjured controls or the male working force (Kraft, Schwab, Salazar, & Brown, 1993). In this population, factor and logistic regression analysis identified seven strictly defined impairments that significantly predicted failure of RTW: post-traumatic epilepsy, paresis, visual field loss, verbal memory loss, visual memory loss, psychological problems, and violent behavior. The seven items describe widely different domains of brain function, suggesting the global nature of RTW as a functional measure. The items were also relatively equipotential in their prediction of RTW, so that a summed score of the number of these seven impairments present was suggested as a practical "Disability Score" (Table 8-6) (Schwab et al., 1993). It was the *number* of items present, more so

Table 8-6. Disability Score and Return to Work

Post-traumatic epilepsy
Paresis
Visual field loss
Verbal memory loss
Visual memory loss
Psychological problems
Violent behavior

than which one, that predicted RTW. Patients with more than any three of these impairments were generally unable to compensate and had much lower work rates. This analysis reemphasizes the remarkable capacity of the young adult brain to compensate for injury, probably by using intact domains of brain function to make up for those that are impaired. Close examination of these factors also shows that most of them are in the cognitive and behavioral domains, as is also true in closed head injured patients. Post-traumatic seizures are more common in PHI than in CHI and may therefore be more specific to this military population than to closed head injured patients.

The RTW rate of 56% for penetrating head injured patients (Schwab et al., 1993) is close to figures provided by other authors regarding survivors of severe closed head injury (Najenson et al., 1980; Najenson et al., 1974; Schalén, Nordström, & Nordström, 1994), although earlier studies showed more discouraging figures of 29% and 22% (Brooks, Campsie, Symington, Beattie, & McKinlay, 1987; Levin, Grossman, Rose, & Teasdale, 1979). Recently, Wehman and colleagues found that 51% of their severe TBI patients were employed at one year, although some of them did so after several job trials (Wehman, West, Kregel, Sherron, & Kreutzer, 1995). Given that all these series report on patients with similar severity, the differences between the earlier and the more optimistic later reports that were generated from rehabilitation-oriented programs may reflect the usefulness of methods such as supported employment. Patients and their families should thus no longer be led to believe that returning to work is impossible (Wehman et al., 1995).

Assessment of Outcome by Consumers of Therapy—Families and Patients

Disability scales cannot measure the convergence between therapists on one side and TBI patients and their families on the other. What actually matters for patients and families is the perceived handicap caused by impairment and disability and its influence on quality of life. Understanding and awareness of the patient's objective residual capacity is crucial for all involved for setting realistic goals.

Families

In the immediate post-traumatic period, the question of life or death dominates. While the patient is still unconscious and if this period becomes prolonged, the uncertainty may lead to anxiety and overt or covert aggression toward the staff (Stern, Sazbon, Becker, & Costeff, 1988).

The surviving severe TBI patient creates a different range of questions for his family, which is a different source of stress. Oddy and colleagues used the Wakefield Depression Scale to measure stress in the family. They found that the worst period of stress for the majority of relatives appeared to be during the first month post-injury and that stress tended to level off by the sixth month and not diminish afterwards (Oddy, Humphrey, & Uttley, 1978a). Female relatives of male severe TBI patients suffered significant psychiatric morbidity when interviewed at home three months after the injury (Livingston, Brooks, & Bond, 1985), and that morbidity was significantly higher when compared to family members of stroke or spinal cord patients (Rosenbaum & Najenson, 1976). Various long-term follow-ups of one to seven years have shown that the burden on families is not lessened with time, mostly because of the residual cognitive and behavioral sequelae. Relatives tended to report increasing disturbances by the patient, probably indicating a higher level of frustration in the family more so than actual deterioration of the patient (Brooks et al., 1986; Brooks et al., 1987; Klonoff, Snow, & Costa, 1986). Several authors have reported on differences in the perceived residual handicaps between TBI patients and their families. There was more agreement regarding physical disabilities, while families tended to report more severe cognitive and behavioral disturbances than patients (Braun, Baribeau, & Ethier, 1988; Goldstein & McCue, 1995). This may reflect denial of illness and the patients' decreased awareness of their impairments and failure to accept disability (Melamed, Groswasser, & Stern, 1992), emphasizing the need for prolonged patient and family care and support.

The Katz Adjustment Scale (KAS) was developed as a set of inventories designed for ". . . objectively assessing the adjustment and social behavior of pre-psychotic and ex-hospital patients in the community" (Katz & Lyerly, 1963). The instrument was to be used to measure patient adjustment over long periods of time, making it useful for long-term follow-up of patients. It was meant to be administered to a "close relative" who could report on the patient. The authors note that "only the patient can report on his own personal comfort and his satisfaction with his level of performance." However, the authors note that when a patient is "highly disturbed," responses to inventories are likely to be less than dependable. A subset of items was identified for patient self-rating.

The instrument was subjected to cluster analysis and was found to produce 12 clusters of items, which the authors labeled *belligerence, verbal expansiveness, negativism, helplessness, suspiciousness, anxiety, withdrawal and retardation, general psychopathology, nervousness, confusion, bizarreness,* and *hyperactivity.* These items and the description of patient symptoms and social behavior fit many of the frequent complaints of TBI patients and their relatives. Not surprisingly, this instrument has been used in some TBI studies, particularly those concerned with long-term follow-up. Adjustments of the KAS for use in TBI patients were proposed by several authors (Goran & Fabiano, 1992; Jackson et al., 1992).

The Sickness Impact Profile (SIP) is a measure of health status comprised of 136 statements measuring functioning in 12 areas of living: sleep and rest, emotional behavior, body care and movement, home management, mobility, social interaction, ambulation, alertness, communication, recreation and pastimes, eating, and work (Bergner, Bobbitt, Cartyer, & Gilson, 1981; Bergner, Bobbitt, Pollard, Martin, & Gilson, 1976). It has been shown to be reliable and valid across demographic and cultural subgroups (Bergner et al., 1981; Bergner et al., 1976). Careful review of the instrument for possible deficiencies in measuring the status of TBI populations led to testing of a modified version of the SIP. However, Temkin and colleagues report that these modifications did not make "differences of practical degree" and so recommended that the "standard Sickness Impact Profile performed well and is recommended for evaluation of day-to-day functioning in head injury studies" (Temkin et al., 1988).

Patients

As already shown, there are numerous studies on treatment, prognosis, outcome, and attitudes of families, and we have attempted to provide an outline of how TBI survival and outcome have been measured for such studies. A closer look reveals that all those measures are linked to society's expectations of the TBI patient, including the cost of survival and treatment and the burden on relatives. The number of studies devoted to the way TBI patients look upon their lives are very few and are based on surveys (Condeluci, Ferris, & Bogdan, 1992). Yet in the long run, measures of the TBI sur-

vivor's perspective and his or her quality of life may be the most important parameters to consider. Since the definition of quality of life is subjective and can best be provided by patients themselves, it is our obligation to try to understand how each patient defines his or her post-traumatic, post-rehabilitation quality of life. Such an attempt was made by Melamed and colleagues (Melamed et al., 1982), who used the Rehabilitation Need and Status Scale (RNSS), suggested by Kravetz (Kravetz, 1973) and later by Kravetz and colleagues (Kravetz, Florian, & Wright, 1985). Each patient was asked to define his position on seven subscales that represent various aspects of psychosocial life (Table 8-7). Return to work (RTW) was highly correlated with the various subjective components of RNSS. Particularly high correlation was found between patients' work (including sheltered work) and their subjective rating of quality of life (Melamed et al., 1982). This suggests that RTW is a valid measurement of outcome following TBI. Furthermore, it enables us to set RTW, which is objective and measurable, as a goal of rehabilitation, knowing its high correlation with the patient's subjective assessment of good quality of life.

Summary

It is not surprising that the largest body of data regarding severe TBI relates to the acute phase. The post-acute phase, which is concerned with quality of life rather than with preserving life, is less dramatic and has therefore attracted less resources and study. The attitudes of patients have been the least heard as they typically could not speak for themselves. This is reflected in the size of the literature on each phase of the rehabilitation process.

The development of standardized measures of TBI severity and outcome, particularly since the

Table 8-7. Rehabilitation Need and Status Scale (RNSS)

1. Physiological need satisfaction
2. Emotional security need satisfaction
3. Family need satisfaction
4. Social need satisfaction
5. Economic self esteem
6. Economic security need satisfaction
7. Vocational self-actualization need satisfaction

introduction of the GCS and GOS, has allowed for a blossoming of clinical research in this field. Interestingly, this has served to emphasize the validity of older measures of severity such as duration of unconsciousness or PTA and of long-term outcome, such as return to work or school. It is important to consider outcome scales in the context in which they were developed and the needs they were intended to address, whether acute, post-acute, or long-term. The most glaring needs in this regard relate to measuring patient preferences, family needs, and overall quality of life after TBI.

References

Andrews PJD, Piper IR, Dearden NM, Miller JD. Secondary insults during intrahospital transport of head-injured patients. *Lancet* 1993;335:327–30.

Baker SP, O'Neill B, Haddon W, Long WB. The injury severity score: a method for describing patients with multiple injuries and evaluation of emergency care. *J Trauma* 1974;14:187–96.

Bergner M, Bobbitt RA, Carter WB, Gilson BS. The Sickness Impact Profile: development and final revision of a health status measure. *Med Care* 1981;19:787–805.

Bergner M, Bobbitt RA, Pollard WA, Martin DP, Gilson BE. The Sickness Impact Profile: validation of a health status measure. *Med Care* 1976;14:57–67.

Bishara SN, Partridge FM, Godfrey HPD, Knight RTG. Post-traumatic amnesia and the Glasgow Coma Scale related to outcome in survivors in a consecutive series of patients with severe closed head injury. *Brain Injury* 1992;4:373–80.

Born JD, Albert A, Hans P, Bonnal J. Relative prognostic value of best motor response and brain stem reflexes in patients with severe head injury. *Neurosurgery* 1985;16:595–601.

Braun CMJ, Baribeau JM, Ethier M. (1988). A prospective investigation comparing patients' and relatives' symptom reports before and after a rehabilitation program for severe closed head injury. *J Neuro Rehab* 1988;2:109–15.

Brooks DN, Aughton ME, Bond MR, Rivzi S. Cognitive sequelae in relationship to early indices of severity of brain damage after severe blunt head injury. *J Neurol Neurosurg Psychiatry* 1980;43:529–34.

Brooks DN, Campsie L, Symington C, Beattie A, McKinlay W. The five year outcome of severe blunt head injury: a relative's view. *J Neurol Neurosurg Psychiatry* 1986;49:764–70.

Brooks DN, Campsie L, Symington C, Beattie A, McKinlay W. The effects of head injury on patients

and relatives within seven years of injury. *J Head Injury Rehab* 1987;2:1–13.

Chichowski KS, Simantel H. *RIC—FAS Version 3 (manual)*. Chicago: Rehabilitation Institute of Chicago, 1992.

Choi SC, Ward JD, Becker DP. Chart for outcome prediction in severe head injury. *J Neurosurg* 1983;59:294–97.

Colohan ART, Alves WM, Gross CR, Torner JC, Mehta VS, Tandon PN, Jane JA. Head injury mortality in two centers with different emergency medical services and intensive care. *J Neurosurg* 1989;71:202–207.

Condeluci A, Ferris LL, Bogdan A. Outcome and value: the survivor's perspective. *J Head Injury Rehab* 1992;7:37–45.

Cope N, Hall KM. Head injury rehabilitation: benefits of early intervention. *Arch Phys Med Rehabil* 1982;63:433–37.

Diller L. *Finding the right treatment combination: changes over the past five years*. Hillside, NJ: Lawrence Erlbaum Associates, Publishers, 1994.

Elliason MR, Topp BW. Predictive validity of Rappaport's Disability Rating Scale in subjects with acute brain injury. *Phys Ther* 1984;64:1357–60.

Epstein AM. The outcome movement—will it get us where we want to go? *New Engl J Med* 1990;323:266–69.

Fleming JM, Maas F. Prognosis of rehabilitation outcome in head injury using the Disability Rating Scale. *Arch Phys Med Rehabil* 1994;75:156–63.

Fryer LJ, Haffey WJ. Cognitive rehabilitation and community readaptation: outcomes from two program models. *J Head Trauma Rehab* 1987;2:51–63.

Gennarelli TA, Spielman GM, Langfitt TW, et al. Influence of type of intracranial lesion on outcome from severe head injury. *J Neurosurg* 1982;56:26–32.

Gentleman D, Dearden M, Midgley S, Maclean D. Guidelines for resuscitation and transfer of patients with serious head injury. *Br Med J* 1993;307:547–52.

Goldstein G, McCue M. Differences between patients and informant functional outcome rating in head-injured individuals. *Intl J Rehab Health* 1995;1:25–35.

Goldstein M. Traumatic brain injury: a silent epidemic. *Ann Neurol* 1990;27:327.

Goran DA, Fabiano RJ. The scaling of the Katz Adjustment Scale in a traumatic brain injury rehabilitation sample. *Brain Injury* 1992;7:219–29.

Gouvier WD, Blanton PD, LePorte KK, Nepomuceno C. Reliability and validity of the Disability Rating Scale and the levels of cognitive functioning scale in monitoring recovery from severe head injury. *Arch Phys Med Rehabil* 1987;68:94–97.

Grafman J, Jonas BS, Martin A, et al. Intellectual function following penetrating head injury in Vietnam veterans. *Brain* 1988;111:169–84.

Groswasser Z, Cohen M. Rehabilitation outcome of combat head injuries: Comparison of October 1973 War and Lebanon War, 1982. *Israel Journal of Medical Sciences* 1985;21:957–61.

Groswasser Z, Lotem M, Mendelson L. Treatment of femoral fractures in patients with craniocerebral injury. *International Surgery* 1982;67:556–58.

Groswasser Z, Mendelson L, Stern JM, Schechter I, Najenson T. Re-evaluation of prognostic parameters in rehabilitation after severe head injury. *Scand J Rehab Med* 1977;9:147–49.

Groswasser Z, Sazbon L. Outcome in 134 patients with prolonged posttraumatic unawareness. Part 2: functional outcome of 72 patients recovering consciousness. *J Neurosurg* 1990;(72):81–84.

Hagen C (ed.). *Language cognitive disorganization following closed head injury: a conceptualization.* New York: Plenum Press, 1982.

Hall K, Cope N, Rappaport M. (1985). Glasgow Outcome Scale and Disability rating scale: comparative usefulness in following recovery in traumatic head injury. *Arch Phys Med Rehabil* 1985;66:35–37.

Hall KM, Hamilton BB, Gordon WA, Zasler ND. (1993). Characteristics and comparisons of functional assessment indices: Disability Rating Scale, Functional Independence Measure, and Functional Assessment Measure. *J Head Trauma Rehab* 1993;8:60–74.

Hall KM, Johnston MV. (1994). Outcomes evaluation in TBI rehabilitation. Part II: Measuring tools for a National Data System. *Arch Phys Med Rehabil* 1994;75:SC75–SC18.

Harvey RF, Jellinek HM. Functional performance assessment: a program approach. *Arch Phys Med Rehabil* 1981;62:456–61.

Ip RY, Dornan J, Schentag C. Traumatic brain injury: factors predicting return to work or school. *Brain Injury* 1995;9:517–32.

Jackson HF, Hopewell CA, Glass CA, Warburg R, Dewey M, Ghadiali E. (1992). The Katz Adjustment Scale: modification for use with victims of traumatic brain and spinal injury. *Brain Injury* 1992;6:109–27.

Jennett B, Bond M. Assessment of outcome after severe brain damage. A practical scale. *Lancet* 1975;I:480–84.

Jennett B, Plum M (1972). Persistent vegetative state after brain damage. *Lancet* 1972;I:734–37.

Jennett B, Teasdale G, Braakman R, Minderhoud J, Knill-Jones R. Predicting outcome in individual patients after severe head injury. *Lancet* 1976;I:1031–34.

Katz MM, Lyerly SB. (1963). Methods for measuring adjustment and social behavior in the community: I. rational, description, discriminative validity and scale development. *Psychological Reports* 1963;13:503–35.

Klauber MR, Marshall LF, Luersen TG, Frankowski R, Tabaddor K, Eisenberg HM. (1989). Determinants of head injury mortality: importance of low risk patient. *Neurosurgery* 1989;24:31–36.

Klauber MR, Marshall LF, Toole BM, Knowlton SL, Bowers SA. Cause of decline in head-injury mortality rate in San Diego County, California. *J Neurosurg* 1985;62:528–31.

Klonoff PS, Snow WG, Costa LD. Determinants of head injury mortality: importance of low risk patient. *Neurosurgery* 1996;(19):735–42.

Kraft JF, Schwab K, Salazar AM, Brown HR. Occupational and educational achievements of head injured Vietnam veterans at 15-year follow-up. *Arch Phys Med Rehabil* 1993;74:596–601.

Kravetz S. Rehabilitation need and status: substance, structure, and process. Unpublished Ph.D., Wisconsin, 1973.

Kravetz S, Florian V, Wright GN. The development of a multifaceted measure of rehabilitation effectiveness: theoretical rationale and scale construction. *Rehab Psych* 1985;30:195–208.

Langfitt TW, Gennarelli TA. Can the outcome from head injury be improved? *J Neurosurg* 1982;56:19–25.

Levati A, Farina ML, Vecchi G, Rossanda M, Marrubini MB. Prognosis of severe head injuries. *J Neurosurg* 1982;57:779–83.

Levin HS, Grossman RG, Rose JE, Teasdale G. Long-term neuropsychological outcome in closed head injury. *J Neurosurg* 1979;50:412–22.

Livingston MG, Brooks DN, Bond MR. Three months after severe head injury: psychiatric and social impact on relatives. *J Neurol Neurosurg Psychiatry* 1985;48:870–75.

Livneh H. Assessing outcome criteria in rehabilitation: a multi-component approach. *Rehab Counseling Bull* 1988:32:72–94.

Lokkenberg AR, Grimes RM. Assessing the influence of non-treatment variables in the study of outcome from severe head injury. *J Neurosurg* 1984;61:254–62.

Luersen TG, Klauber MR, Marshall LF. Outcome from head injury related to patient's age. *J Neurosurgery* 1988;68:409–16.

Lyle DM, Pierce JP, Freeman EA, et al. Clinical course and outcome of severe head injury in Australia. *J Neurosurg* 1986;65:15–18.

Maas AIR, Braakman R, Schouten HJA, Minderhoud JM, van Zommern AH. Agreement between physicians on assessment of outcome following severe head injury. *J Neurosurg* 1983;58:321–25.

Mackay LE, Bernstein BA, Chapman PE, Morgan AS, Milazzo LS. Early intervention in severe head injury: long-term benefits of a formalized program. *Arch Phys Med Rehabil* 1992;73:635–41.

McLean A, Dikman SS, Temkin NR. Psychosocial recovery after head injury. *Arch Phys Med Rehabil* 1993;74:1041–46.

McMordie WR, Barker SL, Paolo TM. Return to work (RTW) after head injury. *Brain Injury* 1990;4:57–69.

Melamed S, Groswasser Z, Stern JM. Acceptance of disability, work congruence and subjective rehabilitation status of traumatic brain injured (TBI) patients. *Brain Injury* 1992;6:233–43.

Melamed S, Stern MJ, Rahmani L, Groswasser Z, Najenson T. Work congruence, behavioural pathology and rehabilitation status of severe craniocerebral injury. In: Lahav E (ed.). *Psychosocial research in rehabilitation.* Tel-Aviv: Ministry of Defense Publishing House, 1982:59–74.

Murray LS, Teasdale GM, Murray GD, et al. Does prediction of outcome alter patient management? *Lancet* 1993;341:1487–91.

Najenson T, Groswasser Z, Mendelson L, Hackett, P. Rehabilitation outcome of brain damaged patients after severe head injury. *Intl Rehab Med* 1080;2:17–22.

Najenson T, Groswasser Z, Stern JM., Schechter I, David C, Berghaus N, Mendelson L. Prognostic factors in rehabilitation after severe head injury. *Scand J Rehab Med* 1975;7:101–105.

Najenson T, Mendelson L, Schechter I, David C, Mintz N, Groswasser Z. Rehabilitation after severe head injury. *Scand J Rehab Med* 1974;6:5–12.

Oddy M, Humphrey M, Uttley D. Stress upon relatives of head injured patients. *J Neurol Neurosurg Psychiatry* 1978a;41:507–13.

Oddy M, Humphrey M, Uttley D. Subjective impairment and social recovery after closed head injury. *J Neurol Neurosurg Psychiatry* 1978b;41:611–16.

Overgaard J, Christensen S, Hvid-Hansen O, Land AM, Hein O, Pedersen K, Tweed W. Prognosis after head injury based on early clinical examination. *Lancet* 1973;II:631–35.

Rao N, Rosenthal M, Cronin-Stubb D, Lambert R, Barnes P, Swanson B. Return to work after rehabilitation following traumatic brain injury. *Brain Injury* 1990;4:49–56.

Rappaport M, Hall KM, Hopkins K, Belleza T, Cope N. Disability rating scale for severe head trauma: coma to community. *Arch Phys Med Rehabil* 1982;63:118–23.

Rappaport M, Herreo-Backe C, Rappaport ML, Winterfield KM. Head injury outcome up to ten years later. *Arch Phys Med Rehabil* 1989;70:885–92.

Roberts AH. Long-term prognosis of severe accidental head injury. *Proc Royal Soc Med* 1976;69:137–40.

Robertson J. Return to work after severe head injury. *International Disability Studies* 1987;9:49–54.

Robotham G. *Acute injuries to the head.* Edinburgh: E&S Livingstone Ltd., 1949.

Rosenbaum M, Najenson T. Changes in life pattern and symptoms of low mood as reported by wives of severely brain injured soldiers. *J Consult Clin Psychol* 1976;44:881–88.

Rusk HA, Block JM, Lowman EW (eds.). *Rehabilitation of the brain injured patient.* Springfield: Charles C. Thomas, 1969.

Russell WR, Smith A. Post-traumatic amnesia in closed head injury. *Arch Neurol* 1961;5:16–29.

Salazar AM, Grafman J, Vance SC, Weingartner H, Dollon JD, Ludlow C. Consciousness and amnesia after penetrating head injury: neurology and anatomy. *Neurology* 1986;36:178–87.

Sazbon L, Groswasser Z. Outcome in 134 patients with prolonged posttraumatic unawareness. Part 1: parameters determining late recovery of consciousness. *J Neurosurg* 1990;72:75–80.

Schalén W, Nordström G, Nordström CH. Economic aspects of capacity to work after severe traumatic brain lesions. *Brain Injury* 1994;8:37–47.

Schwab K, Grafman J, Salazar AM, Kraft J. Residual impairments and work status 15 years after penetrating head injury: report from the Vietnam Head Injury Study. *Neurology* 1993;43:95–103.

Starmark JE, Stålhammar D, Holmgren E. The Reaction Level Scale (RLS85). *Acta Neurochirurgica* 1988;91:12–20.

Stein SG, Spettel C. Head Injury Severity Scale (HISS): a practical classification of closed-head injury. *Brain Injury* 1995;9:437–44.

Stern MJ, Sazbon L, Becker L, Costeff H. Severe behavioural disturbances in families of patients with prolonged coma. *Brain Injury* 1988;2:259–62.

Tate RL, Lulham JM, Broe GA, Strettles B, Pfaff A. Psychosocial outcome for survivors of severe blunt head injury: the results from a consecutive series of 100 patients. *J Neurol Neurosurg Psychiatry* 1989;52:1128–34.

Teasdale G, Jennett B. Assessment of coma and impaired consciousness. *Lancet* 1974;II:81–84.

Teasdale GM. Head injury. *J Neurol Neurosurg Psychiatry* 1995;58:526–39.

Temkin N, McLean A, Dikmen S, Gale J, Bergner M, Almes MJ. Development and evaluation of modification to the Sickness Impact Profile for head injury. *J Clin Epidemiol* 1988;14:47–57.

Uzzell B, Langfitt TW, Dolinkas CA. Influence of injury severity on quality of survival after head injury. *Surg Neurol* 1987;27:419–29.

Vogenthaler DR, Smith KR, Goldfader P. Head injury, a multivariate study: prediction of long-term productivity and independent living outcome. *Brain Injury* 1989;3:369–85.

Vollmer DG, Torner JC, Jane JA, et al. Age and outcome following traumatic coma: why do older patients fare worse? *J Neurosurg* 1991;75:S37–S49.

Wehman PH, West MD, Kregel J, Sherron P, Kreutzer JS. Return to work for persons with severe traumatic brain injury: a data-based approach to program development. *J Brain Injury Rehab* 1995;10:27–39.

Whiteneck G. (1994). Measuring what matters: key rehabilitation outcomes. *Arch Phys Med Rehabil* 1994;75: 1073–76.

Young B, Rapp RP, Norton JA, Haack D, Tibbs PA, Bean JR. Early prediction of outcome in head injured patients. *J Neurosurg* 1981;54:300–303.

Appendix 1

GLASGOW COMA SCALE

Eye Opening		*Score*
None	1	Even to supra-orbital pressure
To pain	2	Pain from sternum/limb/supra-orbital pressure
To speech	3	Non-specific response, not necessarily to command
Spontaneous	4	Eyes open, not necessarily aware

Motor Response		
None	1	To any pain; limbs remain flaccid
Extension	2	Shoulder adducted and shoulder and forearm internally rotated
Flexor response	3	Withdrawal response or assumption of hemiplegic posture
Withdrawal	4	Arm withdraws to pain, shoulder abducts
Localizes pain	5	Arm attempts to remove supra-orbital/chest pressure
Obeys commands	6	Follows simple commands

Verbal Response		
None	1	No verbalization of any type
Incomprehensible	2	Moans/groans, no speech
Inappropriate	3	Intelligible, no sustained sentences
Confused	4	Converses but confused, disoriented
Oriented	5	Aware of time (year, season, month), place person

Reference: Teasdale G, Jennett B, 1974

Appendix 2

GLASGOW-LIEGE SCALE

This scale is added to the Glasgow Coma Scale to give the Glasgow-Liege Scale, yielding additional useful prognostic information. Minimum score is 3; maximum score is 20.

Brain Stem Reflexes

Fronto-orbicular (glabellar)	5	Eye blink with tap
Vertical oculovestibular	4	Vertical eye movement to head flexion/extension or bilateral ice water caloric testing
Pupillary light	3	Direct response, need only be present in one eye
Horizontal oculovestibular	2	Lateral eye movement to head rotation or unilateral cold caloric testing
Oculocardiac	1	Slowing of heart rate to ocular pressure
No response	0	

Reference: Born et. al. 1985

Appendix 3

DISABILITY RATING SCALE (RAPPAPORT)

Arousability, Awareness and Responsivity

Eye Opening	Score	
Spontaneous	0	Eyes open, not necessarily aware
To speech	1	Non-specific response, not necessarily to command
To pain	2	Pain from sternum/limb/supra-orbital pressure
None	3	Even to supra-orbital pressure

Verbal response

Oriented	0	Aware of time (year, season, month), place person
Confused	1	Converses but confused, disoriented
Inappropriate	2	Intelligible, no sustained sentences
Incomprehensible	3	Moans/groans, no speech
None	4	No verbalization of any type

Motor response

0   Obeys commands (follows simple commands)
1   Localizes pain (arm attempts to remove supra-orbital/chest pressure)
2   Withdrawal (arm withdraws to pain, shoulder abducts)
3   Flexor response (withdrawal response or assumption of hemiplegic posture)
4   Extension (shoulder adducted and shoulder and forearm internally rotated)
5   None (to any pain; limbs remain flaccid)

Cognitive Ability for Self-Care Activities

Feeding

0   Complete
1   Partial
2   Minimal
3   None

Toileting
Grooming

0   Complete
1   Partial
2   Minimal
3   None

Dependence on Others
Level of Functioning

0   Completely independent
1   Independent in special environment
2   Mildly dependent (needs limited assistance, nonresident helper)

3   Moderately dependent (needs moderate assistance, person in home)
4   Markedly dependent (needs assistance with all major activities at all times)
5   Totally dependent (24/hr nursing care required)

Psychosocial Adaptability

0   Not restricted
1   Selected jobs competitive
2   Sheltered workshop, noncompetitive
3   Not employable

Appendix 4

RANCHO LOS AMIGOS COGNITIVE SCALE

1. No Response. Patient appears to be in a deep sleep and is completely unresponsive to any stimuli presented to him/her.

2. Generalized Response. Patient reacts inconsistently and nonpurposefully to stimuli in a nonspecific manner. Responses are limited in nature and are often the same regardless of stimulus presented. Responses may be physiological changes, gross body movements, and vocalization. Responses are likely to be delayed. The earliest response is to deep pain.

3. Localized Response. Patient reacts specifically, but inconsistently to stimuli. Responses are directly related to the type of stimulus presented, as in turning head toward a sound or focusing on an object presented. The patient may withdraw an extremity and vocalize when presented with a painful stimulus. May follow simple commands in an inconsistent, delayed manner, such as closing the eyes, hand squeezing, or extending an extremity. Once external stimuli are removed, the patient may lie quietly. He/she may also show a vague awareness of self and body by responding to discomfort by pulling at nasogastric tube, catheter, or resisting restraints. May show a bias toward responding to some persons, especially family and friends, but not to others.

4. Confused-Agitated. Patient is in a heightened state of activity with severely decreased ability to process information. He/she is detached from the present and responds primarily to his/her own internal confusion. Behavior is frequently bizarre and nonpurposeful relative to immediate environment. May cry out or scream out of proportion to stimuli even after removal, may show aggressive behavior, attempt to remove restraints or tube, or crawl out of bed in a purposeful manner. Patient does not discriminate among persons or objects and is unable to cooperate directly with treatment efforts. Verbalization is frequently incoherent or inappropriate to the environment. Confabulation may be present; he/she may be hostile. Gross attention to environment is very brief, and selective attention often nonexistent. Being unaware of present events patient lacks short-term recall and may be reacting to past events. Unable to perform self-care activities such as sitting, reaching, and ambulating as part of his/her agitated state but not as a purposeful act or on request necessarily.

5. Confused-Inappropriate. Patient appears alert and is able to respond to simple commands fairly consistently. However, with increased complexity of commands or lack of any external structure, responses are nonpurposeful, random, or, at best, fragmented toward any desired goal. May show agitated behavior, but not on stimulus. Has gross attention to the environment, is highly distractible, and lacks ability to focus attention to a specific task without frequent redirection. With structure may be able to converse on a very simple level for short periods of time. Verbalization is often inappropriate; confabulation may be triggered by present events. Memory is severely impaired, with confusion of past and present in reaction to ongoing activity. Patient does not initiate functional tasks, and often shows inappropriate use of objects with external direction. May be able to perform previously learned tasks when structured for him/her, but is unable to learn new information. Responds best to self, body, comfort, and often family members. The patient can usually perform self-care activities with assistance and may accomplish feeding with supervision. Management on the unit is often a problem if the patient is physically mobile, as he/she may wander off, either randomly or with vague intention of "going home."

6. Confused-Appropriate. Patient shows goal-directed behavior, but is dependent on external input for direction. Response to discomfort is appropriate and patient is able to tolerate unpleasant stimuli, e.g., NG tube when need is explained. Follows simple directions consistently, and shows carryover for tasks he/she has learned; e.g., self-care. Responses may be incorrect due to memory problems, but are appropriate to the situation. The patient shows increased ability to process information with little or no anticipation or prediction of events. Past memories show more depth and detail than recent memory. The patient may show some awareness of situation by realizing he/she does not know an answer. The patient no longer wanders and is inconsistently oriented to time and place. Selective attention to tasks may be impaired, especially with difficult tasks, and in unstructured settings, but is functional for common daily activities (30 minutes with structure). May show a vague recognition of some staff, has increased awareness of self, family, and basic needs (as food), again in an appropriate manner, in contrast to level 5.

7. Automatic-Appropriate. Patient appears appropriate and oriented within hospital and home settings, goes through daily routine automatically, but frequently robot-like, with minimal-to-absent confusion, but has shallow recall of what he/she has been doing. Shows increased awareness of self, body, family, foods, people, and interaction in the environment. Has superficial awareness of, but lacks insight into, his/her condition, decreased judgment and problem-solving and lacks realistic planning for the future. Shows carryover for new learning, but at a decreased rate. Requires minimal supervision for learning and for safety purposes. With structure, is able to initiate tasks or social and recreational activities in which he/she now has interest. Judgment remains impaired, such that he/she is unable to drive a car.

8. Purposeful-Appropriate. Patient is alert and oriented, is able to recall and integrate past and recent events, and is aware of and responsive to his/her culture. Shows carryover for new learning if acceptable to him/her and his/her life role, and needs no supervision once activities are learned. Within physical capabilities, the patient is independent in home and community skills, including driving. Vocational rehabilitation to determine ability to return as a contributor to society (perhaps in a new capacity) is indicated. May continue to show decreases relative to premorbid abilities in quality and rate of processing, abstract reasoning, tolerance for stress, and judgment in emergencies or unusual circumstances. Social, emotional, and intellectual capacities may continue to be at a decreased level, but patient is functional in society.

CHAPTER 9 Health-Related Quality of Life Scales for Epilepsy

Orrin Devinsky, M.D.,
and Joyce Cramer, M.D.

Epilepsy affects people in different ways. Seizures of the same type demonstrate tremendous clinical variability—from the premonitory, ictal, and post-ictal symptoms to their duration, intensity, frequency, and tendency to cluster. Similarly, antiepileptic drugs affect people differently. Some are exquisitively sensitive to very low doses of "benign" drugs while others tolerate very high doses of several "toxic" medications quite well. However, the effects of epilepsy extend well beyond seizures and side effects. Epilepsy is a disorder that can penetrate the entire social fabric of a person's life. The ways in which seizures and epilepsy impact a person are as idiosyncratic as fingerprints. Although certain issues are paramount—self-esteem, independence, education, driving, employment, and fear of seizures—the relative importance of these and other psychosocial and medical issues varies between patients and over the course of an individual patient's lifetime.

Exploring the full spectrum of issues affecting a patient's quality of life is beyond the scope of routine clinical practice. However, exclusive attention to seizures and medication side effects limits the clinician's ability to help patients. We often focus on achieving a balance between seizures and side effects. However, there is an even more important, dynamic balance between the care delivered for the

epilepsy and the impact of the disorder and its medical care on a person's life. The development and use of quality of life scales in epilepsy will expand our appreciation of how epilepsy affects people and how our therapies impact the lives of patients.

Health-Related Quality of Life

Interest in the effects of disease on the patient's quality of life first began in the late 1940s with Karnovsky's rating scale for cancer patients and has grown exponentially during the past decade. Quality of life measurement has been increasingly reported in clinical trials, nonexperimental outcome studies, cost-utility analyses, and studies of quality of care (Gill & Feinstein, 1994; Spilker, 1990). "Quality of life" encompasses an individual's overall sense of well-being and daily functioning. Health-related quality of life (HRQOL) is commonly divided into three main components: physical health (e.g., general health, daily function, symptoms such as seizures and medication side effects); mental health (e.g., mood, feeling of well-being, perceived stigma); and social health (e.g., social activities and relationships). Although epilepsy heavily impacts economic and environmental factors, these are not usually encompassed by health-related quality of life.

Quality of life issues are especially relevant in chronic disorders such as epilepsy, in which mental and social difficulties extend well outside the usual range of "disease symptoms"(Cramer, 1994). The correlation between the doctor's and patient's assessment of the patient's quality of life is often poor. HRQOL measures can thus provide valuable complementary information to traditional assessments directed at seizure control and adverse antiepileptic drug (AED) effects.

Although HRQOL is achieving increased recognition as a vital measure, its quantification remains a challenge. Validation of HRQOL instruments is especially challenging since no "gold standards" are available. Validation *should* be based on some absolute patient-derived measure, but no such measure is available. Instead, validation is often based on medical outcomes, precisely the domain from which HRQOL sought to lessen its dependence. Items included in HRQOL scales are often derived mainly from "medical experts." However, the patient's opinion of what is important and determining the relative impact of different factors assume higher priority in assessing HRQOL (Gill & Feinstein, 1994).

HRQOL assessments may be generic or targeted toward a specific disease or disorder. Generic instruments assess various functions and issues of well-being regardless of disease state. These instruments can evaluate diverse patient populations. Popular and validated generic HRQOL instruments include the RAND 36-item Health Survey, (Hays et al., 1993), the Sickness Impact Profile (Bergner et al., 1981), and the McMaster Health Index Questionnaire (Sackett et al., 1977). Generic instruments allow for comparisons between patients with different diseases but often lack sensitivity to change or responsiveness to intervention.

Disease-specific instruments assess the unique ways in which a particular disease impacts HRQOL. Such knowledge may be derived from patient interviews, medical and lay literature, expert opinion, or a combination of these sources (Gill & Feinstein, 1994). Problems that are specific to the disease entity under study may be emphasized and weighted according to their relative contribution to the patient's disability. Disease-specific HRQOL instruments are limited by the time of administration and the resulting lack of information with which to make meaningful comparisons between groups with different disorders. One

approach has been to combine a generic core with a disease-specific supplement to provide the benefits of both types of instruments.

Special Issues in Epilepsy

Epilepsy is often a chronic illness that has a heavy impact on the patient's mental, social, and economic well-being. For patients with mild epilepsy—infrequent seizures and minimal or no adverse effects of AEDs—epilepsy still poses difficult problems that can linger long after the last seizure. While most people with epilepsy can achieve a normal or near-normal life, patients with difficult-to-control epilepsy or those who require high doses of one or more AEDs with the associated adverse effects often limit their HRQOL.

Problems Unique to Epilepsy

Outcome measures for epilepsy patients usually include seizure frequency, severity, and morbidity (e.g., seizure-related trauma), as well as AED side effects such as sedation, nausea, and tremor. The traditional medical factors—seizures and AED side effects—are viewed quite differently by patients and doctors. "Occasional" or "mild" seizures and "infrequent" and "tolerable" side effects that may be acceptable to physicians may be quite "unacceptable" to the patient. The gap in patient-doctor communication is often wide. Many doctors would rather not hear about "minor" problems that they may be ill-equipped to handle. In many cases, doctors may be insensitive to complaints that do not match their a priori beliefs (e.g., bothersome lethargy or confusion with low therapeutic doses of a "cognitively benign" AED). Alternatively, patients may want to present a positive picture to the doctor and may have difficulty communicating their actual level of functioning. In either scenario, the physician will remain unaware of important problems.

People with epilepsy have increased rates of psychosocial problems and psychopathology as compared to healthy age-matched adults and patients with many other chronic disorders. After the diagnosis of epilepsy is made, the greatest HRQOL problems often occur during the seizure-free intervals. Medical therapy is measured in years, not months. Medications often need to be taken several times per day and can cause side effects that affect a person's daily life, and the psychological and social consequences of epilepsy are often enormous. People with epilepsy may be restricted in educational, social, transportation, and employment opportunities—limitations that are often both real and perceived. Both the perceived and real stigma and social limitations can have a paralyzing effect on a person's life. For children, parental and societal attitudes often foster low self-esteem, dependence, discrimination, and restrictions. As the children of past generations with epilepsy reach adulthood, those long-standing attitudes toward self and society become fixed and difficult to alter. In considering epilepsy as a chronic burden, one must carefully examine the neglected social, psychological, and behavioral problems as well as the medical issues.

Physical Issues

Seizures increase the risk of physical injuries, including bruises, lacerations, bone fracture and dislocation, burns, and drowning, as well as unexplained death (Hauser & Hesdorffer, 1990). Daily antiepileptic medications reduce seizure frequency and severity but can cause adverse physical effects (e.g., osteopenia, gingival hyperplasia, sedation, nausea, double vision, tremor, hirsutism) and mental effects (e.g., psychomotor slowing, memory impairments), some of which are subtle but chronic (Mattson et al., 1985). HRQOL measures show impairments in people who have systemic or neurologic adverse effects (Devinsky & Cramer, 1993).

Psychological Consequences

People with epilepsy have increased rates of psychiatric disorders, including depression, anxiety, and psychosis, as well as cognitive problems such as impaired short-term memory. Multiple factors can contribute to the behavioral problems and psychopathology in epilepsy, including social, biological, and medication factors. Epilepsy lessens a person's sense of control over his life, contributing to debilitating psychological problems. Fear of public exposure or injury can underlie self-imposed social and vocational restrictions. The behavioral and cognitive problems associated with epilepsy have been extensively reviewed (Devinsky & Theodore, 1991; Smith et al., 1991), and recent studies have assessed these issues using standardized neuropsychological tests and psychiatric questionnaires [e.g., Minnesota Multiphasic Personality Inventory (MMPI) and Beck Depression Scale]. However, these cognitive and behavioral scales do

not directly assess psychosocial functioning or HRQOL.

Social Consequences

The social label of epilepsy can isolate and paralyze an individual. Children and adults with epilepsy often feel removed from their social group and activities. Epilepsy differs from most other medical and neurologic disorders because of legal restrictions and requirements (e.g., notification on driving applications or jobs that may require functions limited by epilepsy). Underemployment is probably the most common problem among adults with epilepsy, with a significant impact on financial well-being and the ability to obtain health insurance. People with epilepsy may fear dating, marriage, or having seizures during sexual activity. There are also well-founded fears of decreased fertility, the need for AEDs and increased seizure frequency during pregnancy, increased rate of birth defects or the possibility of the child having epilepsy, and the dangers of a seizure occurring while caring for a baby.

Early Measures of Psychosocial Outcome

The majority of scales presently available for measuring HRQOL in epilepsy were developed and reported in the 1990s. Most HRQOL scales for epilepsy are profile measures in which multiple scores are generated reflecting different aspects of HRQOL, using Likert scaling. One novel exception is the Repertory Grid Technique used by Trimble and his group, which emphasizes the individual patient's assessment of the relative importance of HRQOL domains in his or her own life.

The Washington Psychosocial Seizure Inventory (WPSI), developed by Dodrill and colleagues in 1980, was the first epilepsy-specific psychosocial measure (Dodrill et al., 1980). This 132-item inventory self-report measure consists of eight psychosocial scales (Family Background; Emotional, Interpersonal, and Vocational Adjustment; Financial Status; Adjustment to the Diagnosis of Seizures and Epilepsy; Satisfaction with Medical Management; and Overall Psychosocial Functioning) and three validity scales. Responses are either yes or no and one can derive subscale scores as well as overall scores. The WPSI can help assess psychosocial outcome in adults and adolescents with epilepsy and compare psychosocial functioning before and after a specific intervention such as epilepsy surgery or a new AED (Dodrill et al., 1993). The adult scale has been used in a variety of studies and evaluations of special populations, such as before and after epilepsy surgery. The adolescent scale (APSI) developed by Batzel and colleagues (1991) can evaluate psychosocial issues in teenagers with epilepsy. A quality of life subscale has been derived from the WPSI based on correlations with the QOLIE-31 (Dodrill & Batzel, 1995).

The Social Effects Scale was developed by Chaplin and colleagues (1990) to investigate social aspects of epilepsy in a wide range of epilepsy patients. It was based on extensive patient interviews. Initially, 21 areas of concern were identified but only 14 were included in the final 42-item version. The questionnaire is completed by the patient using a 5-point Likert scale. Scale reliability, assessed by test-retest method, was only moderate. Validity was established through a comparison of patients' responses and their behavior as observed by medical staff. Further evaluation of the scale is necessary, although the authors have applied the scale successfully in the National General Practice Survey of Epilepsy (Chaplin et al., 1990; Chaplin et al., 1992).

Collings Well-Being Scale (Collings, 1990) was conceived as an assessment of overall well-being. The questionnaire is completed by the patient and assesses the difference between current self-perception and how the patient imagines life would be without epilepsy. The instrument is divided into six subscales: (1) self-esteem (20 seven-point semantic rating items); (2) life fulfillment (20 aspects of life are rated according to importance and then whether each aspect is true of the patient's life; first and second ratings are subtracted to yield fulfillment scores); (3) social and interpersonal difficulties (30 items); (4) general physical health (14 items); (5) worries (11 items); and (6) affect-balance (10 items on positive and negative emotions). In 392 patients (359 with epilepsy and 33 controls), those with active epilepsy showed lower well-being on all subscales than a control group without epilepsy. Visibility of severe seizures and frequency of seizures inversely correlated with well-being. Self-image (perception of self) and epilepsy were most predictive of overall well-being. The Well-Being Scale has not been validated.

Current Outcome Measures in Adults

The Epilepsy Surgery Inventory-55 (ESI-55)

Vickrey and colleagues (1992) devised the ESI-55 (Table 9-1), an epilepsy-specific inventory to assess HRQOL. Using the RAND 36-item Health Survey (SF-36) (Ware & Sherbourne, 1992) as the generic core, they added 19 items related to epilepsy. Fifty-four items comprise 11 unique scales tapping into distinct dimensions of HRQOL. These include health perception (9 items); energy/fatigue (4 items); overall QOL (2 items); emotional well-being (5 items); cognitive functioning (5 items); physical functioning (10 items); pain (2 items); role limitation comprised of emotional (5 items) and memory (5 items); and one item that assesses change in health over the preceding year. Three composite scores (mental health, physical health, and role limitations/cognitive) and a total score can be derived by weighting and summing individual scale scores.

The ESI-55 was originally used to assess HRQOL in 224 patients who had undergone epilepsy surgery to alleviate treatment-refractory seizures (Vickrey et al., 1992). Patients who continued to have seizures after surgery had lower ESI-55 scores (i.e., worse HRQOL) on all 11 scales (p < 0.05) than those who were completely seizure-free. However, these post-surgical patients represent only a small and somewhat skewed group of patients with epilepsy. As a result, some aspects of HRQOL were underrepresented in the ESI-55, particularly with regard to social health, which is assessed using a two-item social function scale. In the early validity testing, the overall ESI-55 score appeared to cluster at the high end, reflecting "best possible quality of life." One advantage of the scale is that scores appear to be capable of detecting change with a reasonable sample size (approximately 19 per treatment group) (Vickrey et al., 1993).

The ESI-55 was recently used as an external standard to differentiate among seven previously published, seizure-based outcome classifications used as outcomes by various groups performing epilepsy surgery (Vickrey et al., 1995). A comparison of the reliability and validity of the ESI-55, WPSI, and the generic Sickness Impact Profile (Bergner et al., 1981) in a population of patients with intractable seizures was recently reported by Langfitt (1995). The author concluded that the ESI-55 and SIP assessed a broader range of QOL func-

Table 9-1.   ESI-55 Scales[1]

Scale	Number of Items
Health perception	9
Energy/fatigue	4
Overall QOL	2
Social function	2
Emotional well-being	5
Cognitive functioning	5
Physical functioning	10
Pain	2
Role limitation:	
Emotional	5
Memory	5
Change in health	1

[1] Vickrey et al., 1992

Permission to use the ESI-55 and scoring manual may be obtained by writing to: RAND, 1700 Main Street, P.O. Box 2138, Santa Monica, CA 90407-2138 (Attention: Contracts and Grant Services). Additional information may be obtained from Dr. Vickrey at that address.

tions compared to the more specific focus of the WPSI on psychological and social adjustment.

The Liverpool Quality of Life Battery

The Liverpool battery (Table 9-2) consists of a series of questionnaires, some developed specifically for epilepsy and some for use in other disorders but successfully validated in people with epilepsy. The battery encompasses numerous measures of physical functioning: seizure severity (Baker et al., 1991), seizure frequency, activities of daily living (Brown & Thomlinson, 1984), social functioning, and psychological functioning (Affect Balance Scale) (Bradburn, 1969), Hospital Anxiety and Depression Scale, (Zigmond & Snaith, 1983), Self-Esteem, (Rosenberg, 1965), and the Mastery Scale (Perlin & Schooler, 1978), in addition to the following original scales: Stigma (Jacoby, 1994), Life Fulfillment (Baker et al., 1994), Impact of Epilepsy Scale (Jacoby et al., 1994), and Adverse Effects Profile. Scores are derived for each scale, with no overall score. The instrument's validity has been established (Baker et al., 1993; Baker et al., 1994; Jacoby, 1994).

The Liverpool battery was originally used to assess the effect on a patient's psychosocial functioning of withdrawing versus not withdrawing from antiepileptic medications (Jacoby et al., 1992). In a 100-patient study of the early version of the battery, anxiety, depression, low self-esteem, low perceived internal control, and unhappiness were common in epilepsy patients (Smith et al., 1991). Interestingly, seizure severity but not frequency appeared to be a major determinant of psychosocial difficulties. In testing a revised version of the battery in 79 patients with severe epilepsy, Baker and colleagues (1993) found that anxiety was common, and significant differences were seen in the ictal seizure subscale, happiness scale, and mastery scale in two treatment groups (drug vs. placebo). Since then Baker and his group have applied quality of life measures in several critical areas of epilepsy, including the assessment of a novel antiepileptic drug in patients with refractory epilepsy (Smith et al., 1993), quality of life and quality of services for a community-based population, efficacy of a novel antiepileptic drug in children with epilepsy and learning disabilities, and psychosocial outcomes of immediate versus delayed treatment in single seizures and early epilepsy. The flexibility of this measure—the group chooses appropriate measures

tailored to answer specific clinical questions—is an advantage, but can result in different measures being selected, making it less useful in making comparisons across studies.

Quality of Life Assessment Schedule

Kendrick and Trimble (1994) based the Quality of Life Assessment Schedule (QOLAS) (Table 9-3) on the theory that people judge their current quality of life relative to past experiences and that of other people. This reflects the increasing recognition that HRQOL measures should be patient-centered, incorporating the patient's perceptions. The scale is completed by a trained interviewer after an extensive interview in which the patient identifies specific issues of importance in their lives, including physical functioning, cognition, emotion, social functioning, and economic/work status.

A repertory-grid technique (Fransella & Bannister, 1977) was used with a Construct Importance Scale in which patients identify 10 issues affecting their quality of life, and rate the issues during follow-up on a scale ranging from 1 ("no problem") to 5 ("it could not be worse"). Two types of outcome measures are calculated: aggregate scores, which give a single index of QOL, and profile scores, which provide information relative to satisfaction with the five key domains assessed (physical, cognitive, emotion, social, and economic). The profiles showed differences between actual (NOW) and desired (LIKE) status. Reliability, validity, and sensitivity of the method was evaluated in 50 patients with chronic epilepsy, retested 4 times in 6 months. It was also administered to 11 patients undergoing surgery for the relief of trigeminal neuralgia. Analyses by gender showed that women and men with epilepsy had similar perceptions about their HRQOL (McGuire-Kendrick, 1991). Women were more concerned about friendship and being free of worries and anxiety than men. Men were more concerned than women about controlling their temper and being married.

This labor-intensive interview method is not feasible for large populations, but can be applied in hospital or research settings in which extended interviews are possible, such as during evaluation for epilepsy surgery. An added advantage of the method is its flexibility. Due to the individualized nature of the assessment, it may be applied to virtually any illness or situation. The original tech-

Table 9-2. The Liverpool Assessment Battery[1]

Scale	Number of Items
Liverpool Seizure Severity Scale	
Perception of Control	8
Ictal/Post Ictal Effects	12
Nottingham Health Profile*	38
SEALS Activities of Daily Living*	19
Social Problems Questionnaire*	33
Hospital Anxiety & Depression Scale	14
Affect Balance Scale	10
Profile of Mood States*	36
Rosenberg Self-Esteem Scale	10
Liverpool Mastery Scale	8
Stigma Scale**	3
Life Fulfillment Scale**	24
Impact of Epilepsy Scale**	8
Adverse Effects Profile**	20

*Deleted from later versions

**Added to later versions

[1]Baker et al., 1993

Additional information may be obtained from Dr. Baker at the Department of Neurosciences, Walton Hospital, Rice Lane, Liverpool L9 1AE, UK.

Table 9-3. QOLAS: Calculating Scores for the Streamlined Repertory Grid Technique*

	Constructs	NOW	LIKE	NOW-LIKE Difference
Phys.	Tiredness	5	1	4
	Nausea	5	1	4
Psych.	Depression	4	1	3
	Anxiety	5	2	3
Soc.	Stigma	4	1	3
	(In)dependence	3	1	2
Work	No promotion	5	1	4
	Choice limited	4	1	3
Cogn.	Memory	3	1	2
	Concentration	2	1	1

Total NOW-LIKE difference is 4 + 4 + 3 + 3 + 3 + 2 + 4 + 3 + 2 + 1 = 29

Profile scores for each domain =
  Phys.   4 + 4 = 8
  Psych.   3 + 3 = 6
  Soc.   3 + 2 = 5
  Work   4 + 3 = 7
  Cogn.   2 + 1 = 3
The scoring system is 1 = no problem; 2 = slight problem; 3 = moderate problem; 4 = big problem; 5 = it could not be worse.

*Additional information may be obtained from Professor Michael Trimble, National Hospital for Neurology, Queens Square, London WC1N 3BG, UK.

nique has been revised and simplified by Selai and Trimble. A semistructured interview is now used to elicit the 10 constructs. The number of elements and scoring system have been simplified and a single score can be calculated by looking at the overall difference between the NOW and LIKE scores. Profile scores for each domain can also be calculated. The validity and sensitivity of the revised version has been assessed by comparing patients starting on new AEDs and comparing scores to the ESI-55 administered to 50 patients awaiting epilepsy surgery (Selai, 1995).

Quality of Life in Epilepsy (QOLIE) Instruments

The QOLIE Development Group expanded on the ESI-55 to create a broad-based instrument for people with a wide range of epilepsy severities. The QOLIE test instrument included the RAND SF-36 as a generic core, with 8 additional multi-item scales. The epilepsy-targeted segment consisted of 48 items derived from patient interviews, literature review, and expert opinion. A final open-ended question encouraged patients to report additional items that affected their quality of life. The resulting instruments include the QOLIE-89 (17 scales, 89 items), the QOLIE-31 (7 scales, 31 items), and the QOLIE-10 screening questionnaire (10 items selected from the 7 scales in the QOLIE-31) (see Table 9-4). The QOLIE-89 and QOLIE-31 showed good reliability and construct validity. Hays and colleagues (1995) examined the agreement between self-reports and proxy reports of quality of life (n = 292) and reported good correlations in patients with low to moderate seizure frequency.

Factor analysis of the 17 scales suggested four dimensions: (1) epilepsy-targeted; (2) cognitive; (3) mental health; and (4) physical health factors. Health care utilization was negatively correlated, whereas education and employment were positively correlated with better QOLIE scores. The mood factor showed high correlation and was a strong predictor of total HRQOL scores, with psychomotor slowing also showing significant relationships (Perrine et al., in press). Patients with less severe epilepsy generally had higher HRQOL scores compared to those with more severe epilepsy (Devinsky et al., 1994). The epilepsy-targeted factor and the seizure worry, health discouragement, and work/driving/social function scales best discrimi-

nated between groups with different epilepsy severities. Negative correlations were found for all four HRQOL factors and overall scores for neurotoxicity and systemic toxicity. Employment also correlated well with the overall score, cognitive and physical health factors. These findings demonstrate the sensitivity of the instrument to differences between groups based on seizure frequency, demographic characteristics, and presence of adverse side effects.

Health-Related Quality of Life Questionnaire for People with Epilepsy (HQLQ-E)

Wagner and associates incorporated the RAND 36-item Health Survey (SF-36) (Ware & Sherbourne, 1992) into the Health-Related Quality of Life Questionnaire for People with Epilepsy (HQLQ-E) (Table 9-5), which contains 31 subscales, including other generic health measures, as well as a symptom checklist (Wagner et al., 1995). The HQLQ-E is a self-administered questionnaire, which takes approximately 40 minutes to complete and was developed for use in clinical trials of antiepileptic medications. Validation testing of a 171-item questionnaire was performed with 136 epilepsy patients who were seizure-free for six months or had active epilepsy. The HQLQ-E items allow for measurement of the impact of seizures as well as AED therapy. Because it contains the SF-36 as a generic core instrument, it also permits comparisons with the SF-36 scale norms. Several domains of HRQOL that are important in epilepsy, such as sleep, stigma, and sexual function, are not assessed in detail in the HQLQ-E. The scales and subscales, number of items per scale, and source for the items are noted.

General HRQOL Assessment by the SF-36

Wagner and colleagues (1993) evaluated general HRQOL in 148 people with epilepsy using the RAND 36-item Health Survey. Scores were compared with the Medical Outcomes Study (MOS) well-population matched for social and demographic factors. Epilepsy patients had significantly lower scores in six of eight domains (all but physical functioning and bodily pain). Patients who had at least one seizure during the week before the assessment had significantly lower scores than

Table 9-4. QOLIE-89[1] and QOLIE-31[2*] Scales and Number of Items in Each Scale

Scale	Number of Items
Health perceptions	6
Seizure worry*	5
Physical function	10
Role limitation—physical	5
Role limitation—emotional	5
Pain	2
Overall quality of Life*	2
Emotional well-being*	5
Energy/fatigue*	4
Attention/concentration*	9
Memory	6
Language	5
Medication effects*	3
Social function, work, driving*	11
Social support	4
Social isolation	2
Health discouragement	2
Sexual function**	1
Change in health	1
Overall Health*, **	1

[1] The QOLIE-89 contains 17 scales with 87 field-tested questions.

[2*] The shorter QOLIE-31 includes items from the 7 scales marked with an asterisk.

** Two additional items were added after validation studies.

The QOLIE-10 contains one or more questions from each of the 7 QOLIE-31 scales.

Permission to use the QOLIE-89 or QOLIE-31 and scoring manuals may be obtained by writing to: RAND, 1700 Main Street, P.O. Box 2138, Santa Monica, CA 90407-2138 (Attention: Contracts and Grant Services). Permission to use the QOLIE-10 may be obtained from Professional Postgraduate Services (400 Plaza Drive, Secaucus, NJ 07094).

For more information about the QOLIE scales, contact Orrin Devinsky or Joyce A. Cramer.

Table 9-5.   Scales, Subscales, Number of Items, and Source of Items of the HQLQ-E*

HQL Scales and Subscales	# of Items1	Source
General HQL—SF-36 Scales		
Physical Functioning	**10**	SF-36 UK version
Role Functioning—Physical	**4**	SF-36 UK version plus 1 new
Augmented Role Functioning—Physical	5	item
Bodily Pain	**2**	SF-36 UK version
General Health Perceptions	**5**	SF-36 UK version plus 1 item from
Current Health	4	the Medical Outcomes Study (MOS)[6]
Health Outlook	1	
Resistance to Illness	1	
Vitality	**4**	SF-36 UK version
Social Functioning	**2**	SF-36 UK version
Role Functioning—Emotional	**3**	SF-36 UK version plus 1 new item
Augmented Role Functioning—Emotional	**4**	
Mental Health	**5**	SF-36 UK version
Change in Health	**1**	SF-36 UK version
General HQL—Additional Scales		
Mental Health	**18**	MH-18 (includes MH-5) plus
Anxiety	4	
Depression	4	
Behavior/Emotional Control	5	1 item from MHI-38
Positive Well-Being	5	
Emotional Ties	4	3 items from UCLA Loneliness Scale
Overall Quality of Life	**1**	MOS
Cognition	**13**	6 item MOS cognition scale plus
Confusion	2	1 item from SIP
Thinking	2	1 item from PERI
Concentration	2	2 items from PERI
Attention	2	1 item from SIP
Memory	1	
Reasoning	1	
Psychomotor Functioning	3	2 items from SI
Epilepsy-Specific HQL Scales		
Mastery	**6**	Pearlin/Schooler Mastery Scale
Impact	**8**	Liverpool Impact Scale
Experience	**13**	New items
Worry	**9**	New items
Agitation	**2**	Health Insurance Study
Distress	**2**	MOS

Table 9-5. *(continued)*

HQL Scales and Subscales	# of Items1	Source
Seizures Severity Scales		
Ictal	**12**	Liverpool Seizure Severity Scale
Percept	**8**	Liverpool Seizure Severity Scale
Symptoms	**16**	New items
Open-Ended Questions	**2**	New items

¹Bold numbers indicate the overall number of items for each major domain. Nonbold numbers indicate number of items for each subscale.

MHI = Mental Health Inventory

SIP = Sickness Impact Profile

PERI = Psychiatric Epidemiology Research Interview

*Development of the HQLQ-E was supported by Schering-Plough International.

patients who were seizure-free for more than one year. Systemic and neurologic toxicity assessment, controlling for the impact of time since the last seizure, revealed that patients with adverse effects (76%) had worse HRQOL in five domains than patients without adverse effects (Wagner et al., 1994).

Vickrey and colleagues (1994) compared scores for a pictorial item and the eight scales of the RAND 36-item Health Survey from epilepsy surgery patients and other medical disorders. After resective surgery, seizure-free patients had generally better scores on all scales, and those with continuing simple partial seizures had HRQOL scores similar to patients with hypertension, heart disease, and diabetes. Patients who continued to have complex partial or tonic-clonic seizures after surgery had poorer emotional well-being and overall HRQOL than all other patient groups except those with depression.

The SF-36 was used in a comparison of self-reported HRQOL in 271 patients with epilepsy, comparing it to another neurologic condition (multiple sclerosis; n = 85), and a nonneurologic but chronic illness (diabetes; n = 555) (Hermann et al., in press). The patients with multiple sclerosis reported significantly worse HRQOL than both epilepsy and diabetes groups (which did not differ from each other) on four scales, reflecting primarily physical limitations. Patients with epilepsy and multiple sclerosis reported significantly lower HRQOL scores than the diabetes group on two scales involving emotional well-being (but again did not differ from one another). The epilepsy group did report better health perceptions than the other two groups. Hermann and colleagues (Hermann et al., in press) concluded that while generic measures appear to be useful in identifying some aspects of HRQOL, disease-targeted supplements may be required to clearly identify the specific effects of epilepsy on HRQOL.

Assessments of Adolescents and Children

HRQOL instruments must be revised or created to address issues specific to the age group under study. Adolescents with epilepsy have special concerns about the feasibility of driving and dating that differ from those of adults. The verbal and intellectual skills of adolescents allow one to directly assess HRQOL through direct patient reporting. In contrast, the assessment of children must often involve interviewing the parent or caregiver, recognizing that the responses might not accurately reflect all the concerns of the child. Children with epilepsy often confront issues of self-esteem and dependence. These issues are probably most important in families with over-protective parents. Dysfunctional families can create serious problems for children with epilepsy, but parents from such families may not accurately report problems. Thus, having parents rate the HRQOL of children with epilepsy can provide a biased perspective. Another issue of concern in families is the impact of a child's epilepsy on siblings and family. In adults epilepsy also has important consequences for the family that have not been formally assessed.

Studying 127 children (8–12 years of age) and their mothers with self-report questionnaires, interviews, and medical records, Austin and colleagues (1992) identified five variables that related to behavior problems: female gender, family stress, family mastery, extended family social support, and seizure frequency. Comparing children (8–12 years of age) with epilepsy to children with asthma, Austin's group (1994) found more compromises in psychological, social, and school domains in the epilepsy group. The magnitude of differences between the two types of illness and other findings suggest that some other factor apart from medical illness is related to poor quality of life for children with epilepsy.

The QOLIE Development Group is currently field-testing an adolescent version of the QOLIE instrument. Work and recreation activities were modified to include school and sports activities, and items were added (e.g., school behavior and family and social relationships) targeted to the age group's needs and concerns. New items were added emphasizing both the degree of difficulty caused by epilepsy and how bothersome the limitation is to the teenager. The present 106-item version is being administered to 240 adolescents between the ages of 11 and 17 with a 2–4 week retest. A parent/proxy is completing a parallel 11-item questionnaire. The scale is divided into three parts: general health, the effects of epilepsy and antiepileptic medications, and feelings about yourself. There is a final open-ended question enabling patients to comment on topics of concern that were not covered in the questionnaire

Conclusions

Quality of life measures are entering the clinic in order to better understand the impact of epilepsy and its treatment on the individual. Medical outcome—seizures and medication side effects—is only one area that needs to be addressed in a person living with epilepsy. Further, the doctor's and patient's perspectives on how seizures and side effects impact a person's life can be quite different. Quality of life questionnaires can be useful in epilepsy clinical trials and medical practice, allowing patients to express their concerns about a variety of issues affecting their lives. Thus, the patient's perspective can provide new information not only about the critical psychological and social issues, but also about the medical outcomes such as seizures and medication side effects that are often viewed one-sidedly by the physician. The newly developed HRQOL for epilepsy instruments need to be further assessed in larger patient groups to define their sensitivity and usefulness

References

Austin JK, Risinger MW, Beckett LA. Correlates of behavior problems in children with epilepsy. *Epilepsia* 1992;33:1115–22.

Austin JK, Smith MS, Risinger MW, McNelis AM. Childhood epilepsy and asthma: comparison of quality of life. *Epilepsia* 1994;35:608–15.

Baker GA, Smith DF, Dewey M, Morrow J, Crawford PM, Chadwick DW. The development of a seizure severity scale as an outcome measure in epilepsy. *Epil Res* 1991;8:245–51.

Baker GA, Smith DF, Dewey M, Jacoby A, Chadwick DW. The development of a health-related quality of life measure for patients with intractable epilepsy. *Epil Res* 1993;16:65–81.

Baker GA, Jacoby A, Smith DF, Dewey ME, Chadwick DW. The development of a novel scale to assess life fulfillment as part of the further refinement of a quality of life model for epilepsy. *Epilepsia* 1994;35:591–96.

Batzel LW, Dodrill CB, Dubinsky BL. An objective method for the assessment of psychosocial problems in adolescents with epilepsy. *Epilepsia* 1991;32:202–11.

Bergner M, Bobbit RA, Carter WB, Gilson BS. The Sickness Impact Profile: development and final revision of a health status measure. *Med Care* 1981;19:787–805.

Bradburn NM. *The structure of psychological well-being*. Chicago: Adline, 1969.

Brown S, Thomlinson LL. Anticonvulsant side effects: a self report questionnaire for use in community surveys. *Br J Clin Pract, Symposium* 1984 (Suppl); 18:147–49.

Chaplin JE, Yepez R, Shorvon S, Floyd M. A quantitative approach to measuring the social effects of epilepsy. *Neuroepidemiology* 1990;9:151–58.

Chaplin JE, Yepez R, Shorvon SD, Floyd M. National General Practice study of epilepsy: the social and psychological effects of a recent diagnosis of epilepsy. *Br Med J* 1992;34;1416–18

Collings JA. Psychosocial well-being and epilepsy: an empirical study. *Epilepsia* 1990;31:418–26.

Cramer JA. Quality of life for people with epilepsy. *Neurol Clin* 1994;12:1–13.

Devinsky O, Vickrey BG, Perrine K, Hermann B, Meador K, Hays RD, Cramer JA. Development of an instrument of health-related quality of life for people with epilepsy. *Neurology* 1994;44(Suppl 2):A141.

Devinsky O, Cramer JA (eds.). Quality of life in epilepsy. *Epilepsia* 1993 (Suppl 4).

Devinsky O, Theodore WH (eds.). *Epilepsy and behavior*. New York: Alan R. Liss, 1991.

Dodrill CB, Arnett JL, Sommerville KW, Sussman NM. Evaluation of the effects of vigabatrin on cognitive abilities and quality of life in epilepsy. *Neurology* 1993;43:2501–2507.

Dodrill CB, Batzel LW. The Washington Psychosocial Seizure Inventory: new developments in the light of the quality of life concept. *Epilepsia* 1995;36(Suppl 3):S220.

Dodrill CB, Batzel LW, Queisser HR, et al. An objective method for the assessment of psychological and social problems among epileptics. *Epilepsia* 1980;21:123–35.

Gill TM, Feinstein AR. A critical appraisal of the quality of quality-of-life measurements. *JAMA* 1994;272:619–26.

Hays RD, Sherbourne C, Mazel E. The RAND 36-item health survey 1.0. *Health Econ* 1993;2:217–27.

Hays RD, Vickrey BG, Hermann BP, et al. Agreement between self reports and proxy reports of quality of life in epilepsy patients. *Qual of Life Res* 1995;4:159–68.

Hauser WA, Hesdorffer DC. *Epilepsy: frequency, causes, and consequences*. New York: Demos, 1990:1–378.

Hermann BP, Vickrey B, Hays RD, Cramer J, Devinsky O, Meador K, Perrine K, Myers LW, Ellison GW. A comparison of health-related quality of life in patients with epilepsy, diabetes, and multiple sclerosis. *Epil Res*, in press.

Fransella F, Bannister D. *A manual for Repertory Grid Technique*. London: Academic Press, 1977.

Jacoby A, Johnson A, Chadwick DM, on behalf of the Medical Research Council Antiepileptic Drug Withdrawal Group. Psychosocial outcomes of antiepileptic drug discontinuation. *Epilepsia* 1992;33:112331.

Jacoby A. Felt versus enacted stigma: a concept revisited. Evidence from a study of people with epilepsy in remission. *Soc Sci Med* 1994;38:269–74.

Jacoby A, Baker GA, Smith DF, Dewey M, Chadwick DW. Measuring the impact of epilepsy: the development of a novel scale. *Epil Res* 1994;16:83–88.

Kendrick AM, Trimble MR. Repertory Grid in the Assessment of Quality of Life in Patients with Epilepsy: The Quality of Life Assessment Schedule. In: Trimble MR, Dodson WE (eds.). *Epilepsy and quality of life*. New York: Raven Press, 1994:151–164.

Langfitt JT. Comparison of the psychometric characteristics of three quality of life measures in intractable epilepsy. *Qual of Life Res* 1995;4:101–14.

Mattson, RH, Cramer, JA, Collins, JF, et al. Comparison of carbamazepine, phenobarbital, phenytoin and primidone in partial and secondarily generalized tonic clonic seizures. *N Engl J Med* 313:145–51, 1985.

McGuire-Kendrick AM. Quality of life in women with epilepsy. In: Trimble MR (ed.). *Women and epilepsy.* London: John Wiley & Sons Ltd., 1991:13–30.

Perlin L, Schooler C. The structure of coping. *J Hlth Soc Behav* 1978;19:2–21.

Perrine K, Hermann BP, Meador KJ, Vickrey BG. Cramer JA, Hays RD, Devinsky O, The relationship of neuropsychological functioning to quality of life in epilepsy. *Arch Neurol* (in press).

Rosenberg M. *Society and the adolescent self-image.* Princeton, NJ: Princeton University Press, 1965.

Sackett DL, Chambers LW, MacPherson AS, et al. The development and application of indices of health: general models and a summary of results. *Am J Pub Health* 1977;67:423–28.

Selai C. Assessment of health-related quality of life based on the repertory grid technique (streamlined method). Presented at the International Epilepsy Conference, Australia, September 1995.

Smith DB, Treiman DM, Trimble MR (eds.). *Neurobehavioral problems in epilepsy.* New York: Raven Press, 1991.

Smith DF, Baker GA, Davies G, et al. Outcomes of add-on treatment with lamotrigine in partial epilepsy. *Epilepsia* 1993;34:312–22.

Smith DF, Baker GA, Dewey M, Jacoby A, Chadwick DW. Seizure frequency, patient-perceived seizure severity and the psychosocial consequences of intractable epilepsy. *Epil Res* 1991;9:231–41.

Spilker B. *Quality of life assessments in clinical trials.* New York: Raven Press, 1990.

Vickrey BG, Hays RD, Engel J, Spritzer K, Rogers WH, Rausch R, Graber J, Brook RH. Outcome assessment for epilepsy surgery: the impact of measuring health-related quality of life. *Ann Neurol* 1995;37:158–66.

Vickrey BG, Hays RD, Graber J, Rausch R, Engel J, Brook RH. A health-related quality of life instrument for patients evaluated for epilepsy surgery. *Med Care* 1992;30:299–319.

Vickrey BG, Hays RD, Rausch R, Sutherling WW, Engel JP, Brook RH. Quality of life of epilepsy surgery patients as compared to outpatients with hypertension, diabetes, heart disease, and/or depressive symptoms. *Epilepsia* 1994;35:597–607.

Vickrey BG, Hays RD, Spritzer KL. Methodological issues in quality of life assessment for epilepsy surgery. In: Chadwick DW, Baker GA, Jacoby A (eds.). *Quality of life and quality of care in epilepsy: Update 1993.* London: Royal Society of Medicine Services Limited, Round Table Series 31. 1993:27–37.

Wagner AK, Bungay KM, Bromfield EB, Ehrenberg BL. Health-related quality of life of adult persons with epilepsy as compared with health-related quality of life of well persons. *Epilepsia* 1993;34 (Suppl 6):5.

Wagner AK, Bungay KM, Bromfield E, Ehrenberg BL. Relationship of health-related quality of life to seizure control and antiepileptic drug side effects. *Epilepsia* 1994.

Wagner AK, Keller SD, Kosinski M, Baker GA, Jacoby A, Hsu MA, Chadwick DW, Ware JE. Advances in methods for assessing the impact of epilepsy and antiepileptic drug therapy on patients' health-related quality of life. *QOL Res* 1995;4:115–34.

Ware JE, Sherbourne CD. A 36-item short form health survey (SF-36). I. Conceptual framework and item selection. *Med Care* 1992;30:473–83.

Zigmond AS, Snaith RP. The hospital anxiety and depression scale. *Acta Psychiatr* 1983;67:361–70.

CHAPTER 10 Rehabilitation Outcome Measures

Linda Coulthard-Morris, M.A.,
Jack S. Burks, M.D.,
and Robert M. Herndon, M.D.

The field of rehabilitation has grown and changed dramatically, shifting from the acute treatment of impairment to the long-term management of disability and handicap. This shift is evident by the large percentage (80%) of health care resources being spent to manage people with chronic diseases (Cluff, 1981). Simultaneously, there is increased pressure from the managed care industry for cost-effectiveness data before therapy reimbursement is granted. These focuses have led to the development of numerous rehabilitation assessment and outcome instruments.

Rehabilitation outcome instruments are rapidly evolving to meet the changing needs of researchers, practitioners, and policy makers in this field. These measures now assess a broad range of outcomes from disability and handicap to quality of life and patient satisfaction. With the increased need for valid and reliable outcome data, there is increased pressure to develop standardized instruments (Stewart, 1990; Johnston, Keith, & Hinderer, 1991; Hinderer & Hinderer, 1993).

For purposes of evaluating and understanding rehabilitation instruments and their meaning, it is important to first understand the technical definitions outlined by the World Health Organization (WHO) on which many of these scales are based (WHO, 1980). In using the WHO model, rehabilitation instruments are classified as measures of impairment, disability, or handicap.

Impairment refers to "... loss or abnormality or psychological, physiological, or anatomical structure or function" (WHO, 1980). Examples of impairments include symptoms like double vision, ataxia, intention tremor, or spasticity.

Disability refers to "... any restriction or lack of ability to perform an activity within the range considered normal for a human being" (WHO, 1980).

Handicap is defined as "... a disadvantage for a given individual that limits or prevents the fulfillment of a role that is normal for that individual" (WHO, 1980). It refers to the social disadvantages that result from the presence of an underlying impairment or disability.

There are numerous measures used in rehabilitation, far too many to be reviewed in this chapter. Here, as elsewhere in this book, the emphasis is on evaluating prevalent standardized instruments while also examining some of the newer measures now being developed and utilized. The instruments in this chapter cover a broad array of rehabilitation outcome needs ranging from functional status to health status. The depth and quality of the more recently constructed health status measures are indicative of the progress the field of rehabilitation medicine has made toward viewing rehabilitation success in more global terms like the quality of the patient's life and how satisfied the patient is with the rehabilitation services provided.

For additional information regarding rehabilitation measures, the reader is referred to the following sources: Bowling, 1991; Christiansen, Schwartz, & Barnes 1993; Granger & Gresham 1984, 1993; McDowell & Newell 1987; Spilker, 1990; Wade, 1992; Wilkin, Hallam, & Doggett, 1992.

Impairment Measures

Impairment may or may not change with rehabilitation. For this reason, impairment measures are probably not the best or the most appropriate outcome in determining rehabilitation success. Compared to disability measures, impairment measures are less sensitive to change (Johnston, Wilerson, & Maney, 1993). Impairment measures are probably most appropriate as a diagnostic and assessment tool. Many impairment instruments are designed for a specific disease population, injury, or condition and as such are reviewed in other chapters of this book.

Disability Measures

According to Bowling (1991), direct, objective tests of disability or functional status such as grip strength or range of movement may not be the best or most reliable indicator of actual performance. Therefore, most disability measures either assess activities of daily living (ADLs) or instrumental activities of daily living (IADLs). ADL instruments measure personal care activities like dressing, eating, bathing, grooming, toileting, and mobility. IADL instruments also assess the patient's ability to adapt to the environment and include such domains as home management, money management, shopping, work, transportation, and social interactions. Determining the ability to perform these activities is part of assessing overall functional status.

Rehabilitation makes its strongest impact in terms of influencing disability as evidenced by the

hundreds of disability instruments available. Unlike impairment measures, disability measures tend to be generic and universally applied to every patient population (Whiteneck, 1994). Disease-specific measures are discussed elsewhere in this book. Probably the most widely used and valued disability measure is the Functional Independence Measure (FIM) developed by Dr. Carl Granger. The FIM is reviewed in Chapter 7.

Two traditionally used and one newer disability instruments are reviewed in this chapter. The well-established measures are the PULSES Profile and the Barthel Index. The novel instrument is the Assessment of Motor and Process Skills (AMPS).

PULSES Profile

The PULSES Profile, developed by Moskowitz and McCann in 1957, has been characterized as the first significant functional assessment instrument to be used widely in the United States (Moskowitz & McCann, 1957). It was originally designed to evaluate the functional change of chronically ill and elderly patients (Moskowitz, 1985). The PULSES Profile is used to assess current physical functioning, to document progress, to predict future physical status, and to help guide treatment intervention (Granger & Greer, 1976). Granger modified the PULSES Profile to include a scoring system and improved rating criteria (Granger, Albrecht, & Hamilton, 1979). In this chapter, the reliability and validity information is based on Granger's version of the PULSES Profile (Table 10-1).

Description

The PULSES Profile is a mixed instrument, assessing both impairment and disability. It consists of six components:

(P) = Physical Condition
(U) = Upper Limb Functions
(L) = Lower Limb Functions
(S) = Sensory Components (speech, vision, hearing)
(E) = Excretory Functions (bowel and bladder)
(S) = Support Factors (mental and emotional status)

The subscales are rated on a 4-point Likert scale from essentially normal (1) to severely disabled and dependent (4). The six components or categories are equally weighted. The total scores on the PULSES Profile range from 6 (fully independent) to 24 (total dependence). A score of 12 or more is indicative of severe disability (Gresham & Labi, 1984).

Psychometric Properties

Reliability

The PULSES Profile has demonstrated high test-retest reliability ($r = 0.87$) and high interrater reliability ($r > 0.95$) (Granger, Albrecht, & Hamilton, 1979).

Validity

A series of validation studies were conducted using severely disabled adults receiving inpatient rehabilitation (review Granger & Gresham, 1984). Results from these studies indicate that the PULSES Profile is a sensitive measure, and it is able to detect functional change before and after rehabilitation. Specifically, the PULSES Profile discharge score was closely correlated with discharge outcome (Granger & Greer, 1976; Granger, Albrecht, & Hamilton, 1979; Granger, Sherwood, & Greer, 1977). Patients who returned home scored significantly lower than those who were referred to long-term institutions. The PULSES Profile has demonstrated concurrent validity by its significant correlation with the Barthel Index ($r = -0.74$ to -0.80, $p < 0.0001$) (Granger, Albrecht, & Hamilton, 1979). (Negative correlations result from the inverse scoring of the two scales).

Administration/Scoring

A trained professional can obtain the PULSES Profile information by reviewing medical records, interview, or observation (Granger, Albrecht, & Hamilton, 1979). It is also simple and brief enough to be self-administered and normally requires about 20 minutes to complete (Law & Letts, 1989). A score of 12 is a useful cut-off point for distinguishing lesser from more marked disability, with 16 or greater indicating severe disability.

Advantages

The PULSES Profile is a short simple measure of global disability for both neurologic and nonneurologic patients. It is a valid, reliable, and sensitive measure of functional abilities and status changes over time.

Disadvantages

There are no apparent disadvantages when used appropriately.

Comments

The PULSES Profile is a good measure of functional impairments relating to general health status, communication skills, and psychosocial support (Granger, Albrecht, & Hamilton, 1979). It is appropriate to use when the impairment type is not specified and a general estimate of functional status is needed (Granger, Albrecht, & Hamilton, 1979). It is probably most relevant for patient populations in which substantial changes in functional status are likely to occur with rehabilitation therapy (Christiansen, Schwartz, & Barnes, 1993).

Barthel Index

The Barthel Index was developed by Mahoney and Barthel in 1965 to assess the functional status and mobility skills of neuromuscular and musculoskeletal patients in Maryland's chronic disease hospitals (Mahoney & Barthel, 1965). The Barthel Index is primarily used to evaluate disability prior to admission and to document progress during inpatient rehabilitation. This measure is one of the best known, highly recommended, and commonly used ADL instruments (Wade, 1992).

Description

The Barthel Index is designed to assess the degree of independence a patient has in performing the various self-care and mobility ADL tasks. Each item measures a discrete ADL task function like bowels, bladder, grooming, toilet use, feeding, transfer, mobility, dressing, stairs, and bathing.

Since its development, two versions of the original Barthel Index have been commonly used. Wade and Collin's version (Collin et al., 1988) contains 10 ADL items and provides a total score that ranges from 0 (total dependence) to 20 (total independence) in 1-point increments (Table 10-2). Granger's version (Granger, 1982) includes 15 ADL items and provides a total score that ranges from 0 (total dependence) to 100 (total independence) in

Table 10-1. PULSES Profile (Adapted)

P—Physical condition: includes diseases of the viscera (cardiovascular, gastrointestinal, urologic, and endocrine) and neurologic disorders:

1. Medical problems sufficiently stable that medical or nursing monitoring is not required more often than 3-month intervals.
2. Medical or nurse monitoring is needed more often than 3-month intervals but not each week.
3. Medical problems are sufficiently unstable as to require regular medical and/or nursing attention at least weekly.
4. Medical problems require intensive medical and/or nursing attention at least daily (excluding personal care assistance only).

U—Upper limb functions: Self-care activities (drink/feed, dress upper/lower, brace/prosthesis, groom, wash, perineal care) dependent mainly upon upper limb function:

1. Independent in self-care without impairment of upper limbs.
2. Independent in self-care with some impairment of upper limbs.
3. Dependent upon assistance or supervision in self-care with or without impairment of upper limbs.
4. Dependent totally in self-care with marked impairment of upper limbs.

L—Lower limb functions: Mobility (transfer chair/toilet/tub or shower, walk, stairs, wheelchair) dependent mainly upon lower limb function:

1. Independent in mobility without impairment of lower limbs.
2. Independent of mobility with some impairment in lower limbs, such as needing ambulatory aids, a brace or prosthesis, or else fully independent in a wheelchair without significant architectural or environmental barriers.
3. Dependent upon assistance or supervision in mobility with or without impairment of lower limbs, or partly independent in a wheelchair, or there are significant architectural or environmental barriers.
4. Dependent totally in mobility with marked impairment of lower limbs.

S—Sensory components: Relating to communication (speech and hearing) and vision:

1. Independent in communication and vision without impairment.
2. Independent in communication and vision with some imairment such as mild dysarthria, mild aphasia, or need for eyeglasses or hearing aid, or needing regular eye medication.
3. Dependent upon assistance, an interpreter, or supervision in communication or vision.
4. Dependent totally in communication or vision.

E—Excretory functions (bladder and bowel):

1. Complete voluntary control of bladder and bowel sphincters.
2. Control of sphincters allows normal social activities despite urgency or need for catheter, appliance, suppositories, etc. Able to care for needs without assistance.
3. Dependent upon assistance in sphincter management or else has accidents occasionally.
4. Frequent wetting or soiling from incontinence or bladder or bowel sphincters.

S—Support factors:

1. Able to fulfill usual roles and perform customary tasks.
2. Must make some modification in usual roles and performance of customary tasks.
3. Dependent upon assistance, supervision, encouragement, or assistance from a public or private agency due to any of the above considerations.
4. Dependent upon long-term institutional care (chronic hospitalization, nursing home, etc.) excluding time-limited hospital for specific evaluation, treatment, or active rehabilitation.

Granger CV, Albrecht GL, Hamilton BB. Outcomes of comprehensive medical rehabilitation: measurement by PULSES Profile and the Barthel Index. *Archives of Physical Medicine and Rehabilitation* 1979;60:145–54. (Granger, Albrecht, & Hamilton, 1979).

Table 10-2.   The Barthel Index (Wade and Collin's Version)

Bowels

0 = incontinent (or needs to be given enemata)
1 = occasional accident (once/week)
2 = continent

Bladder

0 = incontinent, or catheterized and unable to manage
1 = occasional accident (max once per 24 hours)
2 = continent (for over 7 days)

Grooming

0 = needs help with personal care
1 = independent face/hair/teeth/shaving (implements provided)

Toilet use

0 = dependent
1 = needs some help, but can do something alone
2 = independent (on and off, dressing, wiping)

Feeding

0 = unable
1 = needs help cutting, spreading butter, etc.
2 = independent (food provided in reach)

Transfer

0 = unable—no sitting balance
1 = major help (one or two people, physical), can sit
2 = minor help (verbal or physical)
3 = independent

Mobility

0 = immobile
1 = wheel chair independent including corners etc.
2 = walks with help of one person (verbal or physical)
3 = independent (but may use any aid, e.g. stick)

Dressing

0 = dependent
1 = needs help, but can do about half unaided
2 = independent (including buttons, zips, laces, etc.)

Stairs

0 = unable
1 = needs help (verbal, physical, carrying aid)
2 = independent up and down

Bathing

0 = dependent
1 = independent (or in shower)
Total (0–20)

Collin C, Wade DT, Davies S, Horne V. The Barthel ADL Index: a reliability study. *International Disability Studies* 1988;10:61–63.

5-point increments (Table 10-3). The Barthel Index uses ordinal data and the weighting of the items varies.

Psychometric Properties

The original reliability and validity studies were conducted with stroke patients by Wylie and White (1964) and later by Wylie (1967). Since that time the Barthel ADL Index has demonstrated high reliability and validity with many patient populations and different conditions (Granger, Albrecht, & Hamilton, 1979; Mahoney & Barthel, 1965; Collin et al., 1988; Wade & Collin, 1988; Jacelon, 1986).

Reliability

The Barthel Index has demonstrated high test-retest reliability ($r = 0.89$), interrater reliability ($r > 0.95$) (Granger, Albrecht, & Hamilton, 1979), and Cronbach alpha internal consistency ($r = 0.98$) (Shiner et al., 1987).

Validity

This measure has documented predictive and concurrent validity. Predictive validity was demonstrated by successfully predicting mortality among stroke patients (Granger, Albrecht, & Hamilton, 1979). Among patients who survived, intake scores also predicted length of stay and rate of rehabilitation progress. Patients with a discharge Barthel Index score greater than 60 were more likely to go home (Granger & Greer, 1976), were easier to manage, and required less time and effort (Granger, Albrecht, & Hamilton, 1979) than those who scored less than 60 (Granger's version).

Concurrent validity was demonstrated by its significant correlation with the PULSES Profile ($r = -0.74$ to -0.90) (Granger, Albrecht, & Hamilton, 1979). (Note that the negative sign results because the two scales were inversely scored.) The Barthel Index has also documented the ability to discriminate between persons with and without ADL disability and predict level of disability (Law & Letts, 1989).

Administration/Scoring

The Barthel Index can be self-administered (Collin et al., 1988), administered by any health care professional, or administered by telephone (Fortinsky, Granger, & Selzer, 1981). It can be given to the patient, spouse, family member, or nurse, depending on who in your judgment provides the most reliable information. Direct observation may be used but it is not required. Whether the ADL and mobility information is obtained from the patient or from another reliable source, the critical factor is to record what the patient does, not what the patient could do. It is realistic to allow about 20 minutes to complete this measure.

Granger and associates report that a score of 60 is the cut-off point between independence and some dependence (Granger, Albrecht, & Hamilton, 1979). They further state that a score between 40 and 20 indicates severe dependence, and a score of 20 or below indicates total mobility and self-care dependence.

Advantages

The Barthel Index is a reliable and valid instrument of ADLs and mobility. It is simple to administer and easy to score because of its metric-like rating system (Wade & Collin, 1988; Jacelon, 1986). It is a very sensitive measure of functional change and as such an excellent measure for predicting rehabilitation outcomes. The Barthel Index includes bowel and bladder functioning items, which some other ADL measures have overlooked.

Disadvantages

The Barthel Index is not an ordered scale. The weights attributed to each item are somewhat arbitrary and therefore are not linear (Duckworth, 1980). Changes by a given number of points do not reflect equivalent changes in ADL function across different activities (McDowell & Newell, 1987).

As with all ADL measures, the Barthel Index has also been criticized for its definite floor and ceiling effect (Granger, Albrecht, & Hamilton, 1979). In other words, the maximum range of behaviors measured does not include the full range of behavioral changes that can occur with rehabilitation. Some functional changes may occur outside the range allowed by this measure and thus will not be detected or examined (McDowell & Newell, 1987). However, the Barthel Index is sensitive enough to detect when a patient first needs personal assistance, and this makes it a highly useful clinical measure (Wade & Collin, 1988).

While the number of ADL domains accessed appears to be adequate, specific subscale behaviors are not included. For example, dressing is one domain or one item appraised in the original version. In Granger's version, upper and lower extremity dressing was evaluated separately, thus

Table 10-3. Barthel Index (Granger's Version)

Independent		Dependent		
Intact	Limited	Helper	Null	
10	5	1	1	Drink from cup/Feed from dish
5	5	3	0	Dress upper body
5	5	2	0	Dress lower body
0	0	-2	0	Don brace or prosthesis
5	5	0	0	Grooming
4	4	0	0	Wash or bathe
10	10	5	0	Bladder continence
10	10	5	0	Bowel continence
4	4	2	0	Care perineum/cloth at toilet
15	15	7	0	Transfer, chair
6	5	3	0	Transfer, toilet
1	1	0	0	Transfer, tub or shower
15	15	10	0	Walk on level 50 yards or more
10	10	5	0	Up and down stairs, 1 flight
15	5	0	0	Wheelchair/50 yds—if not walking

Barthel Total Score

Granger CV. Health accounting—functional assessment of the long-term patient. In: Kottke FJ, Stillwell GK, Lehmann JF (eds.). *Krusen's handbook of physical medicine and rehabilitation.* Philadelphia: Saunders, 1982.

providing the assessor with additional information. Similarly, some of the items (transfers, feeding, toileting, and dressing) may be interpreted differently by different raters (Collin et al., 1988). Again, in referring to the dressing item, dressing is difficult because *half* could be interpreted as upper or lower *half* of the body is unaided, or *half* the effort and needs help with both halves. Most of the major disadvantages of this instrument are resolved by following the Barthel ADL Index Guidelines (Table 10-4).

Comments

The Barthel Index is intended to only assess a narrow domain, self-care and mobility. The Barthel Index is best suited for assessing and monitoring paralytic patients, i.e., spinal cord or limb amputation patients (Granger, Albrecht, & Hamilton, 1979), and/or patients who have continence and mobility problems (Wade, 1992). It has been criticized for being too limited in focus, for only assessing physical activities and not including other domains like psychological well-being (Bowling, 1991; McDowell & Newell, 1987). It is not recommended for assessing general health status, communication skills, or psychosocial status (Granger, Albrecht, & Hamilton, 1979). However, it is important to remember that it measures what it is designed and intended to measure. If a global or multidimensional measure of health is desired, then an instrument like the Sickness Impact Profile (SIP) would be a good choice.

Assessment of Motor and Process Skills (AMPS)

The Assessment of Motor and Process Skills (AMPS) was developed by Fisher and colleagues (Fisher, 1995). The AMPS is an observational measure of functional competence in instrumental activities of daily living (IADLs). It was designed to guide the occupational therapist in determining the appropriate intervention. More importantly, it attempts to assess why a patient might be having difficulty performing a task. This means that the AMPS simultaneously assesses both the ability to perform various ADL and the underlying motor and process skill capacities used while performing a task. Motor skills have been defined as the observable actions used to move the body during task performance and are considered

related to the underlying postural control, mobility, coordination, and strength. Process skills are considered actions observed during any task performance that are associated with underlying attentional, conceptual, organizational, and adaptive capabilities (Park, Fisher, & Velozo, 1993). Compared to the motor skills scale, the process skills scale is better able to discriminate between patients who are able to independently live in the community than those who need assistance (Fisher, 1995).

Description

The AMPS is a performance-based test. The clinician must observe the patient performing the various IADL tasks. This measure contains two subscales, motor and process skills, with 5 components each (Fisher & Fisher, 1993). The motor skills subscale includes 16 items covering the following 5 areas: posture, mobility, coordination, strength and effort, and energy. The process skills subscale has 20 items covering the following 5 areas: using knowledge, temporal organization, space and objects, adaptation, and energy (Table 10-5).

Psychometric Properties

Several reliability and validity studies have been conducted on a variety of patient populations including multiple sclerosis (Doble et al., 1994), psychiatrically disabled adults (Doble, 1991), elderly (Park, Fisher, & Velozo, 1994), and dementia patients (Nygard et al., 1994).

Reliability

The AMPS has demonstrated moderate to high interrater reliability ranging from $r = 0.74$ (Fisher, 1995) to $r = 0.93$ (Fisher et al., 1992), depending on the study. Cronbach alpha internal consistencies were high (motor tasks $r = 0.83$; motor skill items $r = 0.98$; process tasks $r = 0.98$; and process skill items $r = 0.98$) (Fisher, 1995).

Validity

The concurrent validity study results are summarized in the AMPS test manual (Fisher, 1995). The AMPS has been compared to the Expanded Disability Status Scale (EDSS) ($r = -0.79$ motor scale; $r = -0.55$ process scale), the Functional Independence Measure (FIM) ($r = 0.62$), Broad Independence Scale of the Scales of Independent

Table 10-4.   The Barthel ADL Index Guidelines

1. The Index should be used as a record of what a patient does, NOT as a record of what a patient could do.

2. The main aim is to establish degree of independence from any help, physical or verbal, however minor and for whatever reason.

3. The need for supervision renders the patient NOT independent.

4. A patient's performance should be established using the best available evidence. Asking the patient, friends/relatives, and nurses will be the usual source, but direct observation and common sense are also important. Direct testing is not needed.

5. The performance over the preceding 24–48* hours is usually important, but occasionally longer periods will be relevant.

6. Unconscious patients should score "0" throughout, even if not yet incontinent.

7. Middle categories imply that patient supplies over 50% of the effort.

8. Use of aids to be independent is allowed.

  Bowels (preceding week)

If needs enema from nurse, then "incontinent."*
Occasional = once a week.

  Bladder (preceding 24–48 hours)

Occasional = less than once a day.
A catheterized patient who can completely manage the catheter alone is registered as "continent."

  Grooming (preceding 24–48 hours)

Refers to personal hygiene: doing teeth, fitting false teeth, doing hair, shaving, washing face. Implements* can be provided by helper.

  Toilet use

Should be able to reach toilet/commode, undress sufficiently, clean self, dress, and leave.
With help = can wipe self, and do some other of above.*

  Feeding

Able to eat any normal food (not only soft food). Food cooked and served by others. But not cut up.
Help = food cut up, patient feeds self.*

  Transfer

From bed to chair and back.
Dependent = no sitting balance (unable to sit); two people to lift.
Major help = one strong/skilled, or two normal people. Can sit up.
Minor help = one person easily, OR needs any supervision for safety.

  Mobility

Refers to mobility about house or ward, indoors. May use aid. If in wheelchair, must negotiate corners/doors unaided.
Help = by one, untrained person, including supervision/moral support.

  Dressing

Should be able to select and put on all clothes, which may be adapted.
Half = help with buttons, zips, etc., but can put on some garments alone.*

Table 10-4.   *(continued)*

Stairs

Must carry any walking aid used to be independent.

Bathing

Usually the most difficult activity.

Must get in and out unsupervised, and wash self.

Independent in shower = "independent" if unsupervised/unaided.*

*Items added or modified after study; asterisk at end, whole item added; asterisk in middle, phrase added or clarified.

Collin C, Wade DT, Davies S, Horne V. The Barthel ADL Index: a reliability study. *International Disability Studies* 1988;10:61–63.

Behavior (SIB) ($r = 0.85$ motor scale; $r = 0.71$ process scale), and a few other instruments.

Administration/Scoring

The AMPS can only be administered by a highly trained clinician (Fisher, 1995). The selection of tasks to be performed is based on two criteria. First, based on the clinician's knowledge and judgment, the task selected is one within the patient's ability to perform. Second, the tasks selected must be familiar and routinely performed by the patient.

The clinician rates the patient's performance in two skill areas: ADL motor and ADL process (Park, Fisher, & Velozo, 1993). The motor skill items are rated on a 4-point Likert scale from 4 = competent to 1 = deficit (Table 10-6). Motor and process skill items and the activities performed are calibrated on a linear scale from easiest to hardest (Tables 10-7 and 10-8). Consequently, the motor and process ability score for each patient is based on the skill item difficulty, task challenge, and rater severity (Doble et al., 1994).

Advantages

The AMPS is the first IADL measure specifically designed to simultaneously observe the patient performing various ADL tasks while evaluating underlying motor or process skill deficits. Patients select tasks that are familiar and relevant to them. Having the patient select the tasks avoids the problems inherent in traditional ADL instruments in which every patient performs the same homemaking tasks without regard to gender or familiarity with the task.

According to Pan and Fisher (1994), because the AMPS is designed to simultaneously compare all patients' performance on all task difficulty levels on two single equal-interval scales, motor ability and process ability, the clinician can predict which tasks are going to be difficult and use this information to select the type and order in which to present the tasks.

Another benefit of the AMPS is that it can reliably assess both low and high functioning patients. The AMPS is an individualized test, tailored to assess the patient's current level of functioning. This minimizes the definite ceiling and floor effect problem, a common criticism of most traditional ADL and IADL measures.

Disadvantages

The AMPS is a complex, time-consuming instrument that needs to be administered and scored by a trained professional. An occupational therapist must complete the AMPS workshop and become certified before using this measure. Depending on the clinician's level of experience and the patient's level of disability, administration of the AMPS may require 60 minutes. The amount of time required may also be extended when the assessment is conducted in the patient's home. There is no question that the AMPS is extremely clinically relevant, but its disadvantages will probably limit its global use and applications.

Performance on the AMPS, as with all performance measures, is influenced by many external and emotional factors. The AMPS was specifically designed to control for these external artifacts by selecting familiar tasks and performing the tasks at home if necessary. However, psychological factors like depression and motivation can also influence performance. One solution may be to include a brief psychological status questionnaire along with the AMPS.

Comments

The AMPS is a new generation ADL and IADL assessment instrument whose performance standards will be used to compare future IADLs measures.

Handicap Measures

Ameliorating handicap is one of the primary long-term goals of rehabilitation and yet there are few instruments available to assess this goal (Johnston, Wilerson, & Maney, 1993). Since World War II, the primary focus of rehabilitation has been on reducing disability and improving functional status. With increased political and economic pressure created by the National Disability Act and from the managed care industry for better and more cost-effective medical services, the goals of rehabilitation have expanded to include such domains as quality of life, patient satisfaction, and home and community integration. These changes, along with other focuses including the increased numbers of

Table 10-5. AMPS Motor and Process Skill Items by Group

Motor Skill Items by Group	*Process Skill Items by Group*
Posture	**Using Knowledge**
Stabilizes	Chooses
Aligns	Uses
Positions	Handles
Mobility	Inquires
Walks	Notices
Reaches	**Temporal Organization**
Bends	Initiates
Coordination	Continues
Coordination	Sequences
Manipulates	Terminates
Flows	**Space & Objects**
Strength & Effort	Searches
Moves	Gathers
Transports	Organizes
Lifts	Restores
Calibrates	**Adaptation**
Grips	Accommodates
Energy	Adjusts
Endures	Navigates
Paces	Benefits
	Energy
	Paces
	Attends

Fisher AG. *Assessment of Motor and Process Skills* (rev. ed.). Fort Collins, CO: Three Star Press, 1995.

Table 10-6.   AMPS Skill Item Rating Scale Criteria

Score	Quality of Performance	Impact on Action or Task Progression	Outcome Yielded
4	Competent	Supporting	Good
3	Questionable	Placiong at risk	Uncertain
2	Ineffective	Interfering	Indesirable
1	Deficit	Impeding	Unacceptable

Fisher AG. *Assessment of Motor and Process Skills* (rev. ed.). Fort Collins, CO: Three Star Press, 1995.

Table 10-7. AMPS Motor and Process Skill Item Difficulty Calibration Order

	Motor	*Process*
Easy	Lifts	Uses
	Moves	Attends
	Endures	Handles
	Reaches	Chooses
	Coordinates	Gathers
	Transports	Sequences
	Aligns	Terminates
	Grips	Searches/Locates
	Manipulates	Inquires
	Stabilizes	Navigates
	Flows	Heeds
	Bends	Notices/Responds
	Walks	Organizes
	Calibrates	Continues
	Paces	Paces
	Positions	Adjusts
		Restores
		Initiates
		Benefits
Hard		Accommodates

Fisher AG. *Assessment of Motor and Process Skills* (rev. ed.). Fort Collins, CO: Three Star Press, 1995.

Table 10-8. Sample AMPS Tasks Used to Assess Motor and Process Skills, in Calibration Difficulty Order

	MOTOR	*PROCESS*
Easy	Machine wash laundry	Drink refrigerator
	Drink refrigerator	Make standard bed
	Instant drink	Machine wash laundry
	Fold laundry	Fold laundry
	Wash dishes	Instant drink
	Cottage cheese & fruit salad	Hand wash laundry
	Set table for 1 or 4	Polish shoes
	Hand wash laundry	Water plants
	Ironing/no setup	Set table for 1 or 4
	Juice & cereal	Wash dishes
	Polish shoes	Sweep floor
	Pot of tea	Juice & cereal
	Jam sandwich	Peanut butter/jelly sandwich
	Repot plant	Ironing/no setup
	"	"
	"	"
	"	"
	Egg, toast, & brewed coffee	Grilled cheese sandwich
	Change standard bed	Egg, meat, & brewed coffee
	Mop floor	Omelette, toast, & beverage
	French toast & beverage	Egg, toast, & brewed coffee
Hard	Vacuum	French toast & beverage

Fisher AG. *Assessment of Motor and Process Skills* (rev. ed.). Fort Collins, CO: Three Star Press, 1995.

chronically ill patients, have made handicap an important rehabilitation outcome deserving of additional attention.

Handicap is probably the most comprehensive outcome measure because it incorporates disability, the environment, disadvantage to the person, and social norms (Johnston, Keith, & Hinderer, 1992). The WHO defines handicap to include six domains of role function: orientation, mobility, physical dependence, economic self-sufficiency, occupation, and social integration. Handicap is determined by comparing the expectations of the specific individual to the reference group's expectations within the same cultural, social, economic, and physical environment (Granger, Albrecht, & Hamilton, 1979).

Although handicap measures are broad, it is difficult to judge long-term rehabilitation success based on handicap alone. Handicap is influenced by many factors, including poverty, support, or ethnicity, outside the control of the rehabilitation intervention (Johnston, Keith, & Hinderer, 1992). In general, handicap instruments fail to assess the reasoning behind a particular situation. This failure leads to misinterpretation of rehabilitation outcomes.

In this chapter, three measures of handicap are reviewed: the Craig Handicap Assessment and Reporting Technique (CHART), the Community Integration Questionnaire (CIQ), and the London Handicap Scale.

Craig Handicap Assessment and Reporting Technique (CHART)

The CHART, developed by Whiteneck and colleagues (Whiteneck et al., 1992), is a measure of handicap specifically designed to assess objective, observable behaviors. Although it has been used primarily with spinal cord injury patients, it can be applied to many chronic conditions as well as the general population. Results from CHART studies indicate that mildly impaired spinal cord patients performed their social roles as well as most nondisabled people (Whiteneck et al., 1992).

Description

The CHART contains five subscales—physical independence, mobility, occupation, economic self-sufficiency, and social integration—and consists of 27 items (Table 10-9). The *Physical Independence* subscale assesses the number of hours of assistance

needed. The *Mobility* subscale measures the number of hours of independence within the home and the degree of access to transportation. The *Occupation* subscale measures the number of productive hours spent on activities like homemaking, volunteering, or schooling. The *Social Integration* subscale measures the number and nature of the patient's social relationships. The *Economic Self-Sufficiency* subscale evaluates annual household income and medical expenses.

Psychometric Properties

The psychometric properties of the CHART were obtained on 135 spinal cord injury (SCI) patients who were living in the community. The subjects ranged in age from 16 to 74 years; 16% of the participants were female (Whiteneck et al., 1992).

Reliability

Overall test-retest reliability of the CHART is high ($r = 0.93$) (Whiteneck et al., 1992). High test-retest reliability has been shown on the subscales. In a similar test, good agreement between the patient and proxy (family member or family) was obtained ($r = 0.83$) for the total CHART.

Validity

The validity of the CHART was assessed by having two independent groups classify the participants as being low or high handicapped. Significant differences were obtained between the high and low handicap groups on the overall CHART. Group differences were also found on the physical independence, mobility, occupation, and social integration subscales. Rasch analysis demonstrated that the CHART is a linear scale with a good fit of both items and persons to its data (Whiteneck et al., 1992).

Administration/Scoring

The CHART was designed to be administered in person or by telephone by a trained interviewer, but it can also be self-administered. Items on the CHART are given different weight values, depending on their importance in society. For example, work, school, and homemaking are weighted twice as much as nonrevenue-producing activities such as recreation and volunteer work (Whiteneck et al., 1992). Score totals for each subscale range from 0 (total handicap) to 100 (no handicap). Most nondisabled adults obtain 100 for each subscale (Whiteneck et al., 1988). The subscale totals are added for a maximum overall score of 500. Information regarding the scoring protocol is contained in the user's manual (Whiteneck et al., 1988).

Advantages

The CHART is a short, simple, and objective measure of handicap. It measures the overall effect of handicap, not the cause. This is important because impairment and disability may or may not lead to handicap. As noted by Wade (1992), there is only a general, not specific, relationship between impairment, disability, and handicap. Thus, the CHART is a pure and clean measure that can be used to assess handicap in both patient and general populations.

Although the CHART does not assess the orientation domain included in the WHO definition of handicap, it is a multidimensional measure that appears to give relatively equal importance to the other dimensions of handicap. For example, Boake and High found that the occupation, social integration, and physical independence subscales of the CHART were weighted equally (Boake & High, 1996).

Disadvantages

The physical independence subscale has been criticized for three reasons. First, it assumes that the patient has access to attendant care, and therefore a patient who does not have help would be considered independent (Willer et al., 1993). Second, this subscale does not credit nonphysical assistance, such as when a caregiver provides assistance through supervision (Boake & High, 1996). Finally, the physical independence subscale has the largest ceiling effect of all the subscales, with half of all patients attaining the maximum score possible (Boake & High, 1996).

Comments

The occupation and social integration scales are sensitive to conditions that are likely to change with compensatory interventions and thus would be especially useful in measuring postacute stage of brain injury recovery (Boake & High, 1996).

Community Integration Questionnaire (CIQ)

The CIQ was developed by Willer and associates in accordance with the WHO definition of handicap (Willer et al., 1993). The CIQ is an objective outcome measure of community integration that assesses home integration, social network, and activities.

Description

The CIQ contains 15 items and has 3 subscales: home integration, social integration, and productivity (Table 10-10). The home integration subscale evaluates the degree to which the patient is actively involved in running his or her home. The social integration subscale evaluates the amount of participation in activities outside the home, e.g., shopping, visiting friends, and going to the movies. The productivity subscale examines the degree to which the patient is out of the house during the day engaging in such activities as employment, school, or volunteer work.

Psychometric Properties

The original reliability and validity studies were conducted on moderate to severe brain injury patients who lived in the community (Willer et al., 1993).

Reliability

The CIQ has demonstrated acceptable Cronbach alpha internal consistency ($r = 0.76$) and high test-retest reliability ($r = 0.91$) for the patient and ($r = 0.97$) for the family members' assessment of the patient (Willer et al., 1993). Similarly high test-retest reliability coefficients were obtained for each subscale. High interrater reliability is evident by the high correlation between responses given by the patient and the family member.

Validity

To determine concurrent validity, the CIQ was compared to the CHART. Overall concurrent validity between the CHART and the CIQ was moderate for the patient ($r = 0.62$) and for the family ($r = 0.70$) (Willer et al., 1993). The social integration subscale of the CHART did not correlate significantly with any subscales of the CIQ. Willer and associates believe the low ceiling on the CHART social integration subscale may account for this nonsignificant finding. However, these subscales may not be highly correlated simply because they are assessing different dimensions.

Table 10-9. The CHART

What Assistance Do You Need?

1. How many hours in a typical 24-hour day do you have someone with you to provide assistance? (hours paid/hours unpaid)
2. Not including any regular care as reported above, how many hours in a *typical month* do you occasionally have assistance with such things as grocery shopping, laundry, housekeeping, or infrequent medical needs like catheter changes?
3. Who takes responsibility for instructing and directing your attendants and/or caregivers?

Are You Up and About Regularly?

4. On a *typical day,* how many hours are you out of bed?
5. In a typical *week,* how many days do you get out of your house and go somewhere?
6. In the last *year,* how many nights have you spent away from your home (excluding hospitalizations)? (none); (1–2); (3–4); (5 or more)
7. Can you enter and exit your home without any assistance from someone? (yes) (no)
8. In your home, do you have independent access to your sleeping area, kitchen, bathroom, telephone, and TV (or radio)? (yes) (no)

Is Your Transportation Adequate?

9. Can you use your transportation independently? (yes) (no)
10. Does your transportation allow you to get to all the places you would like to go? (yes) (no)
11. Does your transportation let you get out whenever you want? (yes) (no)
12. Can you use your transportation with little or no advance notice? (yes) (no)

How Do You Spend Your Time?

13. How many hours per week do you spend working in a job for which you get paid?
14. How many hours per week do you spend in school working toward a degree or in an accredited technical training program? (hours in class and studying).
15. How many hours per week do you spend in active homemaking including parenting, housekeeping, and food preparation?
16. How many hours per week do you spend in home maintenance activities such as yard work, house repairs, or home improvement?
17. How many hours per week do you spend in ongoing volunteer work for an organization?
18. How many hour per week do you spend in recreational activities such as sports, exercise, playing cards, or going to movies? Please do not include time spent watching TV or listening to the radio.
19. How many hours per week do you spend in other self-improvement activities such as hobbies or leisure reading? Please do not include time spent watching TV or listening to the radio.

With Whom Do You Spend Time?

20. Do you live alone; or with: a spouse or significant other; children (how many?); other relative (how many?); roommate (how many?); attendant (how many?)
21. If you don't live with a spouse or significant other, are you involved in a romantic relationship? (yes) (no)
22. How many relatives (not in your household) do you visit, phone, or write to at least once a month?
23. How many business or organizational associates do you visit, phone, or write to at least once a month?

Table 10-9.   *(continued)*

24. How many friends (nonrelatives contacted outside business or organizational settings) do you visit, phone, or write to at least once a month?

25. With how many strangers have you initiated a conversation in the last month (for example, to ask information or place an order)? (none); (1–2); (3–5); (6 or more)

What Financial Resources Do You Have?

26. Approximately what was the combined annual income of **all family members in your household?** (Consider all sources including wages and earnings, disability benefits, pensions, and retirement income, income from court settlements, investments and trust funds, child support and alimony, contributions from relatives, and any other source.)

27. Approximately how much did you pay last year for medical care expenses? (Consider any amounts paid by yourself or the family members in your household and **not reimbursed** by insurance or benefits.)

Whiteneck GG, Charlifue SW, Gerhart KA, Overholser JD, Richardson GN. Quantifying handicap: a new measure of long-term rehabilitation outcomes. *Archives of Physical Medicine and Rehabilitation* 1992;73:519–26. Reproduced with permission of Dr. Whiteneck.

Administration/Scoring

The CIQ is a self-administered questionnaire that generally requires less than 10 minutes to complete. The overall score, which represents a summation of the scores from individual questions, ranges from 0 (low integration) to 29 (high integration) for the home, social integration, and productivity subscales. Subscale scores can also be obtained for the CIQ. Each item is weighted equally for each subscale. Additional information regarding the scoring protocol is contained in the user's manual (Willer & Button, 1994).

Advantages

Chronically ill patients often experience fatigue, short-term memory deficits, and poor concentration. The CIQ was specifically designed to combat these difficulties. It is a short, simple self-report measure of handicap that focuses on assessing recent life events.

Disadvantages

As with the CHART, the CIQ is only a behavioral measure of handicap. It asks how much time the patient engages in a particular activity and does not assess whether particular activities or interactions were successful or meaningful.

Comments

The CIQ is a convenient, reliable, and valid measure of handicap that is appropriate to use for assessing both healthy and disabled populations.

London Handicap Scale

The London Handicap Scale was developed by Harwood and associates in 1994 in response to the need for evaluating health care outcomes (Harwood & Gompertz, 1994).

Description

This instrument assesses the six handicap dimensions outlined by the WHO model: mobility, physical independence, occupation, social integration, orientation, and economic self-sufficiency. It contains only six items, with each item representing a handicap domain (Table 10-11).

Psychometric Properties

The original reliability and validity study was conducted with 361 stroke inpatients (Harwood & Gompertz, 1994). Longitudinal data were obtained 12 months after hospital discharge on the 170 survivors. The follow-up questionnaire packet contained measures on handicap, disability, life satisfaction, mood, and perceived health.

Reliability

The London Handicap Scale has documented high test-retest reliability ($r = 0.91$) (Harwood & Gompertz, 1994).

Validity

Construct validity was assessed by comparing the London Handicap Scale to parts 1 and 2 of the Nottingham Health Profile (NHP) (Hunt, McEwan, & McKenna, 1986) and the Barthel Index. A moderate association between the NHP and London Handicap Scale was found ($r = 0.69$).

Administration/Scoring

This short and simple measure can be completed by the patient within a few minutes. The item responses are on a 6-point Likert scale ranging from 1 (no handicap) to 6 (extreme handicap). The overall score ranges from 1 (no handicap) to 0 (maximum handicap) because the matrix of scale weights enables the severity of disadvantages in each dimension to be combined. The scoring manual for the London Handicap Scale is available through the Medical Outcomes Trust (Harwood & Gompertz, 1996).

Advantages

The London Handicap Scale is a simple, easy, and short measure. It covers all the dimensions of handicap outlined in the WHO definition.

Disadvantages

There are two problems associated with the London Handicap Scale. The first problem relates to how concurrent validity was determined. To demonstrate concurrent validity, the London Handicap Scale should have been compared to other measures of handicap like the CIQ or the CHART. The London Handicap Scale was compared to two measures of disability (the NHP and

Table 10-10.   Community Integration Questionnaire (CIQ)

1.   Who usually does shopping for groceries or other necessities in your household?

____ yourself alone
____ yourself and someone else
____ someone else

2.   Who usually prepares meals in your household?

____ yourself alone
____ yourself and someone else
____ someone else

3.   In your home who usually does normal everyday housework?

____ yourself alone
____ yourself and someone else
____ someone else

4.   Who usually cares for the children in your home?

____ yourself alone
____ yourself and someone else
____ someone else
____ not applicable/no children under 17 in the home

5.   Who usually plans social arrangements such as get-togethers with family and friends?

____ yourself alone
____ yourself and someone else
____ someone else

6.   Who usually looks after your personal finances, such as banking or paying bills?

____ yourself alone
____ yourself and someone else
____ someone else

  Can you tell me approximately how many times a month you now
usually participate in the following activities *outside your home*?

7.   SHOPPING

____ Never   ____ 1–4 times   ____ 5 or more

8.   LEISURE ACTIVITIES SUCH AS MOVIES, SPORTS, RESTAURANTS

____ Never   ____ 1–4 times   ____ 5 or more

9.   VISITING FRIENDS OR RELATIVES

____ Never   ____ 1–4 times   ____ 5 or more

10.   When you participate in leisure activities do you usually do this alone or with others?

____ mostly alone
____ mostly with friends who have head injuries
____ mostly with family members
____ mostly with friends who do not have head injuries
____ with a combination of family and friends

Table 10-10. *(continued)*

11. Do you have a best friend with whom you confide?

____ yes
____ no

12. How often do you travel outside the home?

____ almost every day
____ almost every week
____ seldom/never (less than once per week)

13. Please choose the answer below that best corresponds to your current (during the past month) work situation

____ full-time (more than 20 hours per week)
____ part-time (less than or equal to 20 hours per week)
____ not working, but actively looking for work
____ not working, not looking for work
____ not applicable, retired due to age

14. Please choose the answer below that best corresponds to your current (during the past month) school or training program situation:

____ full-time
____ part-time
____ not attending school or training program

15. In the past month, how often did you engage in volunteer activities?

____ never
____ 1–4 times
____ 5 or more

Reproduced with the permission of B. Willer (Willer & Button, 1994).

Barthel Index). It is difficult to draw conclusions about the concurrent validity of a handicap instrument when it is being compared to a disability measure. Research indicates that there is only a general or nonspecific relationship between impairment, disability, and handicap (Wade, 1992; Whute, 1994). Reducing disability through rehabilitation may or may not impact impairment or handicap. This means that the correlates among impairment, disability, and handicap vary. To demonstrate concurrent validity, the London Handicap Scale should have been compared to another measure of handicap. Comparing the London Handicap Scale to disability measures is not the most appropriate way to determine concurrent validity.

Second, the London Handicap Scale assesses each handicap domain with only one item, making the internal consistency of this instrument questionable. As a general rule, five or more items are necessary to define the predictor construct or domain (Nunnally, 1978),

Comments

Although the London Handicap Scale is a fairly recent measure whose first reliability and validity study results look promising, additional psychometric testing is needed. It does appear to be a very useful addition to the few already available measures of handicap.

Health Status Measures

One of the most dramatic changes in the health care field in the last decade has been the recognition, assessment, and treatment of the "whole person." The patient's perception of his or her own physical and psychosocial functioning has became a central theme in the development of the new multidimensional health status instruments. These comprehensive instruments generally incorporate physical, psychological, and social components into a single measure and assess the impact of an illness from the patient's perspective. The measures included in this chapter are the Sickness Impact Profile (SIP), the Short-Form 36 (SF-36), and the Medical Rehabilitation Follow Along (MRFA).

The Sickness Impact Profile (SIP)

The Sickness Impact Profile (SIP) is a well-known, highly recommended, generic health status questionnaire. It was first developed in 1976 (Bergner et al., 1976) and revised in 1981 (Bergner et al., 1981) as a measure of perceived health status. The SIP has been used to fulfill a variety of needs including outcome measure, health survey, program planning, policy formulation, and monitoring patient progress (Wilkin, Hallam, & Doggett, 1992). "It was designed to be broadly applicable across types and severities of illness and across demographic and cultural subgroups" (Bergner et al., 1981, p. 787).

Description

The SIP contains 136 behavioral items that describe changes in a person's behavior or performance due to an illness (Table 10-12) (Skinner, 1996). It evaluates physical and psychosocial functioning and covers 12 content areas: work, recreation, emotion, affect, home life, sleep, rest, eating, ambulation, mobility, communication, and social interaction. The respondents mark items or statements that apply to them on a given day and are related to their health. The British version of the SIP, the Functional Limitations Profile (FLP), contains all the items of the SIP but the wording of some of the items has been changed (Patrick & Peach, 1989).

Psychometric Properties

Reliability

The 136-item version of the SIP has demonstrated high test-retest reliability (0.88 to 0.92) (Bergner et al., 1981). Cronbach coefficient alpha for this version was also high ($r = 0.94$) (Bergner et al., 1981).

Validity

Convergent and divergent validity was assessed by multitrait, multimethod technique. In comparing the SIP to other measures of functional

Table 10-11. The London Handicap Scale

This questionnaire asks six questions about your everyday life. Please answer each question. Tick the box next to the sentence that describes you best. Think about things you have done over the last week. Compare what you can do with what someone like you who is in good health can do.

Getting around (mobility)

Think about how you get from one place to another, using any help, aids or means of transport that you normally have available. Does you health stop you from getting around?

1. Not at all: You go everywhere you want to, no matter how far away.
2. Very slightly: You go most places you want to, but not all.
3. Quite a lot: You get out of the house, but not far away from it.
4. Very much: You don't go outside, but you can move around from room to room indoors.
5. Almost completely: You are confined to a single room, but can move around in it.
6. Completely: You are confined to a bed or a chair. You can not move around at all. There is no one to move you.

Looking after yourself (physical independence)

Think about things like housework, shopping, looking after money, cooking, laundry, getting dressed, washing, shaving, and using the toilet. Does your health stop you from looking after yourself?

1. Not at all: You can do everything yourself.
2. Very slightly: Now and again you need a little help.
3. Quite a lot: You need help with some tasks (such as heavy housework or shopping), but no more than once a day.
4. Very much: You can do some things but you need help more than once a day. You can be left alone safely for a few hours.
5. Almost completely: You need help to be available all the time. You can not be left alone safely.
6. Completely: You need help with everything. You need constant attention, day and night.

Work and leisure (occupation)

Think about things like work (paid or not), housework, gardening, sports, hobbies, going out with friends, traveling, reading, looking after children, watching television, and going on holiday. Does your health limit your work or leisure activities?

1. Not at all: You can do everything you want to do.
2. Very slightly: You can do almost all the things. you want to do.
3. Quite a lot: You find something to do almost all the time, but can not do some things for as long as you would like.
4. Very much: You are unable to do a lot of things, but can find something to do most of the time.
5. Almost completely: You are unable to do most things, but can find something to do some of the time.
6. Completely: You sit all day doing nothing. You can not keep yourself busy or take part in any activities.

Getting on with people (social integration)

Think about family, friends, and people you might meet during a normal day. Does your health stop you from getting on with people?

1. Not at all: You get on well with people, see everyone you want to see, and meet new people.

Table 10-11. *(continued)*

2. Very slightly: You get on well with people, but your social life is slightly limited.
3. Quite a lot: You are fine with people you know well, but you feel uncomfortable with strangers.
4. Very much: You are fine with people you know well, but you have few friends and little contact with neighbors. Dealing with strangers is very hard.
5. Almost completely: Apart from the person who looks after you, you see no one. You have no friends and no visitors.
6. Completely: You don't get on with anyone, not even people who look after you.

Awareness of your surrounds (orientation)

Think about taking in and understanding the world around you, and finding your way around in it. Does your health stop you from understanding the world around you?

1. Not at all: You fully understand the world around you. You see, hear, speak, and think clearly, and your memory is good.
2. Very slightly: You have problems with hearing, speaking, seeing, or your memory, but these do not stop you doing most things.
3. Quite a lot: You have problems with hearing, speaking, seeing, or your memory, which make life difficult a lot of the time, but you understand what is going on.
4. Very much: You have great difficulty understanding what is going on.
5. Almost completely: You are unable to tell where you are or what day it is. You can not look after yourself at all.
6. Completely: You are unconscious, completely unaware of anything going on around you.

Affording the things you need (economic self-sufficiency)

Think about whether health problems have led to any extra expenses, or have caused you to earn less than you would if you were healthy. Are you able to afford the things you need?

1. Yes, easily: You can afford everything you need. You have easily enough money to buy modern labor-saving devices, and anything you may need because of ill-health.
2. Fairly easily: You have just about enough money. It is fairly easy to cope with expenses caused by ill-health.
3. Just about: You are less well-off than other people like you; however, with sacrifices you can get by without help.
4. Not really: You only have enough money to meet your basic needs. You are dependent on state benefits for any extra expenses you have because of ill-health.
5. No: You are dependent on state benefits, or money from other people or charities. You can not afford things you need.
6. Absolutely not: You have no money at all and no state benefits. You are totally dependent on charity for your most basic needs.

Harwood RH, Gompertz SE. Handicap one year after a stroke: validity of a new scale. *Journal of Neurology, Neurosurgery, and Psychiatry* 1994;57:825–29. Copied with permission of the Medical Outcomes Trust.

status (Katz IADL and National Health Interviews Survey) and among different patient populations (hip replacement, arthritis, and hyperthyroidism), high correlations were obtained (Bergner et al., 1981). The psychosocial dimension of the SIP is highly correlated with various psychological measures and appears to be strongly related to depression (Brooks et al., 1990; Temkin et al., 1989).

Administration/Scoring

The SIP can be self- or interviewer-administered and requires 20 to 30 minutes to complete. The SIP can be totaled by the 12 subscales, by broad domains (physical or psychosocial health), or by item (Bowling, 1991). The total score on the SIP ranges from 0 (better health) to 100 (poor health). To calculate the overall SIP score, add the scale values for each item checked across all subscales, divide by the maximum possible score for the SIP, and then multiply by 100 to obtain the total SIP score (Bowling, 1991). Bowling (1991) notes that a normal population generally obtains a SIP score of 2 or 3 and increases to mid-30 for terminally ill cancer and stroke patients (6). Scoring and instructions for the SIP (Skinner, 1996) and the FIP (Patrick & Peach, 1989) are available.

Advantages

Because the SIP focuses on sickness-related behaviors, it can be applied to a large number of patient populations for a number of different purposes, making cross-study comparisons possible. In summarizing the advantages of the SIP, Keith states, "the broad coverage of the SIP, extensive development, and emphasis on current performance make it a candidate for selected applications in rehabilitation" (Keith, 1994, p. 480).

Disadvantages

The SIP has been criticized for two major reasons. First, it has been criticized for its lack of responsiveness or failure to detect change over time in the same individuals (Wilkin, Hallam, & Doggett, 1992). This limitation is particularly important when determining whether or not to use the SIP as a rehabilitation outcome measure. Additional clinical trials and rehabilitation outcome studies using the SIP are needed before definite conclusions can be stated.

The second major disadvantage of the SIP is its length. It has been criticized by several

researchers and practitioners who state that its length is an obstacle to routine use (Wilkin, Hallam, & Doggett, 1992; Keith, 1994). In a 1993 Dutch study on stroke patients, early recovery patients complained that the SIP was too time-consuming and fatiguing (Schuiling, Greidanus, & Meijboom-DeJong, 1993). In response to this complaint, the short-form SIP68 was developed (Table 10-13). The psychometric properties of the SIP68 appear to be comparable to the longer version (Bruin, Diederiks, Witte, Stevens, & Philipsen, 1994; Bruin, Buys, Witte, & Diederiks, 1994; Post, Bruin, Witte, & Schrijvers, 1996). The SIP68 requires additional validation studies before the effectiveness and generalizability of this shorter version can be accomplished.

Comments

The SIP is a standardized general purpose health status questionnaire that is widely used in the United States as an outcome measure. Although the shorter form, the SIP68, is a new instrument that requires additional reliability and validity testing, it may eventually replace the longer version if for no other reason than convenience.

The 36-Item Short-Form (SF-36)

The 36-item short-form (SF-36) was designed to survey the health status of the general population in the Medical Outcomes Study (Stewart & Ware, 1992; Ware & Sherbourne, 1992). It is a multidimensional health questionnaire that captures those features of health that are important to all patients. The SF-36 has been used for health policy evaluations, general populations surveys, clinical research and practice, and other applications using various diverse populations (Ware & Sherbourne, 1992). The utility of the SF-36 as a rehabilitation outcomes instrument has yet to be determined.

Description

The SF-36 Health Survey measures two broad areas of health status (functional status and well-being) (McHorney, Ware, & Raczek, 1993) and includes eight health subscales. The subscales are: (1) physical functioning; (2) social functioning; (3) role limitations because of physical health problems; (4) role limitations because of emotional problems; (5) mental health status

Table 10-12. Sickness Impact Profile Check *only* those statements that you are sure describe you today and are related to your state of health.

Sleep and Rest Subscale

____ 1. I spend much of the day lying down in order to rest.
____ 2. I sit during much of the day.
____ 3. I am sleeping or dozing most of the time—day and night.
____ 4. I lie down more often during the day in order to rest.
____ 5. I sit around half asleep.
____ 6. I sleep less at night, for example, wake up too early, don't fall asleep for a long time, awaken frequently.
____ 7. I sleep or nap more during the day.

Emotion Subscale

____ 1. I say how bad or useless I am, for example, that I am a burden to others.
____ 2. I laugh or cry suddenly.
____ 3. I often moan and groan in pain and discomfort.
____ 4. I have attempted suicide.
____ 5. I act nervous or restless.
____ 6. I keep rubbing or holding areas of my body that hurt or are uncomfortable.
____ 7. I act irritable and impatient with myself, for example, talk badly about myself, swear at myself, blame myself for things that happen.
____ 8. I talk about the future in a hopeless way.
____ 9. I get sudden frights.

Body Care and Movement Subscale

____ 1. I make difficult moves with help, for example, getting into or out of cars or bathtubs.
____ 2. I do not move into or out of bed or chairs by myself but am moved by a person or mechanical aid.
____ 3. I stand only for short periods of time.
____ 4. I do not maintain balance.
____ 5. I move my hands or fingers with some limitation or difficulty.
____ 6. I stand up only with someone's help.
____ 7. I kneel, stoop, or bend down only by holding onto something.
____ 8. I am in a restricted position all the time.
____ 9. I am very clumsy in body movements.
____ 10. I get in and out of bed or chairs by grasping something for support or using a cane or walker.
____ 11. I stay lying down most of the time.
____ 12. I change position frequently.
____ 13. I hold onto something to move myself around in bed.
____ 14. I do not bathe myself completely, for example, I require assistance with bathing.
____ 15. I do not bathe myself at all but am bathed by someone else.
____ 16. I use a bedpan with assistance.
____ 17. I have trouble getting shoes, socks, or stockings up.
____ 18. I do not have control of my bladder.
____ 19. I do not fasten my clothing, for example, require assistance with buttons, zippers, shoelaces.
____ 20. I spend most of the time partly undressed or in pajamas.
____ 21. I do not have control of my bowels.
____ 22. I dress myself but do so very slowly.
____ 23. I get dressed only with someone's help.

Table 10-12.   *(continued)*

Household Management Subscale

_____ 1. I do work around the house only for short periods of time or rest often.

_____ 2. I am doing less of the regular daily work around the house than I would usually do.

_____ 3. I am not doing any of the regular daily work around the house than I would usually do.

_____ 4. I am not doing any of the maintenance or repair work that I would usually do in my home or yard.

_____ 5. I am not doing any of the shopping that I would usually do.

_____ 6. I am not doing any of the house cleaning that I would usually do.

_____ 7. I have difficulty doing handwork, for example, turning faucets, using kitchen gadgets, sewing, and carpentry.

_____ 8. I am not doing any of the clothes washing that I would usually do.

_____ 9. I am not doing heavy work around the house.

_____ 10. I have given up taking care of personal or household business affairs, for example, paying bills, banking, or working on the budget.

Mobility Subscale

_____ 1. I only get about within one building.

_____ 2. I stay in one room.

_____ 3. I am staying in bed more.

_____ 4. I am staying in bed most of the time.

_____ 5. I am not now using public transportation.

_____ 6. I stay at home most of the time.

_____ 7. I am only going to places with rest rooms nearby.

_____ 8. I am not going into town.

_____ 9. I stay away from home only for brief periods of time.

_____ 10. I do not get around in the dark or in unlit places without someone's help.

Social Interaction Subscale

_____ 1. I am going out less to visit people.

_____ 2. I am not going out to visit people at all.

_____ 3. I show less interest in other people's problems, for example, don't listen when they tell me about their problems, don't offer to help.

_____ 4. I often act irritable toward those around me, for example, snap at people, give sharp answers, criticize easily.

_____ 5. I show less affection.

_____ 6. I am doing fewer social activities with groups of people.

_____ 7. I am cutting down the length of visits with friends.

_____ 8. I am avoiding social visits from others.

_____ 9. My sexual activity is decreased.

_____ 10. I often express concern over what might be happening to my health.

_____ 11. I talk less with those around me.

_____ 12. I make many demands, for example, insist that people do things for me, tell me how to do things.

_____ 13. I stay alone much of the time.

_____ 14. I act disagreeable to family members, for example, I act spiteful, I am stubborn.

_____ 15. I have frequent outbursts of anger at family members, for example, strike at them, scream, throw things at them.

_____ 16. I isolate myself as much as I can from the rest of the family.

_____ 17. I am paying less attention to the children.

Table 10-12. *(continued)*

____ 18. I refuse contact with family members, for example, turn away from them.

____ 19. I am not doing the things I usually do to take care of my children or family.

____ 20. I am not joking with family members as I usually do.

Ambulation Subscale

____ 1. I walk shorter distances or stop to rest often.

____ 2. I do not walk up or down hills.

____ 3. I use stairs only with mechanical support, for example, handrail, cane, crutches.

____ 4. I walk up or down stairs only with assistance from someone else.

____ 5. I get around in a wheelchair.

____ 6. I do not walk at all.

____ 7. I walk by myself but with some difficulty, for example, limp, wobble, stumble, have stiff legs.

____ 8. I walk only with help from someone.

____ 9. I go up and down stairs more slowly, for example, one step at a time, stop often.

____ 10. I do not use stairs at all.

____ 11. I get around only by using a walker, crutches, cane, walls, or furniture.

____ 12. I walk more slowly.

Alertness Subscale

____ 1. I am confused and start several actions at a time.

____ 2. I have more minor accidents, for example, drop things, trip and fall, bump into things.

____ 3. I react slowly to things that are said or done.

____ 4. I do not finish things I start.

____ 5. I have difficulty reasoning and starting problems, for example, making plans, making decisions, learning new things.

____ 6. I sometimes behave as if I were confused or disoriented in place or time, for example, where I am, who is around, directions, what day it is.

____ 7. I forget a lot, for example, things that happened recently, where I put things, appointments.

____ 8. I do not keep my attention on any activity for long.

____ 9. I make more mistakes than usual.

____ 10. I have difficulty doing activities involving concentration and thinking.

Communication Subscale

____ 1. I am having trouble writing or typing.

____ 2. I communicate mostly by gestures, for example, moving my head, pointing, sign language.

____ 3. My speech is understood only by a few people who know me well.

____ 4. I often lose control of my voice when I talk, for example, my voice get louder or softer, trembles, changes unexpectedly.

____ 5. I don't write, except to sign my name.

____ 6. I carry on a conversation only when very close to the other person or looking at him/her.

____ 7. I have difficulty speaking, for example, get stuck, stutter, stammer, slur my words.

____ 8. I am understood with difficulty.

____ 9. I do not speak clearly when I am under stress.

Recreation and Pastime Subscale

____ 1. I do my hobbies and recreation for shorter periods of time.

____ 2. I am going out for entertainment less often.

Table 10-12. *(continued)*

____ 3. I am cutting down on some of my usual inactive recreation and pastimes, for example, watching TV, playing cards, reading.

____ 4. I am not doing any of my usual inactive recreation and pastimes, for example, watching TV, playing cards, reading.

____ 5. I am doing more inactive pastimes in place of my other usual activities.

____ 6. I am doing fewer community activities.

____ 7. I am cutting down on some of my usual physical recreation or activities.

____ 8. I am not doing any of my usual physical recreation or activities.

Eating Subscale

____ 1. I am eating much less than usual.

____ 2. I feed myself but only by using specially prepared food or utensils.

____ 3. I am eating special or different food, for example, soft food, bland diet, low-salt, low-fat, low-sugar.

____ 4. I eat no food at all but am taking fluids.

____ 5. I just pick or nibble at my food.

____ 6. I am drinking less fluids.

____ 7. I feed myself with help from someone else.

____ 8. I do not feed myself at all but must be fed.

____ 9. I am eating no food at all; nutrition is taken through tubes or intravenous fluids.

Work Subscale

1. Do you usually do work other than managing your home? ____ YES ____ NO

   If you answered yes, go to question #5 on this subscale.
   If you answered no, answer questions #2 through #4 on this subscale.

2. Are you retired? ____ YES ____ NO

3. If you are retired, was your retirement related to your health? ____ YES ____ NO

4. If you are not retired but are not working, is this related to your health? ____ YES ____ NO

____ 5. I am not working at all. (If you checked this statement, skip all other questions).

____ 6. I am doing part of my job at home.

____ 7. I am not accomplishing as much as usual at work.

____ 8. I often act irritable toward my work associates, for example, snap at them, give sharp answers, criticize easily.

____ 9. I am working shorter hours.

____ 10. I am doing only light work.

____ 11. I work only for short periods of time or take frequent rests.

____ 12. I am working at my usual job but with some changes, for example, using different tools or special aids, trading some tasks with others.

____ 13. I do not do my job as carefully and accurately as usual.

Skinner, A. *The Sickness Impact Profile.* Boston: Medical Outcomes Trust, 1996. Copied with permission of the Medical Outcomes Trust.

Table 10-13.   The SIP68

Somatic Autonomy

1. I get around in a wheelchair.
2. I get dressed only with someone's help.
3. I do not move into or out of bed by myself, but am moved by a person or mechanical aid.
4. I stand up on with someone's help.
5. I do not fasten my clothing, for example, require assistance with buttons, zippers, shoelaces.
6. I do not walk at all.
7. I do not use stairs at all.*
8. I make difficult moves with help, for example, getting into or out of cars, bathtubs.
9. I do not bathe myself completely, for example, require assistance with bathing.
10. I do not bathe myself at all, but am bathed by someone else.
11. I do not have control of my bladder.
12. I am very clumsy in body movements.
13. I do not have control of my bowels.
14. I feed myself with help from someone else.
15. I do not maintain balance.
16. I use bedpan with assistance.
17. I am in a restricted position all the time.

Mobility Control

1. I go up and down stairs more slowly, for example, one step at a time, stop often.*
2. I walk shorter distance or stop to rest often.*
3. I walk more slowly.*
4. I use stairs only with mechanical support, for example, handrail, cane, crutches.
5. I walk by myself but with some difficulty, for example, limp, wobble, stumble, have stiff leg.*
6. I kneel, stoop, or bend down only by holding on to something.*
7. I do not walk up or down hills.*
8. I get in and out of bed or chairs by grasping something for support or using a cane or walker.
9. I stand only for short periods of time.
10. I dress myself, but do so very slowly.
11. I have difficulty doing handwork, for example, turning faucets, using kitchen gadgets, sewing, carpentry.
12. I move my hands or fingers with some limitation or difficulty.

Psychic Autonomy and Communication

1. I have difficulty reasoning and solving problems, for example, making plans, making decisions, learning new things.
2. I have difficulty doing activities involving concentration and thinking.
3. I react slowly to things that are said or done.
4. I make more mistakes than usual.
5. I do not keep my attention on any activity for long.
6. I forget a lot, for example, things that happened recently, where I put things, appointments.
7. I am confused and start several actions at a time.
8. I do not speak clearly when I am under stress.
9. I have difficulty speaking, for example, get stuck, stutter, stammer, slur my words.
10. I do not finish things I start.
11. I am having trouble writing or typing.

Table 10-13.   *(continued)*

Social Behavior

1. My sexual activity is decreased.
2. I am cutting down the length of visits with friends.
3. I am drinking less fluids.
4. I am doing fewer community activities.
5. I am doing fewer social activities with groups of people.
6. I am going out for entertainments less often.
7. I stay away from home only for brief periods of time.
8. I am eating much less than usual.
9. I am not doing heavy work around the house.
10. I do my hobbies and recreation for shorter periods of time.
11. I am doing less of the regular daily work around the house than I would usually do.
12. I am cutting down on some of my usual inactive recreation and pastime, for example, watching TV, playing cards, reading.

Emotional Stability

1. I often act irritable toward those around me, for example, snap at people, give sharp answers, criticize easily.
2. I act disagreeably to family members, for example, I act spiteful, I am stubborn.
3. I have frequent outbursts of anger at family members, for example, strike at them, scream, throw things at them.
4. I act irritable and impatient with myself, for example, talk badly about myself, swear at myself for things that happen.
5. I am not joking with family members as I usually do.
6. I talk less with those around me.

Mobility Range

1. I am not doing any of the shopping that I would usually do.
2. I am not going into town.
3. I am not doing any of the house cleaning that I would usually do.
4. I am not doing any of the regular work around the house.
5. I stay at home most of the time.
6. I am not doing any of the clothes washing that I would usually do.
7. I am not going out to visit people at all.
8. I am getting around only within one building.
9. I have given up taking care of personal or household business affairs, for example, paying bills, banking, working on budget.
10. I do not get around in the dark or in unlit places without someone's help.

*Items assigned a positive score when "I do not walk at all" was scored positively.

Post MWM, Bruni AF de, Witte LP de, Schrijvers A. The SIP68: a measure of health-related functional status in rehabilitation medicine. *Archives of Physical Medicine and Rehabilitation* 1996;77:440–45. Copied with permission of the Medical Outcomes Trust.

Table 10-14.   SF-36 Health Status Questions and Response Categories

1. In general would you say your health is:

   Excellent _____   Very good _____   Good _____   Fair _____   Poor _____

2. **Compared to one year ago,** how would you rate your health in general **now?**

   Much better now than one year ago _____

   Somewhat better now than one year ago _____

   About the same _____

   Somewhat worse now than one year ago _____

   Much worse now than one year ago _____

3. The following items are about activities you might do during a typical day. Does **your health now limit you in these activities?** If so, how much?

   a. **Vigorous activities,** such as running, lifting heavy objects, participating in strenuous sports.

   b. **Moderate activities,** such as moving a table, pushing a vacuum cleaner, bowling, or playing golf

   c. Lifting or carrying groceries

   d. Climbing **several** flights or stairs

   e. Climbing **one** flight of stairs

   f. Bending, kneeling, or stooping

   g. Walking **more than a mile**

   h. Walking **several blocks**

   i. Walking **one block**

   j. Bathing or dressing yourself

   Response categories: Yes, limited a lot; Yes, limited a little; No, not limited at all.

4. During the **past 4 weeks,** have you had any of the following problems with your work or other regular daily activities **as a result of your physical health?**

   a. Cut down the **amount of time** you spent on work or other activities.

   b. **Accomplished less** than you would like

   c. Were limited in the **kind** of work or other activities

   d. Had difficulty performing the work or other activities (for example, it took extra effort)

   Response categories: Yes; No

5. During the **past 4 weeks,** have you had any of the following problems with your work or other regular daily activities **as a result of any emotional problems** (such as feeling depressed or anxious)?

   a. Cut down the **amount of time** you spent on work or other activities

   b. **Accomplished less** than you would like

   c. Didn't do work or other activities as **carefully** as usual

   Response categories: Yes; No

6. During the **past 4 weeks,** to what extent has your **physical health or emotional problems** interfered with your normal social activities with family, friends, neighbors, or groups?

   Response categories: Not at all; Slightly; Moderately; Quite a bit; Extremely.

7. How much **bodily** pain have you had during the **past 4 weeks?**

   Response categories: None; Very mild; Mild; Moderate; Severe; Very severe.

8. During the **past 4 weeks,** how much did **pain** interfere with your normal work (including both work outside the home and housework)?

   Response categories: Not at all; A little bit; Moderately; Quite a bit; Extremely.

Table 10-14.   *(continued)*

9. These questions are about how you feel and how things have been with you **during the past 4 weeks.** For each question, please give the one answer that comes closest to the way you have been feeling. How much of the time during the past 4 weeks

   a. Did you feel full of pep?

   b. Have you been a very nervous person?

   c. Have you felt so down in the dumps that nothing could cheer you up?

   d. Have you felt calm and peaceful?

   e. Did you have a lot of energy?

   f. Have you felt downhearted and blue?

   g. Did you feel worn out?

   h. Have you been a happy person?

   i. Did you feel tired?

   Response categories: All of the time; Most of the time; A good bit of the time; Some of the time; A little of the time; None of the time.

10. During the **past 4 weeks,** how much of the time has your **physical health or emotional problems** interfered with your social activities (like visiting with friends, relatives, etc.)?

    Response categories: All of the time; Most of the time; Some of the time; A little of the time; None of the time.

11. How **TRUE or FALSE** is **each** of the following statements for you?

    a. I seem to get sick a little easier than other people

    b. I am as healthy as anybody I know

    c. I expect my health to get worse

    d. My health is excellent

    Response categories: Definitely true; Mostly true; Don't know; Mostly false; definitely false.

Ware JE, Sherbourne CD. The MOS 36-item short-form health survey (SF-36) I. Conceptual framework and item selection. *Medical Care* 1992;30:473-83. Modified to include response categories. Copied with permission of the Medical Outcomes Trust.

(psychological distress and psychological well-being); (6) bodily pain; (7) vitality (energy/fatigue); and (8) general health perceptions (Table 10-14). The SF-36 consists of 36 items, 35 of which comprise the 8 subscales. One item pertains to perception of change in health over a 1-year period and is scored separately (Ware & Sherbourne, 1992). Table 10-15 contains summary information on the SF-36.

Psychometric Properties

Reliability

Several SF-36 reliability studies have been completed on a variety of groups including working adults (Jenkinson, Coulter, & Wright, 1993), the elderly (Hayes et al., 1995), and a variety of patient populations (Garratt et al., 1993; Brazier et al., 1993; McHorney et al., 1994). Internal consistency reliability coefficients determined by Cronbach alpha range from $r = 0.78$ to a high of $r = 0.93$ across scales (McHorney et al., 1994; Ware et al., 1993). Lower Cronbach alphas were reported on the social functioning subscale in two studies ($r >$ or $= 0.76$) (Jenkinson, Coulter, & Wright, 1993; Brazier et al., 1992). Test-retest reliability ranged from $r = 0.60$ (social functioning) to $r = 0.81$ (physical functioning) (Brazier et al., 1992).

Validity

The SF-36 has demonstrated construct validity by correctly classifying various patients across the eight subscales (Brazier et al., 1992; McHorney, Ware, & Raczek, 1993; McHorney et al., 1992). Convergent and discriminant validity has also been satisfied. The SF-36 and Nottingham Health Profile were highly correlated on related subscale and less correlated on noncomparable dimensions (Ware et al., 1993). Compared to the Nottingham Health Profile, the SF-36 appears to be a more sensitive measure to lower levels of dysfunction and disability (Jenkinson, Coulter, & Wright, 1993). The SF-36 also correctly classified or discriminated between groups with expected health differences (Brazier et al., 1992).

Administration/Scoring

The SF-36 can be reliably administered over the phone, face to face, or self-administered (Weinberger et al., 1996). It is a short questionnaire that generally requires 10 minutes or less to com-

plete. For each subscale, items are coded, totaled, and transformed to a 0 to 100 scale, with 0 representing the worst health and 100 indicating the best health state (Jenkinson, Coulter, & Wright, 1993). Whether or not the SF-36 subscales scores can be totaled into a valid single score index has yet to be tested. The scoring information and instructions are available in the SF-36 Manual (Ware et al., 1993).

Advantages

The major appeal of the SF-36 is that it is short, comprehensive, and easy to administer. The SF-36 is a multidimensional assessment of functional status and emotional well-being that is applicable across many social, demographic, and age groups.

Disadvantages

The SF-36 has been criticized for its ceiling and floor effect (Wade, 1992). The range of health behavior responses are limited, resulting in large numbers of people obtaining the highest score possible (ceiling effect) or the lowest score possible (floor effect). Specifically, ceiling effects were reported for the role limitations and social functioning scales (McHorney et al., 1994).

The utility and performance of the SF-36 varies, depending on the population being assessed. Ziebland found that the SF-36 adequately detected change in health status among homogeneous treatment groups, but heterogeneous group responses were too varied to correctly determine the impact of health interventions in the whole community (Ziebland, 1995). Compared to the SIP and the Nottingham Health Profile (NHP), the SF-36 appears to be less comprehensive and less suitable for the elderly (Hayes et al., 1995). The SF-36 does not include a sleep disturbance subscale and provides only limited coverage of areas like pain, emotional well-being, and physical mobility. Items pertaining to work or vigorous activities were generally not applicable to the elderly. On the other hand, when assessing an active, healthier population, the SF-36 appears to be more sensitive. Compared to the SIP, only the SF-36 discriminated between patients with relatively good physical performance at the three-month follow-up in terms of their ability to work, play sports, and garden (Stucki et al., 1995). These results indicate that the

SF-36 appears to be a more sensitive mobility measure, whereas the SIP is a more comprehensive, global measure of health status.

Keith notes that the lack of reference to degree of assistance is different from traditional rehabilitation measures (Keith, 1994). More importantly, the time frame in which questions are asked on the SF-36 makes assessing change within a short time frame difficult (Keith, 1994).

Comments

The SF-36 is a promising new multidimensional health status questionnaire that is brief and easy to use. It is sensitive enough to detect health differences in the general population. The SF-36 should be combined with a disease-specific questionnaire when assessing a patient population since the SF-36 is a generic questionnaire.

Medical Rehabilitation Follow Along (MRFA)

The Medical Rehabilitation Follow Along (MRFA), developed by Granger, Ottenbacher, Baker, and Sehgal (1995), was specifically designed for the early detection of the functional problems typically experienced and evaluated during outpatient rehabilitation therapy. Unlike the SIP and the SF-36, which were designed to assess the health status of the general population, the MRFA is the first questionnaire to assess the health status changes of various patient populations.

Description

The MRFA was developed using Rasch analysis to construct linear measures that function on an interval level. It combines the best attributes of several existing questionnaires into a single multidimensional health status questionnaire. There are three forms of the MRFA: the Musculoskeletal Form, the Neurological Form, and the Multiple Sclerosis Form. The number of items for each form varies. The Likert scale range also varies, depending on the health status domain being evaluated.

The Musculoskeletal Form of the MRFA consists of 31 patient report items and includes three domains of physical functioning, the experience of pain, and affective well-being. Components include body movement and control, effort, pain-free, a visual analog pain rating scale, placid, and life sat-

isfaction to assess these three domains. The components include items from the Functional Assessment Screening Questionnaire (FASQ), the Oswestry Scale, and the short-form McGill Pain Questionnaire.

The Neurological Form of the MRFA consists of 39 items both clinician rated and patient report items. This form also includes the domains of physical functioning, pain experience, and affective well-being. Cognitive components from the FIM and Mini-Mental Status Exam and an IADL component to supplement selected FIM motor items are also included in this form.

The Multiple Sclerosis Form of the MRFA is similar to the Musculoskeletal Form with the limitations component and screening in the domain of pain experience. Fatigue sphincters, vision, and EDSS components are also included in this form.

Psychometric Properties

Reliability

The initial validation study of the Musculoskeletal Form of the MRFA demonstrated overall high test-retest reliability. Intraclass correlation coefficient (ICC), a reliability coefficient assessing the stability of responses, showed values ranging from $r = 0.74$ to $r = 0.97$ for the physical functioning domain. The ICC values for the items assessing pain and psychological well-being ranged from 0.36 to 0.93 (Granger et al., 1995).

Validity

Validity studies for the musculoskeletal form of the MRFA have been completed using both raw scoring (Baker et al., in press) and Rasch measures (Baker, Granger, & Fiedler, in press). Content, construct, and criterion validity have been addressed in these studies. The results provide support for the validity of inferences made from the raw score scales and Rasch measures of the MRFA for people with musculoskeletal problems. Additional studies are conducted with other types of problems (i.e., multiple sclerosis patients) in outpatient rehabilitation settings.

Administration/Scoring

The MRFA can be self-administered or administered by interviewing the patient in person or over the telephone. Administration of the MRFA

Table 10-15.   SF-36 Health Status Scale Information

Physical functioning	10	21	Limited a lot in performing all physical activities including bathing or dressing	Performs all types of physical activities including the most vigorous without limitations
Role limitations due to physical problems	4	5	Problems with work or other daily activities as a result of physical health	No problems with work or other daily activities as a result of physical health, past 4 weeks
Social functioning	2	9	Extreme and frequent interference with normal social activities due to physical and emotional problems	Performs normal social activities without interference due to physical or emotional problems, past 4 weeks
Bodily pain	2	11	Very severe and extremely limiting pain	No pain or limitations due to pain, past 4 weeks
General mental health	5	26	Feelings of nervousness and depression all of the time	Feels peaceful, happy, and calm all of the time, past 4 weeks
Role limitations due to emotional problems	3	4	Problems with work or other daily activities as a result of emotional problems	No problems with work or other daily activities as a result of emotional problems, past 4 weeks
Vitality	4	21	Feels tired and worn out all of the time	Feels full of pep and energy all of the time, past 4 weeks
General health perceptions	5	21	Believes personal health is poor and likely to get worse	Believes personal health is excellent

Wade JE, Sherbourne CD. The MOS 36-item short-form health survey (SF-36). *Medical Care* 1992;30:473–83. Copied with permission of the Medical Outcomes Trust.

over the telephone can be difficult if the patient does not have the answer sheet to view. The Likert scale for each health domain or subscale varies, which can be confusing. Clinician rated components of the Neurological Form can be completed with input from the patient or caregiver. The Mini-Mental State component requires questioning by the clinician. Completion of the Musculoskeletal Form of the MRFA requires 7 to 16 minutes (Granger et al., 1995).

Each domain or subscale on the MRFA Form is scored separately. All scoring is from 0 to 100, where a higher score represents better functioning, less pain, less EDSS disability, less emotional distress, and so on. Additional scoring information can be obtained by contacting the instrument developer, Dr. Granger.

Advantages

The MRFA is the first health status instrument specifically designed to assess the type of problems experienced by outpatients receiving rehabilitation therapy. It is also the first outpatient rehabilitation instrument designed for early detection of functional problems in an effort to prevent secondary complications. Because it was specifically designed to assess rehabilitation outcomes, the responsiveness of this measure is likely to be high.

Disadvantages

It is important to note that the Multiple Sclerosis Form of the MRFA is only appropriate to use when assessing benign or mild multiple sclerosis (MS) patients. The Neurological Form of the MRFA is best used when assessing all types of MS (benign, relapsing-remitting, and primary/secondary chronic progressive) or when both ambulatory and wheelchair-bound MS patients are being evaluated.

Comments

Although the reliability and validity studies have not been completed, the MRFA is the first outpatient rehabilitation measure to assess disability, handicap, and general health status with an emphasis on prevention or early detection of secondary problems. The sensitivity or responsiveness of the MRFA still needs to established and will be particularly important to the utility of this instrument since the ability to detect change and demonstrate improvement with rehabilitation therapy is the primary purpose of this instrument.

Summary

The standardized instruments described in this chapter represent a cross-section of the types of rehabilitation outcome measures being widely used today. Although thousands of rehabilitation instruments exist, these measures are considered among the best disability, handicap, and health status instruments available. As the field of rehabilitation medicine progresses, the method of assessing treatment outcomes is changing, shifting from physician-driven assessment of functional status to patient-driven assessment of general health status. More patient completed measures of quality of life, psychological well-being, and patient satisfaction can be expected in the future.

References

Baker JG, Granger CV, Fiedler RC. A brief outpatient functional assessment measure: validity using Rasch measures. *Am J Phys Med Rehabil* (in press).

Baker JG, Granger CV, Ottenbacher KJ. Validity of a brief outpatient functional assessment measure. *Am J Phys Med Rehabil* (in press).

Bergner M, Bobbitt RA, Carter WB, Gilson BS. The Sickness Impact Profile: development and final revision of a health status measure. *Med Care* 1981;19:787–805.

Bergner M, Bobbitt RA, Kressel S, Pollard WE, Gilson BS, Morris JR. The Sickness Impact Profile: conceptual formulation and methodology for the development of a health status measure. *Intl J Health Services* 1976;6:393–415.

Boake C, High WM. Functional outcome from traumatic brain injury. *Am J Phys Med Rehabil* 1996;75:105–13.

Bowling A. *Measuring health: a review of quality of life measurement scales.* Philadelphia: Open University Press, 1991.

Brazier JE, Harper R, Jones NMB, O'Cathain A, Thomas KJ, Usherwood T, Westlake L. Validating the SF-36 health survey questionnaire: new outcome measure for primary care. *Br Med J* 1992;305:160–64.

Brooks WB, Jordan JS, Divine GW, Smith KS, Neelon FA. The impact of psychologic factors on measurement of functional status: assessment of the Sickness Impact Profile. *Med Care* 1990;28:793–804.

Bruin AF de, Buys M, Witte LP de, Diederiks JPM. The Sickness Impact Profile: SIP68, a short generic version. *J Clin Epidemiology* 1994;47:863–871.

Bruin AF de, Diederiks JPM, Witte LP de, Stevens FCJ, Philipsen H. The development of a short generic version of the Sickness Impact Profile. *J Clin Epidemiology* 1994;47:407–18.

Christiansen CH, Schwartz RK, Barnes KJ. Self-care: evaluation and management. In: DeLisa JB, Gans BM, Currie D (eds.). *Rehabilitation medicine: principles and practice.* Philadelphia: Lippincott, 1993:178–200.

Cluff L. Chronic diseases, function and quality care. *J Chronic Disability* 1981;34:299–304.

Collin C, Wade DT, Davies S, Horne V. The Barthel ADL Index: a reliability study. *International Disability Studies* 1988;10:61–63.

Doble S. Test-retest and inter-rater reliability of a process skills assessment. *Occup Ther J Res* 1991;11:8–23. Duckworth D. The measurement of disability by means of summed ADL indices. *Intl Rehab Med* 1980;l2:194–98.

Doble SE, Fisk JD, Fisher AG, Ritvo PG, Murray TJ. Functional competence of community-dwelling person with multiple sclerosis using the assessment of motor and process skills. *Arch Phys Med Rehabil* 1994;75:843–51.

Fisher AG. Assessment of motor and process skills (rev. ed.). Fort Collins, CO: Three Star Press, 1995.

Fisher AG, Liu Y, Velozo CA, Pan AW. Cross-cultural assessment of process skills. *Am J Occup Ther* 1992;46:876–85.

Fisher WP, Fisher AG. Applications of Rasch analysis to studies in occupational therapy. *Phys Med Rehab Clin N Am* 1993;4:551–69.

Fortinsky RH, Granger CV, Selzer, GB. The use of function assessment in understanding home care needs. *Med Care* 1981;19:489–97.

Garratt AM, Ruta DA, Abdalla MI, Buckingham JK, Russell IT. The SF 36 health survey questionnaire: an outcome measure suitable for routine use within the NHS? *Br Med J* 1993;306:1440–44.

Granger CV. Health accounting—functional assessment of the long-term patient. In Kottke FJ, Stillwell GK, Lehmann JF (eds.). *Krusen's handbook of physical medicine and rehabilitation.* Philadelphia: Saunders, 1982.

Granger CV, Albrecht GL, Hamilton BB. Outcomes of comprehensive medical rehabilitation: measurement of PULSES Profile and the Barthel Index. *Arch Phys Med Rehabil* 1979;60:145–54.

Granger CV, Greer DS. Functional status measurement and medical rehabilitation outcomes. *Arch Phys Med Rehabil* 1976;57:103–109.

Granger CV, Gresham GE. *Functional assessment in rehabilitation medicine.* Baltimore: Williams & Wilkins, 1984.

Granger CV, Gresham GE. Functional assessment in rehabilitation medicine: introduction and brief background. *Phys Med Rehab Clin N Am* 1993;4:417–23.

Granger CV, Ottenbacher KJ, Baker JG, Sehgal A. Reliability of a brief outpatient functional outcome assessment measure. *Am J Phys Med Rehabil* 1995;74:469–75.

Granger CV, Sherwood CC, Greer DS. Functional status measures in a comprehensive stroke care program. *Arch Phys Med Rehabil* 1977;58:555–61.

Gresham GE, Labi MLC. Functional assessment instruments currently available for documenting outcomes in rehabilitation medicine. In: Granger CV, Gresham GE (eds.). *Functional assessment in rehabilitation medicine.* Baltimore: Williams & Wilkins, 1984:65–85.

Harwood RH, Gompertz SE. Handicap one year after a stroke: validity of a new scale. *J Neurol Neurosurg Psychiatry* 1994;57:825–29.

Harwood RH, Gompertz SE. *The London Handicap Scale Scoring Manual.* Medical Outcomes Trust, 20 Park Plaza, Suite 1014, Boston, Massachusetts 02116, 1996.

Hayes V, Morris J, Wolfe C, Morgan M. The SF-36 health survey questionnaire: is it suitable for use with older adults? *Age and Ageing* 1995;24:120–25.

Hinderer SR, Hinderer KA. Quantitative methods of evaluation. In DeLisa J, Gans B, Currie D (eds.). *Rehabilitation medicine: principles and practice.* Philadelphia: Lippincott, 1993:96–121.

Hunt SM, McEwan J, McKenna SP. *Measuring health status.* London: Croom Helm, 1986.

Jacelon CA. The Barthel Index and other indices of functional ability. *Rehab Nurs* 1986;11:9–11.

Jenkinson C, Coulter A, Wright L. Short form 36 (SF 36) health survey questionnaire: normative data for adults of working age. *Br Med J* 1993;306:1437–40.

Johnston MV, Keith RA, Hinderer SR. Measurement standards for interdisciplinary medical rehabilitation. *Arch Phys Med Rehabil* 1992;73:S3–S23.

Johnston MV, Wilerson DL, Maney M. Evaluation of the quality and outcomes of medical rehabilitation programs. In: DeLisa JB, Gans BM, Currie D (eds.). *Rehabilitation medicine: principles and practice.* Philadelphia: Lippincott, 1993:240–68.

Keith RA. Functional status and health status. *Arch Phys Med Rehabil* 1994;75:478–83.

Law M, Letts L. A critical review of scales of activities of daily living. *Am J Occup Ther* 1989;43:522-28.

Mahoney FI, Barthel DW. Functional evaluation: the Barthel Index. *MD State Med J* 1965;14:61–65.

McDowell I, Newell C. *Measuring health: a guide to rating scales and questionnaires.* New York: Oxford University Press, 1987.

McHorney CA, Ware JE, Lu JFR, Sherbourne CD. The MOS 36-Item Short-Form Health survey (SF-36): III. Tests of data quality, scaling assumptions, and reliability across diverse patient groups. *Med Care* 1994;32:40–66.

McHorney CA, Ware JE, Raczek AE. The MOS 36-Item Short-Form Health Survey (SF-36): II. Psychometric and clinical tests of validity in measuring physical and mental health constructs. *Med Care* 1993;31:247–63.

McHorney CA, Ware JE, Rogers W, Raczek AE, Lu JFR. The validity of relative precision of MOS short-and long-form health status scales and Darmouth COOP charts: results from the medical outcomes study. *Med Care* 1992;30(Suppl):MS253–265.

Moskowitz E. PULSES Profile in retrospect. *Arch Phys Med Rehabil* 1985;66:647–48.

Moskowitz E, McCann CB. Classification of disability in the chronically ill and aging. *J Chron Dis* 1957;5:342–46.

Nunnally JC. *Psychometric theory*. New York: McGraw-Hill, 1978.

Nygard L, Bernspang B, Fisher AG, Winblad B. Comparing motor and process ability of persons with suspected dementia in home and clinic setting. *Am J Occup Ther* 1994;48:689–96.

Pan AW, Fisher AG. The assessment of motor and process skills of persons with psychiatric disorders. *Am J Occup Ther* 1994;48:775–80.

Park S, Fisher AG, Velozo CA. Using the assessment of motor and process skills to compare occupational performance between clinic and home settings. *Am J Occup Ther* 1993;48:697–709.

Patrick DL, Peach H. *Disablement in the community*. Oxford: Oxford University Press, 1989.

Post MWM, Bruni AF de, Witte LP de, Schrijvers A. The SIP68: a measure of health-related functional status in rehabilitation medicine. *Arch Phys Med Rehabil* 1996;77:440–45.

Schuling J, Greidanus J, Meijboom-De Jong B. Measuring functional status of stroke patients with the Sickness Impact Profile. *Disability Rehab* 1993;15:19–23.

Shiner D, Gross CR, Bronstein, KS, Licata-Gehr EE, Eden DT, Cabrera AR, Fishman IG, Roth AA, Barwick JA, Kunitz SC. Reliability of the activities of daily living scale and its use in telephone interview. *Arch Phys Med Rehabil* 1987;68:723–28.

Skinner A. *The Sickness Impact Profile Scoring Manual*. Medical Outcomes Trust, 20 Park Plaza, Suite 1014, Boston, Massachusetts 02116, 1996.

Spilker B. *Quality of life assessments in clinical trials*. New York: Raven Press, 1990.

Stewart AL. Psychometric considerations in functional status instruments. In: WONCA Classification Committee (ed.). *Functional status measurement in primary care*. New York: Springer-Verlag, 1990:3–26.

Stewart AL, Ware JE. *Measuring functioning and well-being*. Durham: Duke University Press, 1992.

Stucki G, Liang MH, Phillips C, Katz JN. The Short Form-36 is preferable to the SIP as a generic health status measure in patients undergoing elective total hip arthroplasty. *Arthritis Care & Research* 1995;8:174–81.

Temkin NR, Dikmen S, Machamer J, McLean A. General versus disease-specific measures: further work on the Sickness Impact Profile for head injury. *Med Care* 1989;27:S44–53.

Wade DT. *Measurement in neurological rehabilitation*. New York: Oxford Medical Publications, 1992.

Wade DT, Collin C. The Barthel ADL Index: a standard measure of physical disability? *Intl Disability Studies* 1988;10:64–67.

Ware JE, Sherbourne CD. The MOS 36-Item Short-Form Health Survey (SF-36) I. Conceptual framework and item selection. *Med Care* 1992;30:473–83.

Ware JE, Snow KK, Kosinski M, Gandeck B. *SF-36 Health Survey Manual and Interpretation Guide*. Boston: The Health Institute, New England Medical Center, 1993.

Weinberger M, Oddone EZ, Samsa GP, Landsman PB. Are health-related quality-of-life measures affected by the mode of administration? *J Clin Epidemiology* 1996;49:135–40.

Whiteneck GG. Measuring what matters: key rehabilitation outcomes. *Arch Phys Med Rehabil* 1994;75:1073–76.

Whiteneck GG, Charlifue SW, Gerhart KA, Overholser JD, Richardson GN: *Guide for Use of the CHART: Craig Handicap Assessment and Reporting Technique*. Englewood, CO, Craig Hospital, 1988.

Whiteneck GG, Charlifue SW, Gerhart KA, Overholser JD, Richardson GN. Quantifying handicap: a new measure of long-term rehabilitation outcomes. *Arch Phys Med Rehabil* 1992;73:519–26.

Whyte J. Toward a methodology for rehabilitation research. *Am J Phys Med Rehabil* 1994;73:428-35.

Wilkin D, Hallam L, Doggett MA. *Measures of need and outcome for primary health care*. Oxford: Oxford University Press, 1992.

Willer B, Button J. *Community Integration Scoring Manual*. Ontario Brain Injury Association, P.O. Box 2338, St. Catharines, Ontario, Canada L2M 7M7, 1994.

Willer B, Rosethal M, Kreutzer JS, Gordon WA, Rempel R. Assessment of community integration following rehabilitation for traumatic brain injury. *J Head Trauma Rehab* 1993;8:75–85.

World Health Organization. *International Classification of Impairment, Disabilities, Handicaps*. Geneva: World Health Organization, 1980.

Wylie CM. Measuring and results of rehabilitation of patients with stroke. *Public Health Reports* 1967;82:893–98.

Wylie CM, White BK. A measure of disability. *Archives of Environmental Health* 1964;8:834–39.

Ziebland S. The short form 36 health status questionnaire: clues from the Oxford region's normative data about its usefulness in measuring health gain in population surveys. *Journal of Epidemiology & Community Health* 1995;49:102–105.

Index